CHRIS BEAT CANCER

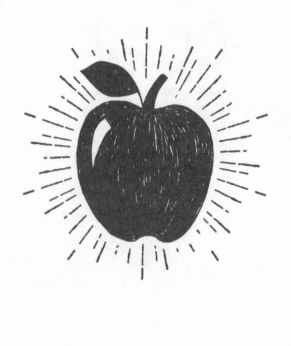

CHRIS BEAT CANCER

A COMPREHENSIVE PLAN FOR HEALING NATURALLY

CHRIS WARK

HAY HOUSE, INC.
Carlsbad, California • New York City
London • Sydney • New Delhi

Published in the United States by: Hay House, Inc.: www.hayhouse.com®
Published in Australia by: Hay House Australia Pty. Ltd.: www.hayhouse.com.au
Published in the United Kingdom by: Hay House UK, Ltd.: www.hayhouse.co.uk
Published in India by: Hay House Publishers India: www.hayhouse.co.in

Indexer: Joan Shapiro
Cover design: theBookDesigners
Interior design: Charles McStravick

Cataloging-in-Publication Data is on file with the Library of Congress

Hardcover ISBN: 978-1-4019-5611-0
E-book ISBN: 978-1-4019-5612-7
Audiobook ISBN: 978-1-4019-5614-1
10 9 8 7 6 5 4 3 2 1
1st edition, September 2018

PRINTED IN THE UNITED STATES OF AMERICA

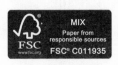

This book is dedicated to:

MY FELLOW MEMBERS OF THE CANCER CLUB,
who have found themselves on an unexpected journey
and courageously face fear, suffering, and uncertainty
every day while choosing to take massive action
to survive and thrive.

MY PARENTS, DAVID AND CATHARINE WARK,
who love me, encourage me, believe in me,
and have always been there for me. Always.

MY WIFE, MICAH,
who said yes to me, stood by me through everything,
and gave me a beautiful family. You are the love of my life
and my best friend in the whole wide world.

MY DAUGHTERS, MARIN AND MACKENZIE,
who are the greatest joys of my life,
are my proudest accomplishments, and have me
wrapped around their little fingers.

CONTENTS

INTRODUCTION

IT WAS EARLY MORNING and light from a streetlamp was illuminating the edges of the window blinds in our bedroom. Dakota, our blue-eyed husky mix, had her head down, resting on her paws, but her eyes were open. She peered up at me with a look like *What do you think you're doing?*

I was trying to get out of the bedroom without waking up my wife, Micah, who, for all her wonderful qualities, is not a morning person and would no doubt greet being woken up by me with the same level of enthusiasm as a hibernating bear. I gently eased myself out of bed, tiptoed across the bedroom, and slowly slid the closet door open. The wheels squeaked sharply on the track, which was almost ear-piercing in the silence.

I held my breath, grabbed my shoes and clothes, and quickly moved toward the door, motioning for Dakota to follow me. She shook her fur, clinking the tags on her collar, and stampeded across the floor. Micah stirred in her sleep and rolled over.

Outside in the frigid February air, I sucked in a huge breath and held it until I felt the pressure of my heart pumping in my chest and head. Then I let it out, feeling my lungs deflate, and I started to jog down the street. My body felt awkward and uncoordinated, like the tin man. My joints, muscles, and tendons were all still working together, just not very well. The icy, cracked, uneven sidewalk was intimidating and hazardous, but after a minute of hobble-jogging down the hill, things began to loosen up and my confidence grew.

I turned east. The sun was cresting the tree line at the far edge of a parking lot. It was warm on my face, and glorious.

I picked up my pace, stretching my legs with each step until I reached full extension. Then I kicked it into high gear, sprinting toward the light. My legs felt wobbly and dangerous, as if they could fly off my body at any moment. I focused to keep them under control. My heart was pounding, my lungs began to ache, and my legs were burning, but I kept on. As I cut across the parking lot, tears streamed from the corners of my eyes. The wind pounded and whooshed in my ears. I felt alive again. I was running as if my life depended on it. "I'm going to live," I said out loud to myself. "I'm going to live."

Framing cancer as a battle or a fight presents a misunderstanding of the disease. Cancer cells are not alien invaders. Cancer cells are your cells with your DNA. Cancer is not just in you, it *is* you. The presence of cancerous tumors is the result of a breakdown in the normal functioning of your body. Damaged cells mutate and begin to behave abnormally, and the systems designed to identify and eliminate those mutant cells fail, allowing them to rapidly divide and corrupt surrounding tissue with lesions and tumors. Cancer is a condition created by the body that the body can resolve, if given the proper nutrition and care.

Chris Beat Cancer was the name I chose for my blog many years ago because it was catchy, easy to remember, and immediately understood. It is the nickname by which I am identified by readers of said blog as well as my followers on social media, and by default it was the obvious title for this book. But years of research and reflection have changed my perspective. While it is true that cancerous cells need to either die or revert back to normal, I no longer view cancer as an enemy to be beaten or defeated, or a battle to be won or lost. Cancer is not something you fight. It is something you heal.

Introduction

The purpose of this book is to tell you my story, explain the methods that I and many others have successfully used to heal, and share what I've learned about the power of nutrition and lifestyle medicine as well as the pitfalls of the cancer industry. I've compiled the most important information from my own experience and 14 years of independent research. Much of this information is ignored and/or rejected by the conventional medical community despite mountainous volumes of scientific validation and empirical evidence. As you will see, the research is well documented in this book and freely available for further investigation.

Over the years, I've met people from all over the world who have healed cancer naturally without any medical intervention, and people who have healed cancer after conventional treatments failed and they were sent home to die. These people are not special. They are not superhuman. They are just like you. Thanks to the internet and social media, I have been able to find these people and compare their strategies. I've interviewed many of them, and if you take the time to learn from them and compare the methods they used, you will find common threads that cannot be ignored. The cancer healing revolution is under way. The tipping point is coming.

I'm not a doctor or a scientist. I'm just a guy who chose nutrition and natural, nontoxic therapies over chemo. I was relatively clueless about health and the human body when I was diagnosed, but I devoured as much information as I could find and learned some extraordinary things that changed my life and restored my health. Everything I did, you can do too.

You can change your life. But changing your life often requires a paradigm shif and re-education. We all go through life with various levels of selective ignorance, especially about health and medicine. Ignorance is bliss, but knowledge requires accountability. The reality is that sometimes we just don't want to know certain things because knowing means we will have to make difficult decisions.

Once your eyes are opened, you can't go back. And once you discover that there are many paths you can take to healing, it can be exciting. But it can also create confusion, fear, doubt, and distress.

When my daughters were little, we got a black-and-white kitten we named Cash. When Cash was about three months old, I took him outside to play with us in the front yard. A soon as I stepped outside, he tensed up and dug his claws into my arm. I rubbed his head and stroked his fur, trying to get him to relax, but it wasn't happening.

When I put him down on the grass, he made a beeline for the bushes. And each time I coaxed him out and carried him over to the open grass again, he darted back into the bushes to hide. I realized that Cash was experiencing information overload from all the new sights, sounds, and smells of the outside world. He was instinctively protecting himself from the unknown.

We started taking him outside daily, and after several weeks of cautious exploration, Cash was climbing trees, stalking birds, chasing squirrels, standing up to neighborhood dogs, and napping in the sun, fearless.

The world of health and healing may be completely new territory for you, but don't be afraid. Just step out into the unknown, take it all in, and absorb as much information as you can. You have the power to learn and grow, to deduce the truth, and to discover the right path to restore your life and health.

This information is available to anyone who wants it, but you must be a seeker of knowledge. Anyone who is closed off to new ideas and thinks they know it all, or that doctors know it all, cannot be helped.

The first cancer patient I had the opportunity to share my experience and convictions with was a dear friend named Kathy. I spoke to her at length about why I chose nutrition and natural therapies to build up my body and support healing instead of treatments that would cause more harm. At the end of a long conversation she said, "Chris, I know you're right. I just know you're right. I shouldn't be doing chemo. Deep down I don't feel good about it. Chemo is horrible—it's poisoning my body. Everything you are saying makes so much sense . . ." But she was exhausted physically, mentally, and emotionally and faced an enormous amount of pressure from her family and doctors. In spite of her intuition and instincts, she continued with conventional treatments.

The rest of Kathy's story is typical. The chemotherapy reduced her cancer initially, but within a few months the cancer came back much worse. She was given more aggressive treatments that destroyed her health. In less than a year, she was gone. She left behind a husband and three teenage daughters. Every time I see someone suffer and die after enduring countless rounds of brutal cancer treatments while others are healing, it strengthens my resolve to share this message of hope. True hope. That cancer can be healed.

There is a common misconception that those in the natural health community are anti-science, but this is not the case. I love science. I get excited about scientific research, especially nutritional science, and I will be citing a lot of scientific research in this book. But it is important that we view science in the proper light. Science is not truth. It is an attempt to discover truth. If science were truth, it would always be right. However, not unlike news stories today, there are countless published scientific studies that contradict each other. This has led to a growing mistrust of science in the public eye.

A true scientist is a perpetual truth seeker driven by curiosity and a thirst for knowledge—one who, however passionate about their conclusions and beliefs, maintains an open mind and is always, graciously and with humility, willing to reconsider new evidence; admit that they may be have been wrong; and change their position. Unfortunately, throughout human history the scientific community has been persistently infected with the disease of dogma disguised as skepticism, arrogantly holding fast to established scientific truths of the day, only to be proven false by the discoveries of their successors.

Scientific knowledge is ever evolving, ever expanding, and is rarely ever "settled." As I write this, one of the biggest headlines in the world is that researchers are claiming to have discovered a "new organ" in the human body called the interstitium, and members of the scientific community are now debating whether or not to call it an organ.

When it comes to published science, the people involved matter. Despite the appearance of legitimacy, publishing a scientific study in a peer-reviewed academic journal does not necessarily make it accurate, true, or trustworthy. Scientific research can easily be misunderstood, manipulated, or manufactured. Millions of dollars have been and will be spent funding scientific studies simply to further an agenda, like the infamous studies funded by the tobacco industry that "proved" cigarettes did not cause cancer—until, years later, unbiased scientific studies proved they did.

When confronted with scientific research, before accepting or rejecting its conclusion, at the very least it's important to consider who funded it and who stands to benefit from its findings. Generally speaking, studies conducted by independent research-ers without conflicts of interest, with no ties to industry, and with conclusions that cannot be monetized tend to be more trustworthy than, say, drug studies funded by the companies that make the drugs. But there are always exceptions. Bad science can persist for many years, but I do believe that good science, like truth, will win in the end. All of which is to say that I have done my best in this book to highlight compelling scientific evidence, good science from a variety of sources, to help you get closer to the truth and to empower you to make informed decisions—the best decisions for you—to transform your life and restore your health.

INTO THE JUNGLE

Health is not valued till sickness comes.

— DR. THOMAS FULLER

BY THE TIME I TURNED 26, I had graduated college, married the love of my life, bought 30 rental properties, started a new band with plans to record an album and tour, and just received a call-back to be a potential cast member on a reality show on NBC. Things were going pretty well. As a kid I had always felt I was destined for greatness, and my dreams of proving myself to the world were becoming real. I bounced out of bed every morning thrilled about life. I couldn't wait to see what the future had in store. I felt invincible. Little did I know that five months later all my big plans would take a backseat to survival.

Micah and I met in the 11th grade. She had been dating my friend Russ over the summer, but she and I hadn't met. Micah had a blonde streak in her black hair. She wore Vans. And she had a patch on her backpack of one of my favorite bands, The Cure. I knew she was cool, so I sat by her in history class. It was easy to make her laugh, so much so that the teacher often separated us to opposite sides of the room. A few months later, Micah and Russ broke up, but she and I stayed friends. We ran around in the same social circles and would often see each other on the weekends at local rock and punk shows.

After high school Micah and I both went to the University of Tennessee–Knoxville for our freshman year. Most of our friends were pledging fraternities and sororities, but neither of us were interested in Greek life, so we ended up hanging out a lot. One thing led to another, and by the end of the first semester, we were officially a couple. Six years later, on Valentine's Day, I proposed to her. Three months after that, I graduated from the University of Memphis with a business degree and no job prospects.

Our wedding was set for September. Micah was working full-time and living on her own, and I had moved back in with my parents and was working part-time folding clothes and unlocking fitting rooms at J.Crew. With a wedding date looming, I was feeling the pressure to find a job worthy of my degree and get my act together. After a few interviews, I took a job at a financial planning firm. I had a great mentor, developed some valuable client relationships, and made enough money to get by, but I had a nagging feeling that I was in the wrong profession. I enjoyed helping people, but I wasn't passionate about insurance and investments. It was fun to put on a suit and tie every day, but it kind of felt like a costume.

One day, while sitting in a weekly staff meeting and listening to my boss talk about investment strategies and watching him wipe his leaky eye with his tie for the umpteenth time, I realized there wasn't anyone in the room I aspired to be. I just couldn't see myself staying in a profession I didn't love for the rest of my life only for the money.

I'd been fantasizing about being a professional real estate investor since college, and at the peak of my dissatisfaction in the financial industry, I bought four rental properties in 30 days. It was trial by fire, but I loved everything about it. I loved hunting down deals and finding them before my competitors.

I loved negotiating to get the best price. I loved the renovation process. I loved the idea of building a business that could eventually get me out of the rat race and give me financial freedom. By the end of that year, Micah and I owned 17 rental properties and I quit financial planning to pursue real estate full-time. Thanks to the guidance of a few generous mentors and the infamous bubble-producing federal loan programs, Micah and I were able to buy 31 houses in just two years. I was having a blast and making a name for myself in the Memphis real estate community.

During that time, I started singing and playing guitar in a new band called Arma Secreta (Portuguese for *secret weapon*) with my longtime friend/drummer/now brother-in-law Brad Bean. I was a realist and didn't expect to make much money off my art, and it had been four years since my last serious band. Now, finally, I was playing shows again and Arma Secreta soon picked up speed.

That summer, another good friend named Clay Hurley told me about a new reality show that NBC was casting. He thought it was right up my alley and offered to help me produce an audition tape, so we made one. The casting team liked my audition and asked me to come to Nashville for an on-camera interview. I dusted off my suit and tie, drove to Nashville, and met two of the producers in a hotel room. I felt like the interview went really well until the end, when one of the producers said, "Okay, Chris, now I want you to look directly into the camera and tell Donald Trump why you think you are the next Apprentice."

The question caught me completely off guard because I had no idea what this brand-new show was about, other than that it involved working for real estate tycoon Donald Trump. And I was really uncomfortable talking directly into the camera. So I said something stupid like, "Hi, Donald. I'm a really big fan of your books . . ." The rest is an embarrassing blur. At the time, I was disappointed that I didn't get another callback but not that surprised. And being an *Apprentice* reject turned out to be a blessing in disguise because I had a pesky little problem.

There was a dull aching in my abdomen that would come and go randomly. It was deep and vague. I felt it, but I couldn't quite put my finger on it. There were also sudden twinges of sharp pain that would make me break out in a cold sweat. I remember thinking, *Whoa, what the heck was that? That's not normal . . . hopefully it's nothing.* This eventually progressed to *Uh-oh, there it is again.* Being busy and a stereotypical male not wanting to go to the doctor, I ignored it for many months, thinking it was probably an ulcer and would get better. My body was trying to tell me something, but I wasn't listening.

I've always believed that the human body is designed to heal itself. In this case, I assumed mine eventually would because it always had, but for some reason this time it didn't. The pain gradually got worse. Also, my stool was dark, and sometimes there was a little blood in it. I often woke up in the middle of the night in a cold sweat with aching pain and an urge to go to the bathroom. In the morning, I woke up feeling fine, which is part of the reason I kept putting off seeing a doctor.

Digestive system diseases are especially terrible because they take all the joy out of food. When food becomes a source of pain, you stop eating and your body begins to waste away. At six-feet-two and 150 pounds, I was already thin; I didn't have any extra weight to lose. Most days the pain started an hour or so after dinner, and sometimes I felt it after lunch.

The pain progressed. Eventually, after I spent several nights balled up on the couch after dinner, Micah convinced me to see a doctor. I had blood work and X-rays done, but they couldn't find anything other than slight anemia, and I was misdiagnosed with an ulcer. When the ulcer medicine didn't help, the gastroenterologist decided to do a colonoscopy and an endoscopy (aka upper and lower GI), which means he stuck a camera scope "where the sun don't shine" to have a look around, and then he stuck another one down my throat.

When I regained consciousness, Micah was there beside me. We were in a small room with a curtain for a door, and I was still lying on the gurney. The doctor came in, accompanied by a nurse, and told us he had found a golf ball–sized tumor in my large intestine, and that they were sending a biopsy to the lab to test it for cancer.

I was still groggy from the anesthesia, and my brain was running at half speed. The scene felt like a dream that I didn't understand. And I was too confused to be upset. Micah began sobbing on the shoulder of the nurse, who was the mother of one of our close friends from church. She was a godsend, a tremendous comfort in that moment, and the first of many providential appointments on my cancer journey.

The next day, the phone rang around 7 A.M. It was the doctor calling to tell me I had cancer. He said, "We've got to get you into surgery and get this thing out of you before it spreads. A surgeon will be calling you to schedule surgery as soon as possible." And that was the moment the fear became real and my life came to a grinding halt. It was two days before Christmas. I was 26 years old. And I had cancer.

Of course, my first reaction was *Really? This is my life? I'm the young guy with cancer? Terrific.* The cancer diagnosis made me feel helpless, vulnerable, and weak. Not to mention the fact that I had colorectal cancer, which in my mind might as well be called butt cancer because you know that's what everyone is thinking. And on top of that, this was an old people's disease. I was now the young guy with old people's butt cancer. Spectacular. I had been reduced to an object of pity and sympathy and I didn't like that at all. Humble pie served. Ego destroyed.

When we told our friends and family, they were all shocked. Most were at a loss for words and didn't know how to react. I didn't either.

Before the diagnosis I felt like I was in control, directing the course of my life. But control is an illusion. Sooner or later we all find ourselves face-to-face with circumstances that remind us how fragile life is, and in difficult situations that are beyond our control. This is true desperation.

My wife and I are Christians. We love Jesus. We believe that He is everything He claimed to be. The son of God and the savior of the world. And we believe that the Bible is God's word, eternal truth. At the time of my diagnosis, we were members of a small nondenominational church and I played in the worship band on Sunday mornings.

But my faith was shaken. I couldn't help but think, *God, why is this happening to me? Why am I the one with cancer? I'm one of the good guys, and I'm actually trying do something good with my life!* It begged the classic question "Why do bad things happen to good people?" As I wrestled with this, I remembered Romans 8:28 (NASB):

> And we know that God causes all things to work together for good to those who love God, to those who are called according to His purpose.

I didn't understand why cancer was happening to me, but I knew that God was in control and I chose to believe that He would ultimately work this bad thing out for my good. The next Sunday we stood up in front of our church and told them the news. Nervous and choked up, I quoted Psalms 34:19 (NIV) as a banner over my situation:

> The righteous person may have many troubles, but the LORD delivers him from them all.

The surgeon who was supposed to call me to schedule surgery forgot to call. This turned out to be another blessing. During this time my father mentioned my situation to a co-worker who called in a favor and got me in to see another gastroenterologist for a second opinion. He saw me right away and referred me to an abdominal surgeon who was considered to be the best in Memphis.

I met with the new surgeon, and we scheduled surgery to remove the tumor with a routine colon resection using laparoscopic surgery. The surgeon explained he would only make a few small incisions, just big enough for a camera and his instruments. I asked him how many times he had done this type of surgery. He said, "Hundreds." Good enough. The only other detail I remember from our meeting was how pink and fleshy his hands were, a stark contrast to the pale skin on his arms. I thought, *Man, he must wash his hands a lot.*

There was a heaviness, a sense of sadness and dread that permeated our family Christmas gatherings that year. I tried to act normally, but I was extremely self-conscious. Everyone knew I was sick but most folks didn't bring it up. What was there to say? I was the cancerous elephant in the room.

The day before surgery, I wasn't allowed to eat any solid food except for Jell-O. Micah and I went to a Chinese buffet for lunch after church. She had a plate of delicious-smelling food. I had three different colors of Jell-O. As instructed, I drank a ridiculous amount of a polyethylene glycol solution called GoLYTELY to clean me out that night. It definitely did. Let's just say it was a wild ride and it did not "go lightly."

NEW YEAR'S EVE EVE

On the big day, Micah and I arrived at the hospital bright and early at 7 A.M. to check in for surgery. The woman who admitted me had a note pinned up in her cubicle.

Psalm 23

The Lord is my Shepherd. *That's Relationship!*

I shall not want. *That's Supply!*

He makes me to lie down in green pastures. *That's Rest!*

He leads me beside the still waters. *That's Refreshment!*

He restores my soul. *That's Healing!*

He leads me in the paths of righteousness.
That's Guidance!

For His name sake. *That's Purpose!*

Yea, though I walk through the valley of the
shadow of death . . . *That's Testing!*

I will fear no evil. *That's Protection!*

For You are with me. *That's Faithfulness!*

Your rod and Your staff they comfort me.
That's Discipline!

You prepare a table before me in the presence
of my enemies. *That's Hope!*

You anoint my head with oil. *That's Consecration!*

My cup overflows. *That's Abundance!*

Surely goodness and mercy will follow me
all the days of my life. *That's Blessing!*

And I will dwell in the house of the Lord . . .
That's Security!

Forever. *That's Eternity!*

— AUTHOR UNKNOWN

Her note was such a huge encouragement to me in that moment. I asked her to make a copy of it for me and she did. I still don't know her name, but I thank God for giving us that sweet woman in the admissions office.

After I checked in, they took me to the pre-surgery holding area, where I stripped down, put on a hospital gown, laid on a gurney, and got hooked up to an IV. Doctors, nurses, and hospital staff scuffled about wearing blue covers over their shoes to keep the floors clean. They were just going about their normal, cancer-free lives. I was jealous of them.

Eventually my number came up. Two nurses rolled me down the hall. I was lying flat on my back watching the ceiling lights pass overhead. We turned a corner and I felt the temperature drop.

"They keep the operating rooms colder to prevent the spread of germs," one of the nurses said mechanically. A set of double doors parted to reveal an operating room with six people in full surgical gear: gloves, mask, gown, goggles. All I could see were their eyes, and all eyes were on me. It was creepy. I laughed to myself as they began preparing to sedate me. *These people are all about to see me naked.*

At that moment, I had peace. I knew God was in control. I wasn't afraid. I put my trust in Him, and I was prepared to meet Him if I didn't wake up. The anesthesiologist leaned over and said, "Are you ready?"

"I'm ready."

I took a deep breath and closed my eyes.

After surgery, I woke up in the post-op holding area. My wife and mother-in-law were there with me. I was heavily medicated and tried to speak but could only moan and grunt. I had instructed my wife to bring my video camera to me immediately after surgery so I could document what I might not remember. I somehow managed to turn the camera on and record myself in my weakest, most vulnerable state for a few seconds before turning it off and passing out again. (You can see this at www.chrisbeatcancer.com/surgeryvideo.)

"WAKE UP, SON. WE'VE GOT TO GET YOU ONTO THIS BED"

A series of thoughts slowly bubbled through my pain-medicated brain:

Where am I? Hospital room . . . Surgery . . .
Someone's talking to me . . .

A nurse was trying to get me off the gurney and onto a bed. As I attempted to roll over, I felt as if my guts were being held together by a string and could explode with the slightest flex of my abs. I was in a panic, afraid to move, and the nurse was talking to me like I should just hop from one bed to the other like a kid in a hotel room. With the help of several people, I slowly inched myself onto the bed and passed out again.

The first night was hellish, one of the worst of my life. All I wanted to do was sleep, but I couldn't get any rest because every hour a nurse had to come in and wake me up to do things like take my temperature, check my blood pressure, and turn me over. Thankfully, the nurse assigned to us was an angel. Every time she came into the room, I felt an amazing peaceful presence.

The next day, a nurse changed my bandage. When she pulled it off, I looked down and was surprised to see a six-inch vertical incision going right down the middle of my stomach. The doctor had cut all the way through my abdominal muscles, which explained the sensation I had of my guts exploding. I was simultaneously confused and amused by it.

"Heeeeey, they cut my belly button in half," I said in a dopey slur.

NEW YEAR'S EVE

The surgeon came in and explained that the cancer was worse than they thought. When he put the scope in and looked around, he didn't like what he saw, so he decided to open me up with a large incision. It appeared that the cancer may have spread from the tumor to surrounding lymph nodes. He removed 49 lymph nodes. Four of them tested positive for cancer. I was now stage IIIC. Later that day, an oncologist was brought into my room and introduced to me. I was told that as soon as I recovered from surgery, I would need 9 to 12 months of chemotherapy in order to prevent a recurrence.

At one point during my stay, a med student came in with the attending physician as he made his rounds. He was thin, his skin was pale and yellow, and he had dark circles under his eyes. He looked like a zombie. I thought to myself, *Man, this guy looks worse than I do.*

At this point in my cancer journey, I had accepted that I would do whatever the doctors recommended. I assumed they had my best interest in mind and would take great care of me. But two things happened in the hospital that began to erode my confidence in conventional medicine. The first one was lunch.

The first meal they served me in the hospital after having a third of my large intestine cut out was the worst cafeteria food imaginable: a sloppy joe. Ground up mystery meat stewed in ketchup and slopped onto a burger bun. Don't look for a sloppy joe on a restaurant menu; you won't find it. This mouthwatering delicacy is exclusively available to summer camp goers, soldiers, inmates, and to my surprise, me, the cancer patient.

The heavy pain medication plus the fact that I hadn't eaten in several days did little to soften the blow of this obvious assassination attempt. I asked my wife, "Shouldn't they be giving me something healthier than this? I'm pretty sure this is like the last thing I should be eating right now."

A key indicator that there are no complications with intestinal surgery is a successful bowel movement. And in order to have a bowel movement, you need to eat. Rather than send the sloppy joe back only to have it replaced by something equally terrible like meatloaf, I begrudgingly accepted my fate and ingested the sloppy joe. The next day I had the strangest, scariest bowel movement ever, while standing up in the shower. Good news, everyone: my plumbing is working! Bad news—somebody needs to clean the shower. For the record, that was the first and last time that has ever happened.

After five days and four luxurious nights in the hospital, they gave me permission to go home. The surgeon came by my room to check on me one last time. I was concerned that I might eat the wrong thing and screw the whole surgery up, so I asked him if there were any foods I needed to avoid while my intestines were healing. He replied, "Nah, just don't lift anything heavier than a beer." I chuckled nervously. His dismissive joke and the horrible hospital/prison food were my first indications that the medical establishment did not place much emphasis on nutrition. I was confused by the obvious disconnect between health care and health food. Something didn't add up.

After they released me from the hospital, I went back home to recuperate. Our immediate family and church family were an amazing blessing to us, bringing us meals, praying with us and for us, and helping with anything we needed. I was on heavy pain medication and spent the first week lying on the couch watching movies and sleeping. My friend Brad Stanfill brought me a bunch of videos to watch, including a tape of *Reno 911!* episodes. I hadn't seen it before and I laughed so hard during the first episode that I had to turn it off. I learned an important life lesson that day: abdominal surgery and comedy do not mix.

I stayed on the pain medication for the first week or so but couldn't finish it. I was tired of feeling doped up and instinctively felt like it might be interfering with my healing. Years later, I discovered studies suggesting that opioid-based painkillers like morphine can stimulate the growth and spread of cancer.[1] I also learned that 1 in 10 cancer patients who were prescribed highly addictive opioid painkillers after a surgery like mine become long-term users.[2] My instincts were correct. As I sobered up, I began to think about my life. I wondered what the next year was going to be like for me as a cancer patient. I wondered how much time I had left. I wondered whether I was going to be able to have children. I wondered what my life story would be. Would I live to a ripe old age and see my grandchildren grow up, or would I die young?

I had initially accepted that I would do chemotherapy, but I was developing an internal resistance to the idea. Call it instinct, intuition, or a gut feeling; I didn't have a sense of peace about it. It's important to note that up to this point, I was even more clueless than the typical clueless cancer patient. I had no personal experience with cancer. I had never had any friends or family members diagnosed with cancer, and I knew very little about chemotherapy, except that it was highly toxic and supposedly killed cancer cells. And that it makes you sick, and your hair falls out, and you look like you are dying. The sickest-looking people I had ever seen in my life were cancer patients, but the only two connections I had to cancer were remote. My pastor was a non-Hodgkin's lymphoma survivor, but he had gone through treatment a few years before we met him. And there was another man at our church who had cancer. He was in the printing business and used to play the drums on Sunday mornings before he got sick. People spoke of him often, but I had never met him. I only saw him once, on a Sunday morning. He was bald and his body was emaciated. His clothes hung loosely on his bony frame. His skin was yellow, his eyes were sunken in, and he was obviously weak. He was wearing a surgical mask over his nose and mouth. I couldn't imagine what it was like to be in his condition. He died soon after I saw him, but that one encounter made a dramatic impression on me.

The more I thought about chemotherapy, the less I wanted to do it. The idea of poisoning my way back to health didn't make sense to me, but I was deeply conflicted. So my wife and I prayed about it. I thanked God for everything He had done in my life. I asked Him to heal me, and I asked that if there was another way besides chemotherapy, He would reveal it to me.

Two days later, a book arrived on my doorstep, sent to me by a business acquaintance of my father who lived in Alaska. I started reading the book that day and learned that the author discovered he had colon cancer in 1976. He had seen his mother and many church members suffer and die after undergoing cancer treatment. So he decided to opt out of treatment and radically change his diet and lifestyle. One year after he began juicing and eating a raw-food diet, his cancer was gone. No surgery, no chemotherapy, no radiation. And he was still alive and in excellent health almost 30 years later.

The more I read, the more excited I became. It gave me a new perspective on health, nutrition, cancer, and the cancer treatment industry. His story gave me hope that healing was possible. I thought if he could heal his colon cancer, maybe I could too. That was when I made the decision to take control of my situation, radically change my diet and lifestyle, and do everything I could to support health and healing in my body.

I was so excited and full of faith that I couldn't wait to tell everyone I knew. I called my wife at work and told her I wanted to heal naturally and that I didn't want to do chemo. She thought I had lost my mind. My wife's family is telepathic, so as soon as you tell one person something, everyone knows. Well-meaning family members were soon calling and saying things like, "You have to do what the doctor says. They're using the best therapies available. Don't you think if there was something better they would know about it? Alternative therapies don't work. I know someone who tried that and they died . . ."

This was a new kind of pressure I wasn't expecting. Almost everyone I knew, including my wife, was insisting that I do chemo. Of course, I don't fault them for it. These people loved me and wanted me to live. They were sincerely trying to help but were unknowingly creating a lot more confusion and anxiety. I had prayed and received what I thought was a clear answer, but now everyone was trying to talk me out of it.

So like most cancer patients, in order to appease everyone around me, I reluctantly agreed to go see the oncologist. My appointment was on January 14, 2004. The parking lot to the West Clinic was packed, and so was the waiting room. When Micah and I sat down, I sized up the other cancer patients, curious whether there was anyone else in the cancer club I could relate to. There wasn't. Everyone was two to three times my age. It was surreal. A bunch of old folks and me, the 26-year-old rock dude with shaggy hair and a handlebar mustache. I thought, *God, I don't belong here.*

The TV in the waiting room was on, and one of the guests on the morning show was 89-year-old health and fitness expert Jack LaLanne. Jack came out full of vigor and talked passionately about how our modern diet of processed food was the cause of disease and how a diet of fruits, vegetables, and juicing could transform your health. He said, "If man made it, don't eat it!"

Later they called my name and moved us to a smaller waiting room for additional waiting, and then to a private room where we got to wait some more. Eventually, the oncologist came in. His demeanor was cold and robotic. He gave me what felt like a boilerplate cancer-patient pitch and told me I had a 60 percent chance of living five years if I did chemotherapy, odds that weren't much better than a coin toss. I asked him about a raw-food diet, which I had adopted one week prior, and he told me that I couldn't do it because it would "fight the chemo." I asked him if there were any alternative therapies available. At that moment his demeanor changed; he looked at me dead in the eye and said, "There are none. If you don't do chemotherapy, you are insane."

Instantly I was overcome with fear, and the rest of our appointment was a blur. His tone was arrogant and condescending, and the more he talked the more helpless I felt. I wanted to get up and run out of there but I couldn't. In the midst of his diatribe, he said something that seemed really out of place. He said, "Look, I'm not saying this because I need your business . . ."

When our visit concluded, I felt hypnotized. He had convinced me. And on my way out I made an appointment to have a port installed in a few weeks, the next step before starting chemo. My faith was shattered. I was depressed, discouraged, and afraid. Micah and I sat in her car in the parking lot and cried.

Over the next few weeks I prayed hard and thought hard, desperate for encouragement and direction. I thought about the unhealthy food in the hospital. I thought about chemotherapy making me sicker. I thought about the book that had been sent to me. I thought about Jack LaLanne on TV in the waiting room.

I thought about everything the oncologist had said and how he had treated me. And I realized that God had answered my prayer. I had asked for another way and He had given me one. There were two paths before me, and I had to choose one.

To my left, was a wide, brightly lit road leading to a modern train station where everyone was boarding a beautiful, comfortable, state-of-the-art express train—the chemo train. If I chose that option, I would be surrounded by love and support. People would be cheering me on, raising money, and running races for me. All my needs would be met. But as shiny and attractive as everything seemed to be, I knew that as soon as I got on that train the suffering would begin. And I knew that once I got on, it would be hard to get off. And no one could tell me where I was going. Would they drop me off in Wellville? Or would they kick me off at the end of the line to die, telling me, "There's nothing more we can do"? And if I died, everyone would call me brave, strong, courageous—a fighter, a warrior.

To my right was an overgrown path into the jungle that I had to hack my way through in the dark. There was an official sign posted that said, "Do not enter," and everyone was telling me not to go that way. I knew if I chose that path, no one would understand. I would lose my support, and I would have to go through the journey alone. And if I didn't make it out, if I died on that path, I would be the stubborn fool who refused chemo and my legacy would be reduced to a cautionary tale: "Don't do what Chris did."

Both options were terrifying.

The chemo port installation date loomed larger with each passing day and so did my fear and anxiety. I couldn't shake my internal resistance to it. When the port day finally arrived, I made my choice and was a no-show for the appointment. I naïvely thought that would be the end of it, but the cancer clinic wasn't giving up that easily. They began calling my house and leaving messages trying to get me to reschedule. There were many days when I would come home to a blinking light on the answering machine but avoided pushing play because I didn't want to hear another message. Then they sent me a certified letter that said:

Dear Mr. Wark,

I have been unable to reach you by phone to inform you that your doctor is concerned regarding your missed appointment. Close monitoring of your cancer status is medically necessary to help prevent any life-threatening events from occurring. Please call me to discuss any concerns you might have.

— Robyn

GROUNDHOG DAYS

My first year of cancer was a lot like the movie *Groundhog Day* because every day felt like the same day. Every morning the sun came in through the blinds. I woke up, warm and cozy in bed, feeling good. Then I remembered I had cancer. A wave of fear and cold sweat washed over me. I wondered if I was getting worse or getting better. I got up and became distracted by the demands of the day and forgot about cancer for a little while. But it seemed like every time I turned on the radio or television I heard the word "cancer," and with it came a fresh dose of fear and anxiety.

Despite my fear, I stuck to the plan and continued reading and researching as much as I could about nutrition and natural therapies that might help my body heal. And that's where my mom came in. Enter Catharine Wark. Mom's been into healthy stuff for as long as I can remember. When I was a kid, she bought whole-grain bread instead of white bread, granola instead of Lucky Charms, and natural stir-it-up peanut butter instead of sugary Peter Pan. She froze yogurt and juice to make popsicles, and

I can't remember a time when we didn't have sprouts, kefir, or wheat germ in the fridge.

I never paid much attention to what my mother was reading, but every month there was a new stack of books on her bedside table, and over the years she had amassed an impressive library devoted to health, nutrition, natural medicine, and alternative cancer therapies. Usually people with chronic health problems are the ones driven to research natural methods, but my mom never had any health problems. She was into prevention. In my quest for knowledge, I was continually finding out about more books I wanted to read, only to discover she already had them. For over three decades, she had unknowingly stored up all these books for me. And in the beginning, she was the only person who understood and supported my decision.

During this time, I was also desperate to find other people, real people, who had healed their cancer naturally. The more I looked, the more I found. There was very little information online, but there was an underground network of information that my mom had tapped into through books and videos from alternative cancer doctors, survivors, and researchers. Each new discovery got me more excited about the healing adventure that lay before me.

My mom knew a clinical nutritionist who specialized in holistic health and suggested that I go see him. A few days later a buddy from church brought him up as well. Divine signal received, loud and clear. At that time, the nutritiounist had a modest two-room office in East Memphis. The first time I met him, he was wearing a loose-fitting, beachy button-up shirt, khakis, and clogs. He was a one-man operation, a stark contrast to the multimillion-dollar cancer clinic I'd been in the day before. And his office felt different, peaceful. He was the first person to tell me I was doing the right thing by radically changing my diet to raw food and juicing to support my body's ability to heal. That was a huge validation and a massive confidence booster.

Holistic practitioners are typically not covered by insurance and working with him involved blood tests, saliva tests, urine and stool tests, hair analysis, and lots of supplementation. It wasn't cheap, but it wasn't crazy expensive either. He was looking at the big picture and trying to help me get to the root cause of my disease by correcting nutritional deficiencies, detoxifying my body, and improving my digestion as well as my adrenal and immune function.

My nutritionist referred me to Dr. Roy Page, a surgical oncologist in his 70s who had come out of retirement because he didn't like being retired and wanted to help more people. Dr. Page had spent a lifetime treating cancer patients with destructive and ineffective conventional therapies and in his later years began to integrate nontoxic therapies into his practice. He also supported my decision not to do chemotherapy, which was another powerful confirmation and confidence booster. Dr. Page checked my blood work every month, administered nutritional IV therapy, and ordered a few scans for me along the way.

My team was assembled and my healing plan was in motion, but the first year was tough. There were many days when I was afraid. Like any cancer patient, I was hoping for the best and fearing the worst. The "scanxiety" would build and build until the test results came back. Even though I really liked Dr. Page, I couldn't stand being at the hospital. I felt like a lab rat and couldn't wait to get out. I always left his office on a natural high, skipping down three flights of stairs and bursting outside into the sunlight and fresh air. A few days later, I'd get a call with the results, and Dr. Page was always just as excited as I was. Another good report and a big sigh of relief—thank you, Jesus! Gradually, with each good report came more encouragement, hope, and optimism.

Cancer has a way of cutting a clear dividing line between the important and the unimportant in your life. And I realized that most of the things I cared about before cancer weren't important to me anymore. What mattered to me now was my life and health, taking care of my wife, and starting a family. I really wanted to be a dad, but my cancer diagnosis threatened to postpone fatherhood indefinitely. I was acutely aware of my own mortality and that I might die sometime within the next 10 years. I asked Micah if she would be willing to start a family with me, and she made one of the most courageous decisions of anyone I know. She said yes, knowing she might have to bury me one day and raise our child without me. That's how much she loved me. During my hospital stay, she never left my side. When I wasn't asleep she would squeeze into the bed and watch marathons of *MythBusters* and *American Chopper* with me.

We found out Micah was pregnant four months after my diagnosis, but when we told family members the reactions were mixed. Some were excited and others were concerned about the timing. But good timing or not, this baby was coming. One year after my cancer diagnosis, I was back in the hospital. But this time I was holding our beautiful little baby girl in my arms. We named her Marin Elizabeth, and I now had someone else to live for.

In the years that followed, I did what most cancer survivors do. I distanced myself from cancer. I didn't want to think about it or talk about it. I just wanted to get back to living a normal life. I continued investing in real estate, flipping houses, and doing custom home renovations. Our second daughter, Mackenzie Rae, was born in June 2008, a week after I turned 31. My band, Arma Secreta, recorded and released two records, *A Century's Remains* and *Dependent Lividity*, and played hundreds of shows in the Midwest and on the East Coast.

Eventually my story got around and people were constantly asking me about my health—why I didn't do chemo and what I did instead—and I realized that I had something important to share with the world.

Seven years after my diagnosis, I started a blog called *Chris Beat Cancer* to give people inspiration, encouragement, and resources on healing and preventing cancer with nutrition and natural, nontoxic therapies. I created the site to be what I wished had existed for me back when I was lost and confused. I knew there were people out there just like me, with a fresh cancer diagnosis looking for answers. As the blog gained exposure, messages began to come in from people all over the world who had healed cancer without conventional treatment or after conventional treatment had failed them, including stage IV cancers. I began interviewing them and sharing their stories on chrisbeatcancer.com, and I realized how important it was to show the world that cancer can be healed and that real people are doing it.

My decision to "go public" with a blog completely changed the course of my life. I've had the opportunity tell my story many times on radio, television, and film. I was featured in the award-winning documentary film *The C Word* and on *The Truth About Cancer* series. I've been a part of online summits like The Food Revolution and Food Matters, and I've had the privilege of traveling to and speaking in places I never dreamed of, including London, Moscow, and even Cambodia. Sharing information that can help people heal and prevent cancer as well as navigate cancer treatment has become my life's work.

The five-year relative survival rate for stage IIIC colon cancer is 53 percent.[3] Young adult patients (under 40) have a 28 percent higher risk of cancer progressing and spreading during a one-year follow-up, and are 30 percent more likely to die from cancer.[4,5] According to the National Cancer Institute, stage III colon cancer patients with one to three involved lymph nodes have significantly better survival than those with four or more involved nodes.[6,7] I had four. Furthermore, a meta-analysis of studies found that colon cancer patients with tumors on the left side have better survival rates.[8,9] Mine was on the right.

Even though the odds of long-term survival were stacked against me, this year I celebrate my 15-year "cancerversary." I am so thankful to be alive. God is good. I put my trust in Him, and He led me in the path of healing.

I want to be very clear that I am not "lucky" or special. I am just a regular guy who listened to his instincts, stepped out in faith, and took massive action to help his body heal. I eliminated everything in my life that may have contributed to my disease, and changed the internal terrain of my body—making it a place where cancer could not thrive. What I did, I believe anyone can do, including you.

I'm going to show you what I've learned in the last 15 years of researching nutritional science, the cancer industry, and people who have healed cancer.

You will discover where conventional medicine went wrong, why the cancer industry has failed to win the war on cancer, and how you can avoid the common perils and pitfalls of cancer treatment. You will also learn the exact steps I took to radically change my life and heal. These actionable diet and lifestyle strategies are not unique to my journey. They are common threads among everyone I know who has healed cancer. Wherever you are in your health journey, whether you are trying to heal or prevent cancer, these are strategies you can implement in your life right now. So let's begin.

SURVIVAL OF THE SICKEST

The problem is not to find the answer;
it's to face the answer.

— TERENCE MCKENNA

IN 2010, RESEARCH SCIENTISTS Professor Rosalie David and Professor Michael Zimmerman published a study on the origins of cancer. They examined nearly a thousand mummies from ancient Egypt and South America, as well as fossils and ancient medical texts, looking for evidence of cancer in our ancestors. They only found five cases of tumors out of a thousand mummies, and only one of those tumors was thought to be malignant.[1]

The earliest scientific literature describing what we now call cancer is dated thousands of years later. Notes dating back to the 1600s described operations for breast and other cancers. In 1761, snuff users were documented to have nasal cancer. Chimney sweeps were developing scrotal cancer in 1775. Hodgkin's disease was first noted in 1832. Some have asserted that the discovery of cancer in a few mummies dispels the notion that cancer is a "man-made disease," but that's not what the expression implies. The incidence of cancer has exploded as a result of the significant changes humanity has made to the world in which we live, and the way we live in it.

Perhaps the most fundamentally misunderstood aspect of cancer is that it is not a singular disease. The term "cancer" is a catch-all term for a broad array of unique diseases in the body that can eventually lead to uncontrolled cell growth. There are over 200 different types of cancer, which is why there will never be a singular "cure" for cancer.

THE PLAGUE OF PROGRESS

Even though cancer is not a singular disease, there is a singular point in history where the incidence of cancer began to snowball: the Industrial Revolution. Factories were built to mass-produce everything: fossil fuels, building materials, textiles, furniture, food, chemicals, and all sorts of exciting innovations. The Industrial Revolution paved the way for all the modern conveniences we enjoy today, including electricity, cars, planes, computers, and smartphones, but it also produced an unfortunate by-product: industrial pollution. Many of the chemicals used in the production of modern goods are highly toxic, and many production processes create toxic waste by-products that have polluted our air, water, soil, food—and our bodies. It's estimated that as many as one in five cancers are caused by environmental pollution.[2]

Air pollution from planes, trains, and motor vehicles, as well as home heating and industrial exhaust, is linked to all sorts of chronic diseases. Exhaust from diesel engines is known to cause lung cancer.[3] Even if you don't breathe polluted air, the pollution can still find its way into your body. Coal-burning power plants spew mercury-laden exhaust fumes into the air, which eventually end up in our water supply and in the flesh of fish we eat, especially in predators like tuna. For decades, factories have quietly polluted our environment with toxic cancer-causing waste like polychlorinated biphenyl (PCB) and hexavalent chromium (think *Erin Brockovich*).

Geographical areas where cancer rates are particularly high due to pollution are known as cancer clusters, and these clusters are usually industrial areas. In 2013 researchers at Emory University found an increased risk of non-Hodgkin's lymphoma among people who lived near factories that released benzene into the environment.[4] Benzene is used in the production of plastics, nylons, resins, and other materials such as lubricants, dyes, cleaners, and pesticides. The closer the people lived to benzene-releasing factories, the higher their risk.

In the United States, there are over 80,000 chemicals registered with the Environmental Protection Agency (EPA) for use in food production, cosmetics, prescription drugs, household cleaners, lawn care, agriculture, and more. These chemicals are in nearly every man-made product you buy, including makeup, plastics, paints, stains, varnishes, fabric dyes, and flame retardants. Full safety test data is available for a small percentage of these chemicals, but over half of them have no safety testing data at all.

Many of these chemicals are considered to be harmless in small amounts, but this is based on the assumption that everyone will only be exposed in small, isolated doses. What isn't taken into account is the synergistic toxicity created by exposure to thousands of these chemicals over one's lifetime.

In 2015, a task force of 174 scientists from 28 countries identified 50 common chemicals considered to be harmless at low doses but that could become carcinogenic when combined with other "harmless" chemicals. Some of the chemicals identified include triclosan in antibacterial soap; phthalates in plastics; titanium dioxide used in sunscreen; and acrylamide, which is found in french fries, coffee, some cereals, bread crust, and roasted nuts. According to cancer biologist and study author Dr. Hemad Yasaei of Brunel University in London, "This research backs up the idea that chemicals not considered harmful by themselves are combining and accumulating in our bodies to trigger cancer and might lie behind the global cancer epidemic we are witnessing."[5]

When you consider all of the chemicals in our environment, as well as those added to our food and in products we use every day, it can be a bit overwhelming. We are swimming in a toxic soup with a risk that is impossible to calculate.

THE POWER OF YOUR CHOICES

"We're all going to die sometime" is a popular bad habit justifier employed by people who don't think that their diet and lifestyle choices matter. But your choices do matter. It is now estimated that 70 percent of premature deaths from preventable diseases in the United States are attributed to three factors: poor nutrition, lack of physical activity, and tobacco use.[6,7] And when it comes to cancer, a recent study published in *Nature* estimated that as many as 70 to 90 percent of cancers are caused by diet, lifestyle, and environmental factors.[8]

It should be noted that before death come years of chronic disease and disability. According to a RAND Corporation study, 60 percent of Americans have at least one chronic condition and 40 percent have multiple chronic conditions. Nearly 150 million Americans are living with at least one chronic condition; around 100 million of us have more than one. And nearly 30 million Americans are living with five chronic conditions or more.[9] Our top killer chronic diseases—cardiovascular disease, cancer, and type 2 diabetes—are for the most part not genetic. They are not caused by bad luck or bad genes. They are directly connected to our choices. Your choices have the power to create health or disease in your body.

ONCE UPON A TIME IN THE WEST

Before we continue, I would like to clarify some terms you will see throughout this book. The Industrial Revolution is a product of Western civilization, which is why industrialized countries are also referred to as Western nations. The diet consumed by industrialized Western nations is known as the Western diet, and the chronic noninfectious diseases common to these nations—like heart disease, diabetes, and many cancers—are known as Western diseases or diseases of affluence. The Western diet is characterized as being high in animal products, especially red meat and dairy; high in refined sugar, saturated fat, junk food, and processed food; and low in fresh fruits, vegetables, legumes, nuts, seeds, and whole grains. The Western diet has its roots in the United States but in the last half century has been exported around the world, and today it has little to do with geography. For example, most European countries are located in the Eastern hemisphere but are considered to be Western nations eating a Western diet and getting Western diseases.

EVERYBODY THINKS THEY ARE HEALTHY

Fewer than 3 percent of Americans are considered to be living a healthy lifestyle, which is made up of four factors: eating five servings of fruits and vegetables daily, getting regular daily exercise, not being overweight, and not smoking.[10,11]

Thanks to a lifetime of food industry marketing, most of us have been conditioned to believe that we eat pretty healthy. The surprising reality is that only about 10 percent of Americans are eating the recommended amount of fruit and vegetables per day.[12] Americans eat an average of 1.7 servings of vegetables per day. Only 2 percent of the American diet is whole fruits, and 3 percent of it is vegetables other than potatoes. Another 3 percent of it is beans and nuts, and 4 percent of it is whole grains like oats, barley, whole wheat, and brown rice.[13,14,15]

Nineteen percent of the American diet consists of foods made from highly processed grains like white flour and corn starch, such as white bread, bagels, muffins, and tortilla chips. Seventeen percent comes from added sugars in soda, candy, and processed food, and 23 percent comes from added fats like butter and margarine, as well as shortening and oils from corn, canola, and soybeans, which are widely used in processed and fried foods and are predominantly made from genetically modified crops.

The remaining 26 percent of the American diet consists of meat, dairy, and eggs, the health benefits of which are widely (and hotly) debated. If you consider animal foods to be healthy, the typical American diet might be about 38 percent healthy and 62 percent unhealthy. If you view animal products as unhealthy, the average American's diet is around 12 percent healthy and 88 percent unhealthy. This doesn't take into account the difference between organic, pasture-raised animal products and those that come from commercial factory farms, which divides the debate further. Either way, both positions offer insight as to why the Western diet has led to industrialized nations suffering from chronic Western diseases in epidemic proportions.

A study published in 2018 offered key insight into how highly processed food may cause inflammation in the body and make the immune system more aggressive over time. Mice fed a high-calorie, high-fat, high-sugar, Western fast-food diet for a month were found to have high levels of immune system activity and inflammation in their bodies, surprisingly similar to how the body responds to a bacterial infection. After the mice were put back on their normal diet for four weeks, the inflammation went away, but some of the genetic switches in their immune cells stayed on, keeping their immune systems on high alert with a tendency to overreact to small stimuli with stronger inflammatory responses.[16] An overly aggressive immune system triggered by the Western diet could be the missing link behind why so many people suffer from chronic inflammation, which makes your body a breeding ground for cancer.

Another 2018 study found that every 10 percent increase in consumption of ultra-processed foods increases your cancer risk by 12 percent.[17] Ultra-processed foods include sugary drinks, processed baked goods, sugary cereals, salty snack foods, reconstituted meat products, and ready meals like instant noodles and soups and TV dinners. The scary reality is that more than half the foods Americans and U.K. citizens eat is ultra-processed, which gives us roughly a 60 percent increase in cancer risk compared to people around the world who don't eat a Western diet loaded with ultra-processed food. Even just one sugary soft drink per day has been linked to an increase in risk of 11 different cancers, including breast, kidney, liver, colorectal, and pancreatic cancer.[18]

OUR LEADING CAUSES OF DEATH

The Western diet causes Western diseases like heart disease, cancer, and diabetes. Heart disease is the leading cause of disease death in the U.S., killing about 595,000 people annually. Cancer is close behind, killing about 580,000 people per year. Cancer is already the leading cause of death in 22 states and is expected to take the number one spot in the U.S. in the coming years. The vast majority of incidences of these killer diseases are not caused by bad luck or bad genes. They are the direct result of our daily diet and lifestyle choices compounded over time. Lung cancer is the number one cancer killer for men and women, and smoking causes roughly 90 percent of lung cancers and at least 30 percent of other cancers, including digestive cancers, head and neck cancers, ovarian cancer, and leukemia.

Smoking also increases your risk for liver, cervical, breast, prostate, and skin cancer because when you smoke, carcinogenic toxins circulate and pollute your entire body. Along with causing cardiovascular disease, smoking is the number one cause of cancer and cancer death. The good news is that you can reduce your risk of lung cancer by roughly 90 percent by not smoking.

Like smoking, alcohol is also classified as a Group 1 carcinogen. Alcohol is responsible for over 5 percent of new cancer cases each year and nearly 6 percent of cancer deaths worldwide. The highest cancer risk is in heavy long-term drinkers who also smoke, but the latest research indicates even just one drink per day for women and two drinks per day for men increases risk over one's lifetime.[19]

LADIES AND GENTLEMEN, WE ARE FAT

We have an unlimited supply of food, and our calorie consumption has increased significantly over time. According to the USDA, the average American ate 3,400 calories per day in 1909. Today the average American eats roughly 4,000 calories per day, 600 more calories per day than we were eating 100 years ago. Two-thirds of American adults and nearly 30 percent of boys and girls under age 20 are overweight or obese. Millennials are on track to be the fattest generation in recorded human history by the time they reach middle age.[20] According to recent estimates, half of Americans don't get enough physical activity, and over one-third of us are actually classified as "physically inactive,"[21] mostly the obese third. Obesity kills roughly 110,000 Americans each year; it is the second leading cause of cancer behind smoking, and it is quickly approaching the number one spot.

Obesity causes over 600,000 cancers each year, roughly 40 percent of all cancers.[22] Excess body weight contributes to insulin resistance, abnormal hormone levels, chronic inflammation, decreased immune function, and significantly increases your risk for 13 different cancers, including colorectal, endometrial, ovarian, pancreatic, thyroid, and postmenopausal breast cancers.[23]

For decades, doctors have advised patients to maintain a healthy weight and keep their body mass index (BMI) in a normal range (between 18.5 and 25) in order to reduce their risk of obesity-related diseases and cancers. But a normal BMI doesn't necessarily mean health when chronic disease is the norm. Surprising new research published in 2018 revealed that having a high percentage of body fat can double a woman's risk for invasive estrogen-positive breast cancer even if she has a normal weight and a normal BMI.[24] Visceral fat, also known as belly fat, which is deposited around abdominal organs such as the liver, pancreas, and intestines, may be the biggest troublemaker. Belly fat produces a protein called fibroblast growth factor-2 (FGF2), which has been demonstrated to drive certain vulnerable skin and mammary cells to transform into cancerous cells.[25]

Excess body fat is primarily caused by poor diet and lifestyle choices, specifically a high-calorie diet with too much white sugar, white flour, refined oils, and animal foods and a lack of exercise.

Our top two causes of cancer come from what we are putting in our mouths—cigarettes and unhealthy food.

AN EXPLOSION OF INACTIVITY

Along with our unhealthy diets, modern conveniences have led to a sedentary lifestyle for modern earthlings compared to our ancestors, who walked everywhere and did physical work every day. They grew crops, hunted for food, raised livestock, ran from tigers, climbed trees, built shelter, danced around the fire, and crafted their tools, clothes, and furniture by hand. They were strong, fit, and rarely overweight, with the exception of the rich.

Now let's compare that to a typical day for someone in a first-world country. After lying down all night, we get up and get ready for the day. We bathe and get dressed. Then we sit down to eat breakfast. Then we sit in a car, bus, or train that carries us to work. Once at work, we sit at our desk to do said work. A few hours later, we get up to eat lunch. Then we find somewhere to sit down and eat it. Some of us eat lunch right there at our desks without getting up at all. After lunch, we do some more sitting at work. Then we have a seat in a car, bus, or train to travel home from work. When we get home, we have a nice sit-down dinner followed by some sitting on the couch or in bed to watch TV and/or surf the internet until bedtime, when we lie down for the night.

Granted, not everyone is *that* sedentary, but many of us are. The bottom line is that we just aren't moving our bottoms enough. On average, we Americans spend roughly 15.5 of our 16 to 17 waking hours each day sitting. Prolonged sitting significantly increases your risk of heart disease, diabetes, and cancer. According to epidemiologist Dr. Christine Friedenreich, physical inactivity is linked to as many as 49,000 cases of breast cancer, 43,000 cases of colon cancer, 37,000 cases of lung cancer, 30,000 cases of prostate cancer, 12,000 cases of endometrial cancer, and 1,800 cases of ovarian cancer. All totaled, prolonged sitting is estimated to contribute to 173,000 cases of cancer per year. Three to six hours per week (30 to 60 minutes per day) of moderate to vigorous exercise, ranging from walking to intense aerobic exercise, has been linked in numerous studies to a 20 to 40 percent reduction in cancer risk for 13 types of cancer.[26,27]

THE FOOD FACTOR

Over the last century, the quality of our food and the quantity that we are eating have changed drastically. Our overall carbohydrate intake has come down about 4 percent, but the types of carbohydrates we eat are very different. In the early 1900s, most of our carbohydrates were from whole foods like grains, beans, and potatoes. Today most of our carbohydrates are from refined foods like white flour, sugar, corn syrup, sugary drinks, potato chips, and french fries. We're also eating about 20 percent more animal protein than we were in 1909 and 60 percent more fat, primarily from oils.

Polyunsaturated fats in our diet, from corn, soybean, and sunflower oils and fatty fish are up 340 percent. Monounsaturated fats from olive, peanut, safflower, and sesame oils are up 70 percent. And saturated fat, mainly from butter and lard in animal foods, is up 20 percent. We are also eating roughly 10 percent more cholesterol. All totaled, our fat consumption has increased 60 percent from oils and animal foods in the last 100 years.[28]

Fresh food has been replaced by fast food. A hundred years ago, giant supermarkets and restaurant chains didn't exist, and it was common for a household to keep a vegetable garden and livestock for food. Today this practice is a rarity in the Western world, and the food that most people assume is healthy has been hijacked.

Food manufacturers strip food of its nutritional value and then add unnatural chemical ingredients, including artificial flavors, colors, additives, preservatives, and texture enhancers, as well as refined sugar and salt, hydrogenated oils, and trans fats.

The food industry has replaced natural ingredients with artificial ones to increase the profit margin and shelf life of their products. Simply put, artificial strawberry flavor is much cheaper than real strawberries.

Caramel coloring, produced with ammonia, is one of the most widely used food colorings in the world. It is used in colas, beer, sauces, and more, and it has been identified as a carcinogen. The state of California requires food manufacturers to put a warning label on food that contains more than 29 micrograms of caramel coloring.[29]

Agricultural giants are growing produce with toxic chemical fertilizers, pesticides, and herbicides. Many fruits and vegetables are picked before they are ripe and then artificially ripened with ethylene gas. These GMOs (genetically modified organisms) are genetically engineered with DNA from bacteria, viruses, or other plants and animals to withstand toxic herbicides like glyphosate (found in Roundup) and to produce their own insecticide.

Numerous studies have shown that GMO foods can be toxic or allergenic, and hazardous to people and animals that eat them, and many developed nations do not consider GMOs to be safe. Over 60 countries, including Australia, Japan, and the European Union, have significant restrictions and/or outright bans on the production and sale of GMOs. Unfortunately, in the U.S. it's a different story. U.S.-grown alfalfa, canola, corn, papaya, soy, sugar beets, zucchini, and yellow summer squash are predominantly genetically modified.

THE MYSTERY MEAT MACHINE

The vast majority of our meat today comes from factory farms where livestock are fed grain-based feed, injected with growth hormones, and given antibiotics to help prevent sickness while living in cramped, unsanitary conditions.

Commercial dairy cows are injected with recombinant bovine growth hormone (rBGH) under the brand name Posilac. This is a genetically engineered hormone introduced by Monsanto in 1995 that increases milk production in dairy cows by about 20 percent. rBGH also increases insulin-like growth factor 1 (IGF-1) in cow's milk. Elevated levels of IGF-1 can promote cancer in humans, specifically endometrial, prostate, breast, pancreatic, and colon cancer.[30] A European Commission report stated that "avoidance of rBGH dairy products in favor of natural products would be the most practical and immediate dietary intervention to . . . (achieve) the goal of preventing cancer."[31] rBGH has been banned in all 25 European Union countries, as well as in Canada, Japan, Australia, and New Zealand, but not the United States.

BREAD IS DEAD

A major source of calories in the Western diet comes from white flour and white bread, but nutritionally speaking, bread—specifically white bread—is dead. Whole organic grains, including whole wheat, are health-promoting staple foods consumed by the longest-living people on earth, and contain phytonutrients known to have protective effects against several types of cancer, especially colon cancer.[32] But when whole wheat is refined into white flour, it is stripped of 25 naturally occurring nutrients and then "enriched" by adding back only 5 isolated nutrients that were removed. Then chemical additives and preservatives are added to make the bread fluffier and increase its shelf life.

White flour is an unhealthy food, and we're eating it at nearly every meal. We're eating cereal, toast, muffins, biscuits, bagels, pancakes, and waffles for breakfast, and we're eating sandwich bread, burger buns, tortillas, pizza, pasta, and rolls for lunch and dinner. And let's not forget snacks and desserts like crackers, cookies, cakes, and pies. White flour converts to sugar in your bloodstream and gives you energy, which is good. But unlike whole-food carbohydrates (fruits, veggies, and whole grains), it lacks beneficial phytonutrients and antioxidants, which neutralize the toxic free radical by-products of cell metabolism. White flour and white sugar are empty calories, and a diet rich in empty calories will eventually make you fat and sick.

To make matters worse, conventionally grown wheat is sprayed with glyphosate (the active ingredient in Roundup) to control weeds and help dry it out 7 to 10 days before harvest. A 2009 article in the journal *Toxicology* cited evidence that glyphosate-based herbicides are endocrine disrupters at trace amounts of just 0.5 parts per million (ppm) and are liver toxic at 5 ppm in humans.[33] Gluten-free foods are all the rage these days, but gluten may not be the real problem for many folks. A 2013 article in *Interdisciplinary Toxicology* reported that the incidence of gluten intolerance, celiac disease, and irritable bowel syndrome has risen in direct proportion to the increased spraying of glyphosate on conventionally grown grains including wheat, rice, seeds, beans, peas, sugar cane, sweet potatoes, and sugar beets.[34] In 2015 the World Health Organization International Agency for Research on Cancer classified glyphosate as "probably carcinogenic to humans." Glyphosate is not only sprayed on genetically modified "Roundup-ready" corn, canola, and soybeans, but it is also sprayed on many types of conventionally grown non-GMO grains and vegetables to dry them out before harvest, including wheat, millet, flax, rye, buckwheat, barley, oats, beans, peas, lentils, corn, potatoes, and more.

MERCURY RISING

Mercury is the only naturally liquid metal on earth and is also classified as a "heavy metal." But despite its unique awesomeness, mercury is also a neurotoxin that has been linked to immune system suppression and a host of physical problems including brain damage, autism, Alzheimer's, amyotrophic lateral sclerosis, multiple sclerosis, cancer, and other chronic diseases. Very small amounts of mercury can damage the brain, nervous system, heart, lungs, liver, kidneys, thyroid, pituitary and adrenal glands, blood cells, enzymes, and hormones.

Mercury is a naturally occurring element that is all around us in our environment, but industrial pollution has doubled that amount. The majority of mercury pollution is spewed into the air by coal-fired power plants. From there it finds its way into the soil, rivers, lakes, oceans, and our food supply.

Fish and shellfish absorb mercury and store it in their fatty tissues. Mercury works its way up the food chain in a process called biomagnification as large fish eat smaller fish. The longer a fish lives, the more toxins like mercury it absorbs, and when you eat that fish you absorb it all. Almost all fish contain trace amounts of mercury, but the most contaminated fish are the predators at the top of the food chain, such as tuna, swordfish, shark, king mackerel, and tilefish. Mercury consumption from fish has been linked to brain and nervous system damage in unborn babies and young children, and has been found to cause cancer in rodents.[35]

FISHY FOOD

In 2003 the Environmental Working Group (EWG) released results of the extensive tests of cancer-causing PCB levels in farmed salmon consumed in the United States. EWG bought the salmon from local grocery stores and found 7 in 10 fish to be so contaminated with PCBs that they raised cancer-risk concerns, based on the health standards of the EPA.[36]

PCBs were banned in the U.S. in 1976 and have been linked to cancer and impaired fetal brain development. PCBs are stored in fatty tissue. Farmed salmon are fed fish meal that tends to be high in PCBs. As a result, farm-raised salmon has roughly 50 percent more fat than wild caught and averages 5 to 10 times more PCBs than wild-caught salmon.

Various species of wild fish have also been found to be contaminated with nanoparticles from the breakdown of plastics in our environment. These nanoparticles are able to cross the blood-brain barrier and cause brain damage and behavioral disorders in fish. Their effect on humans is not yet known.

WE ARE OVERFED BUT UNDERNOURISHED

We're stuffed, but we're starving. We're getting plenty of macronutrients (protein, fat, and carbs), but not nearly enough micronutrients like vitamins, minerals, enzymes, antioxidants, and the thousands of protective anti-cancer phytonutrients in plants, such as polyphenols, flavonoids, and carotenoids; allicin in garlic and onions; quercetin in apples; curcumin in turmeric; apigenin in celery; sulforaphane and indole-3-carbinol in broccoli; catechins in green tea; and ellagic acid in berries. These compounds are known to prevent cancers from forming, prevent tumors from growing, prevent cancer cells from spreading, and even directly cause cancer cell death. Fewer than 2 percent of Americans are getting the recommended minimum daily intake of potassium (4700mg).[37]

BURGER KINGS (AND QUEENS)

If you examine the life spans of the kings of Europe throughout history, you will see that many of them had short life spans. Rich people got rich people disease. Wealthy people got gout, heart disease, diabetes, and cancer because of their diets, which today would also be considered "whole foods" and "organic." Our wealthiest ancestors were also often obese. At one point in history, obesity was a status symbol, a sign of wealth, and obese women were considered the most beautiful because obesity implied a higher socioeconomic status and a life of leisure.

Kings and queens eat whatever they want, whenever they want. They can afford to eat three or more times per day, and they can eat expensive delicacies like meats and cheeses at every meal. Kings and queens can eat the finest, richest foods every day, foods rich in fat, sugar, salt, butter, cream, and oils. They have access to all the wine, beer, and spirits they desire. A king's diet is not a healthy diet. And it is no longer reserved for the wealthy. Today most Americans eat a diet high in animal products and sugar. Even worse, we're eating factory-farmed animal products and processed food loaded with man-made artificial additives, preservatives, flavors, and colors, as well as genetically modified food.

Historically, for the poor, meat was a luxury and typically only consumed on special occasions. Poor folks ate mostly plant foods like fruits, vegetables, legumes, and whole grains. This is still true today in undeveloped parts of the world. But in industrialized nations, thanks to large-scale factory farming and government subsidies that keep the prices of meat and sugar cheap, people can eat as much meat and sugar as they want. We are eating animal products and processed sugar at every meal and between meals. In the last century, processed sugar consumption has increased from about 4 pounds per person per year to roughly 100 pounds. That means the average person is eating about a pound of processed sugar every three days. We are eating about twice as much meat (6 times more chicken) and 25 times more sugar than our great-grandparents did in the early 1900s.[38]

If we keep eating the way we're eating, we're going to keep getting the diseases we're getting. If you eat a king's diet, you're going to get a king's diseases.

IS CANCER CONTAGIOUS?

According to the International Agency for Research on Cancer, 18 to 20 percent of cancers are linked to infections from cancer-causing viruses, such as hepatitis B and C, human immunodeficiency virus (HIV), some types of human papillomavirus (HPV), Epstein-Barr, and lesser known viruses like human T cell lymphotropic virus, Merkel cell polyomavirus, Kaposi sarcoma herpes virus, and bovine leukemia virus (BLV).[39]

Epstein-Barr virus, which has infected 95 percent of adults, has been found to cause Burkitt's lymphoma, Hodgkin's and non-Hodgkin's lymphoma, T cell lymphoma, nasopharyngeal cancer, and some cases of stomach cancer.[40]

Acute lymphoblastic leukemia, the most common form of childhood leukemia, has been linked to congenital cytomegalovirus (CMV), a form of herpes that can be passed from mother to child during childbirth. According to a study published in 2016, children born with congenital CMV are roughly four to six times more likely to develop ALL between two and six years old.[41] Fifty to eighty percent of American adults are infected with CMV by age 40, and one out of three pregnant women passes the virus to her unborn child.[42]

BLV is a cancer-causing virus found in cow's milk and meat. When milk supplies were tested in 2007, researchers discovered that 83 percent of small dairy farms and 100 percent of large dairy farms were found to be infected with bovine leukemia virus.[43] A human study found that 74 percent of subjects had antibodies indicating they had been previously exposed to BLV.[44] Pasteurization is thought to render BLV harmless in dairy products, but humans can also contract it from eating undercooked beef.[45]

In 2014, researchers identified BLV DNA in 44 percent of breast cancer tissue samples removed by surgery.[46] In 2015, they conducted another study to determine whether there was a link between BLV DNA in breast tissue and breast cancer, and concluded that the presence of BLV DNA in breast cancer tissue was strongly associated with diagnosed and histologically confirmed breast cancer. As many as 37 percent of breast cancer cases may be attributable to BLV exposure.[47]

Some viruses can't be avoided, but if you engage in risky behavior, such as unprotected sex or sharing needles with intravenous drugs, your odds of contracting multiple cancer-causing viruses are much higher. If your immune system is strong, your risk of developing cancer from viral infections is low, but viruses can lie dormant in your body for many years and then flare up if your immune system becomes weakened or suppressed for a prolonged period of time. This is why the factors in your life that you can control, like your diet, lifestyle, environment, and stress, are so important. A healthy body keeps infections in check.

CANCER RATES VARY GREATLY

The top cancers in Western nations are lung, colon, breast, and prostate cancer. In 1955, the death rate for pancreatic cancer, leukemia, and lymphomas was three to four times lower in Japan than in the United States, and the death rate for colon, prostate, breast, and ovarian cancers was five to ten times lower. This was at a time when animal products accounted for less than 5 percent of the Japanese diet.[48]

The Japan of 1955 was not an anomaly. Even today there are many parts of the world with much lower rates of cancer than are found in Western industrialized nations. Mexico has half the overall cancer rates of the United States. There are dozens of countries with a third of the overall cancer rates of the U.S.[49] In specific regions, and for specific cancers, it's even lower. The rate of colon cancer is over 60 times lower in native Africans than in African Americans.[50] The native Africans don't have a genetic advantage. They have a dietary advantage. They're not eating a Western diet, known to cause colon cancer.

To sum it up, we're sick. In the last 100 years, the incidence of chronic diseases such as cancer, heart disease, and diabetes has exploded in Western industrialized nations. It is clear that we have multiple factors working against us, including environmental pollution, a diet high in processed food and animal products, and a sedentary lifestyle. Scientists and researchers have identified the major causes of and contributors to chronic Western diseases, yet we are doing very little to prevent them. If you have a chronic disease like cancer or you are serious about prevention, the best thing you can do to promote health and healing in your body is to systematically identify and eliminate all of the cancer causers in your life and return to living as closely to nature as possible. True health care is self-care, taking care of yourself, but unfortunately, the medical and pharmaceutical industries have hijacked the words "health care" to put a rosy spin on what they do, which is most accurately described as sick care. In the following chapters, you'll see how sick the health-care industry has become.

DOCTOR'S ORDERS

I firmly believe that if the whole materia medica, as now used,
could be sunk to the bottom of the sea,
it would be better for mankind—and all the worse for the fishes.

— OLIVER WENDELL HOLMES

PRIMUM NON NOCERE. FIRST, DO NO HARM. This foundational principle of medical ethics dates back to Hippocrates, the father of modern medicine. From the Hippocratic Corpus in *Epidemics*: "The physician must . . . have two special objects in view with regard to disease, namely, to do good or to do no harm." If the methods involved in attempting to cure could produce more suffering than the disease itself, it's better to do nothing than to do something that can potentially hurt a patient.

Most of us assume the best treatment options are the ones our doctor recommends, but treating disease (not curing disease) is a trillion-dollar-per-year global industry. Treating disease makes doctors and drug companies a lot of money. The medical industry needs a steady stream of sick people to stay in business. I'm not implying that they want us to be sick or that they deliberately keep us sick, but the truth is that the medical industry benefits from our sickness. The sicker we all get, the more money they make.

Doctors are humans just like the rest of us, and sometimes humans are lazy, irresponsible, and negligent. I'm not demonizing doctors. There are many doctors who have had a positive impact on my life and to whom I owe a huge debt of gratitude. But let's be realistic. Earning a medical degree does not make you an ethical or moral person. There are good people and bad people in the world. Doctors are no exception. Some doctors care more about people, and some care more about money. Sometimes their priorities change over time. And sometimes it's hard to tell the difference.

Can you imagine being falsely diagnosed with cancer and then treated with multiple rounds of chemo? That is exactly what happened to the patients of Dr. Farid Fata in Michigan. Affectionately known as "Dr. Death," Fata was the perpetrator of one of the largest health-care frauds in American history. Over a six-year period, he falsely diagnosed or intentionally overtreated 553 people, fraudulently billed Medicare to the tune of $34 million dollars, laundered money, and engaged in a kickback scheme. Fata was busted in 2013, pleaded guilty, and was sentenced to 45 years in prison. And many of his patients/victims liked him and believed he was a good doctor. We have been conditioned to regard doctors as saintly, even superhuman. But they are not. They have the same flaws and problems as everyone else.

Being a doctor is a much harder job than most people realize. So hard that doctors have a higher rate of suicide than the general population. Male physicians have a 70 percent higher rate and female physicians have a 250 percent higher rate of suicide than everyone else.[1] Suicide is one of the leading causes of death for medical residents.[2] On a related note, more than 1 in 10 physicians develop drug and/or alcohol problems during their careers.[3] As scary as the implications of this are, let's not forget that sober doctors make mistakes too. But even if all doctors were saints and incapable of error, we would still have the same problem because for the most part, the problem is not doctors; it is our medical system, which is heavily influenced—some would say controlled—by the pharmaceutical industry.

DEATH BY MEDICINE

The third leading cause of death in the U.S. is a term most people have never heard of: iatrogenesis. That is death as a result of medical treatment. In 2000, a *JAMA* article reported that 225,000 Americans were dying each year from medical treatments.[4] Little has changed since then. In 2016, medical safety researchers at Johns Hopkins estimated that more than 250,000 deaths per year were due to medical errors.[5]

Here is an approximate break down of the iatrogenic deaths in the U.S. each year:

➤ Over 12,000 people die from unnecessary surgery.

➤ Over 7,000 people die from medication errors or negligence in hospitals.

➤ Over 20,000 people die from other hospital errors, like surgical errors.

➤ Over 90,000 people die from hospital-acquired infections.

➤ Over 127,000 people die from non-error prescription drug reactions.

Non-error prescription drug reactions are now the fourth leading cause of death in the United States. That's non-error. Every year over 127,000 people who are taking the correct doses of drugs prescribed to them by their doctors are dying from reactions to those drugs.[6,7]

Some experts believe that these numbers are inaccurately low because of unreliable "cause of death" reporting. Hospitals and doctors have a financial incentive (i.e., lawsuit avoidance) not to admit that they accidentally or unintentionally kill people, which is why they may decide to label a patient's cause of death as heart failure instead of heart failure from a drug reaction, or death from "cancer" instead of chemo toxicity.

One paper estimated that the number of medical deaths might be greater than 400,000 per year.[8] Another paper, entitled "Death by Medicine" and authored by Gary Null, Ph.D., Carolyn Dean, M.D., Martin Feldman, M.D., and colleagues, calculated the total number of iatrogenic deaths to be over three times higher than industry estimates, at 783,936 per year.[9,10] If their findings are correct, medical treatment is actually the number one killer of Americans. Even the seemingly harmless saline IV bags used in hospitals have been identified as contributors to kidney failure and death. Researchers estimate that 50,000 to 75,000 deaths could be prevented in the U.S. each year simply by replacing saline IV bags with balanced fluids such as lactated Ringer's solution or Plasma-Lyte A, which more closely mirror blood plasma and include electrolytes such as potassium and magnesium.[11] Your local hospital may be more dangerous than skid row, and the all too common scenario for patients who survive the gauntlet of medical treatment is that they find themselves trapped in a medical spin cycle of unnecessary tests, drugs, and procedures thanks to our epidemic of overdiagnosis and overtreatment.

DIAGNOSIS EPIDEMIC

Each year, tens of thousands of people, mostly women, undergo potentially harmful, unnecessary, and sometimes disfiguring treatments for precancerous conditions known as "incidentalomas." These are slow-growing, nonaggressive, indolent cancers or lesions that are unlikely to ever cause any harm. In 2014, Canadian researchers dropped a bombshell on the breast cancer industry via the *British Medical Journal* (*BMJ*). Their 25-year study of nearly 90,000 women ages 45 to 59 found that mammograms made no difference in the breast cancer death rate when compared to physical breast exams.[12] For every woman saved by breast cancer screening, 10 women will be treated unnecessarily. According to a 2012 study published in *The New England Journal of Medicine*, mammograms have overdiagnosed 1.3 million women in the United States in the last 30 years.[13] It's estimated that for every breast cancer death prevented by a mammogram, there are one to three deaths caused by unnecessary treatments given to overdiagnosed women. This includes death from things like drug reactions or from the long-term effects of radiation therapy, which increases a women's risk for lung cancer and heart disease.

Since 1975, the number of new papillary thyroid cancer cases has nearly tripled, but the death rate has remained the same, at 0.5 per 100,000 people. The vast majority of these thyroid cancers were not life threatening, and thousands of people have been treated unnecessarily. Many have had their thyroids completely removed and now have no choice but to take hormone replacement drugs for the rest of their lives. In a 2014 *JAMA* paper, Louise Davies, M.D., found that the increase in thyroid cancer in women was nearly four times greater than in men and concluded, "There is an ongoing epidemic of thyroid cancer in the United States. The epidemiology of the increased incidence, however, suggests that it is not an epidemic of disease but rather an epidemic of diagnosis."[14]

Overdiagnosis and overtreatment for nonthreatening conditions liberally labeled as cancer have become such a serious issue that a panel of experts, including some of the top scientists in cancer research from the National Cancer Institute, published an article in *JAMA* taking the firm stance that increased screening has not improved the cancer death rate.[15] They also recommended redefining what medical conditions should even be called "cancer." Their opinion is that conditions such as ductal carcinoma in situ (DCIS), prostatic intraepithelial neoplasia, and lesions detected during breast, thyroid, lung, esophagus (Barrett's), and other cancer screenings should be reclassified as IDLE (indolent lesions of epithelial origin), removing all connection to cancer. In short, what many doctors are calling "cancer" today may, in the near future, be simply described as "a lesion that is not likely to spread." In response to the overdiagnosis problem, the American

Cancer Society updated its mammogram screening recommendations in 2018, pushing the starting age from 40 to 45, due to the high incidence of false positives for women under 45.

Another overdiagnosis revelation came from a 2013 study published in *JAMA*, which found that the lung cancer diagnosis rate was 11 percent higher with CT scans over X-rays, and that one in five lung tumors found on CT scans are indolent—growing so slowly that they are unlikely to cause a patient any problems at all. The study also reported that 320 patients have to get a CT screening to prevent one cancer death, and suggested that for every 10 lives saved by CT lung cancer screening, almost 14 people will have been diagnosed with a lung cancer that would never have caused any harm.[16] This indicates that as many as 2 of every 10 lung cancer patients are suffering financially, emotionally, and physically, and in some cases dying from side effects of unnecessary treatments. Lung cancer is the number one cancer killer, with a five-year survival rate of only about 17 percent, and many five-year survivors still have cancer. The small percentage of lung cancer patients who are permanently "cured" may only be so because they were misdiagnosed and treated for a disease that was not life threatening to begin with.

If you are diagnosed with cancer in the United States, your doctor can only prescribe a combination of surgery, drugs, and radiation. That's the "standard of care" in which every patient is essentially treated the same way. In most cases, your doctor is not allowed to prescribe a change in diet or lifestyle or any other natural or nontoxic therapy as a first-line therapy if you have been diagnosed with cancer. They can recommend dietary and lifestyle interventions and other therapies as "complementary" but often do not. And even though many doctors will acknowledge that the body is capable of healing itself, there are pervasive ignorance and arrogance in the medical community, which scoffs at natural healing methods, including evidence-based nutrition and lifestyle medicine.

The medical industry tends to view cancer in a linear fashion, like an unstoppable train. The assumption is that if you have cancer, your body is incapable of healing it. But there is actually a medical term for cancers that go away on their own. It's called spontaneous remission. In 1993, The Institute of Noetic Sciences published *Spontaneous Remission: An Annotated Bibliography*, documenting 3,500 medically reported spontaneous remissions from 800 medical journals in 20 different languages. After interviewing and studying many of these patients, Dr. Kelly Turner wrote a phenomenal book on the subject called *Radical Remission*. When cancer goes away on its own, the industry calls it spontaneous remission, but there's another word for it: *healing*. The body creates cancer and the body can heal it.

THE FEAR FACTORY

Many patients are told by their doctors that nothing they did contributed to their condition, that it was just "bad luck" or genetics. If you believe that you are powerless and there is nothing you can do to help yourself and promote health and healing in your body, then medical procedures and pharmaceutical drugs are your only hope.

Once cancer patients are convinced that oncology is their only hope, doctors often use fear to motivate them to take immediate action. They want to get you onto the conveyor belt as quickly as possible. And once you are strapped on, it is very difficult to get off. Fear is one of the strongest motivators there is, especially the fear of dying. When Micah and I met with the first oncologist, his message was clear. If I didn't do what he said, I was going to die. He was my only hope and nothing else would help me. I was terrified when I left the cancer clinic, and I began second-guessing my nutritional approach. Had I not already started to read and research on my own, I probably would have done what most cancer patients do: reluctantly show up for chemo out of fear.

COMMUNICATION BREAKDOWN

A 2012 study showed that 70 to 80 percent of terminal lung and colorectal cancer patients surveyed thought that the treatments they were receiving were likely to cure them, when in fact the patients were only given chemo as palliative care to "buy some time" or "improve their quality of life," with no intention of curing their cancer.[17]

When doctors were questioned about their failure to communicate the difference between curative and palliative care, a common excuse was "It's hard to tell patients that you can't cure their cancer." Doctors also have a financial incentive not to tell patients the whole truth. If oncologists told every terminal cancer patient that chemotherapy was not likely to cure them, and detailed how harmful and damaging the side effects would be, they would risk losing a lot of patients and a lot of income. Oncologists often use convoluted terminology, medical jargon, and positive-sounding words like "benefit," "successful," "effective," and "working" to describe cancer treatment, but what those words mean to a patient and to an oncologist are very different things.

It's common for patients to hear things like "Your type of cancer has shown to respond favorably to (insert drug therapy here)" or "This treatment has been shown to be effective and works well with your type of cancer." When a chemo drug is described as effective, beneficial, working, or successful, it usually only means the drug might shrink a tumor, or reduce the number of cancer cells in your body temporarily. If shrinkage happens, your cancer is "responding" to treatment. After treatment, it's not unusual for tumors to start growing again at a more aggressive pace. That's when the patient realizes that the "successful treatment" that shrank their tumor for a few months didn't produce the kind of success they were hoping for—curing their cancer.

To convolute further, the benefits of chemotherapy drugs are typically stated using relative risk percentages instead of absolute risk, or overall survival risk. This makes treatments appear more attractive. For example, let's say that after surgery a patient has a

6 percent risk of recurrence within five years, and the patient is told that the recommended chemo regimen has been shown to reduce her absolute or overall risk of recurrence from 6 percent to 3 percent. That patient might be inclined to pass on chemotherapy because her risk of recurrence after surgery is already low at only 6 percent.

But this same therapy that reduces absolute risk of recurrence from 6 percent to 3 percent can also be described as reducing relative risk of recurrence by 50 percent, which sounds huge. This is often how pharmaceutical sales reps sell new drugs to physicians, who in turn use the same statistics and language to sell drugs to patients. When a doctor tells a patient that a drug therapy can reduce her risk of recurrence by 50 percent, she will be far more inclined to say yes to treatment, not knowing that she is only reducing her absolute risk from 6 percent to 3 percent. But even if an oncologist does disclose the overall survival risk, most patients still have no idea what that means. Because it's all about context.

Your doctor tells you, "This combination of drugs is the most effective, and has been shown to increase overall survival in patients with your type of cancer." That sounds positive, but here's the terminology twist: "increasing overall survival" does not mean anyone actually survived. It may only mean that some patients lived a few weeks or a few months longer on that combo of drugs compared to another combo before dying. Furthermore, living an extra two months while being poisoned, sick, bedridden, and in and out of the hospital is not what most people would call living: more like living hell.

Even the term "remission" can be deceptive. Some oncologists use the term remission without distinguishing between partial remission and complete remission. Partial remission means the tumor shrunk partially. Complete remission means that cancer lesions, tumors, or cells are not detectable by scans or tests at a singular point in time, usually immediately after a round of treatments is complete. It's not uncommon for a cancer patient to achieve complete remission after being "successfully treated" with surgery, chemo, and radiation, only to have new tumors form soon thereafter because the underlying causes of cancer were not addressed.

In a recent study, researchers reported that complete remission rates were 76.5 percent for a subset of obese patients with acute myeloid leukemia. Remarkable, right? Not so fast. If you read a bit further, the authors disclose that the average survival of these patients was only 14 months.[18] Complete remission often only means that tumors are gone temporarily, not that cancer is cured. It takes years to determine whether a complete remission will become a permanent cure. Yet it is perfectly acceptable for an oncologist to tell an obese leukemia patient that chemotherapy treatment for AML achieves complete remission in 76 percent of cases. What patient wouldn't agree to a treatment with a 76 percent remission rate? To the patient, a 76 percent remission rate means a 76 percent *cure* rate. But the oncologist knows the cancer is likely to come back after treatment and that the patient will probably die in one to two years. And they may not disclose that to the patient because "It's hard to tell patients you can't cure their cancer."

DOES TREATMENT REALLY EXTEND LIFE?

Over many decades, the cancer industry has developed a unique way of rebranding its failures as successes. To you and me, a successful treatment means being cured of cancer with no recurrence. Complete long-term restoration of health is success. Sickness and death are failure. In the cancer industry, success is measured in a variety of ways that are all designed to reflect positively on the industry. Tiny improvements are heralded as huge successes. One of these is "life extension." If you live a few months longer than your prognosis, which is a guess based on averages, then your treatment "worked" and was a "success," even if you die. Many studies demonstrating life extension of a drug therapy do not have control groups of patients who did no therapy at all.

In 1992, Dr. Ulrich Abel at the University of Heidelberg, Germany, published a comprehensive 92-page analysis of every available clinical trial and publication examining the value of chemotherapy in treating advanced epithelial cancers, also known as carcinomas. These are responsible for more than 80 percent of cancer deaths worldwide, including nearly all malignant tumors of the head, neck, lung, breast, bladder, colon, rectum, pancreas, ovary, cervix, and liver. His research also included surveying hundreds of oncologists around the world. A condensed version of his analysis, which included 140 citations, was published as an article in *Biomedicine & Pharmacotherapy*. Here's an excerpt from Abel's summary:

> Apart from lung cancer, in particular small cell lung cancer, there is no direct evidence that chemotherapy prolongs survival in patients with advanced carcinoma. . . . Many oncologists take it for granted that response to therapy prolongs survival, an opinion which is based on fallacy and which is not supported by clinical studies. . . . With few exceptions, there is no good scientific basis for the application of chemotherapy in symptom-free patients with advanced epithelial malignancy.[19]

Abel's exhaustive and virtually irrefutable research made little to no measurable impact on the cancer industry's standard of care in the years that followed.

In the United States, cancer is the second leading cause of death behind heart disease, and is predicted to be number one soon as it is now the leading cause of death in 22 states. Despite the many innovations in drugs and treatments in the last half century, the cancer industry has not improved the death rate for most cancers, especially epithelial solid tumor cancers. Lung cancer is the number one cancer killer in the U.S., claiming roughly 150,000 people each year. Today, decades after Abel's analysis, standard chemo treatment for non–small cell lung cancer, which is 85 to 90 percent of lung cancers, costs over $40,000 and may only give a patient an extra two months of life. More than half of people with lung cancer die within one year of being diagnosed.[20,21] The average survival of untreated lung cancer patients is seven months.[22]

Defenders of oncology are quick to dismiss older studies such as Abel's as irrelevant due to the development of new drugs and improvements in treatment methods, while conveniently neglecting to mention that some of the most popular chemotherapy drugs used today are between 20 and 60 years old. Here's a list of ten of the most commonly prescribed chemo drugs and when they were developed:

➤ Methotrexate —1950s

➤ Fluorouracil (5-FU)—1957

➤ Cyclophosphamide (Cytoxan, Neosar)—1959

➤ Doxorubicin (Adriamycin)—1960s

➤ Cisplatin (Platinol)—1978

➤ Gemcitabine (Gemzar)—1980s

➤ Etoposide (Eposin, Etopophos, VePesid, VP-16)—1983

➤ Chlorambucil (Leukeran)—pre-1984

➤ Docetaxel (Taxotere, Docecad)—1992

➤ Paclitaxel (Taxol, Abraxane)—1992

In 2013 a study reported that the proportion of patients in the Netherlands with metastatic gastric cancer increased from 24 percent in 1990 to 44 percent in 2011. The use of palliative chemotherapy to treat it increased from 5 percent to 36 percent during this time period, with "a strong increase" after 2006.[23] In this time period, the metastatic gastric cancer rate doubled and the use of chemo for it increased sevenfold, but the average overall survival only increased from 15 weeks in 1990 to 17 weeks in 2011. Twenty-one years of advancements in cancer treatment might get you an extra two weeks of life if you have metastatic gastric cancer. Yet the authors of the study still found a way to put a positive spin on the results by stating that "overall survival remained stable."

A study published in *JAMA* in 2015 reported that giving chemotherapy to end-stage cancer patients with fewer than six months to live did not improve their survival or their quality of life. The sickest patients had no benefit and those who weren't as sick suffered more. The patients who opted out of chemo lived just as long and had better quality of life than those who took the chemo.[24]

Unfortunately, Hippocrates's principle "First, do no harm" has been abandoned by the cancer industry, and treatments are often prescribed despite the certainty of severe physical damage and life-threatening risk to the patient. Most chemotherapy drugs have the potential to cause substantial harm and are often given to the point of overwhelming toxicity, with an all too common end result of death, especially for metastatic solid tumor cancers. So if studies and statistics have shown the same underwhelming results time and time again, why in the world would conventional medicine continue prescribing treatments that don't permanently cure most cancers?

MAKING
A KILLING

Good health makes a lot of sense,
but it doesn't make a lot of dollars.
— DR. ANDREW SAUL

IN 1897 SCIENTISTS AT BAYER began experimenting with acetyl-
salicylic acid, an extract from the bark of the willow tree, known
for centuries to be a pain reliever. They discovered a new way to
synthesize it, patented the formula, and two years later began selling it as aspirin. And the rest is history. Aspirin quickly became
the biggest drug in the world and ushered in a new era of pharmaceutical medicine, which is now a trillion-dollar industry. Pharmaceutical companies make money by creating unique drugs that
can be patented and sold at high profits for many years with no
competition. Over the past century, the pharmaceutical industry has infiltrated every aspect of medicine and exerts enormous
influence over the health-care industry, or what is known as the
medical-industrial complex.

"The medical profession is being bought by the pharmaceutical industry, not only in terms of the practice of medicine, but also in terms of teaching and research. The academic institutions of this country are allowing themselves to be the paid agents of the pharmaceutical industry. I think it's disgraceful."

— DR. ARNOLD S. RELMAN,
former editor-in-chief of *The New England Journal of Medicine*, who coined the term "medical-industrial complex"

In the United States, medical doctors get their educations and earn their degrees at institutions funded by drug companies. Doctors are certified by the American Medical Association (AMA), which receives funding from the drug companies. Doctors prescribe drugs approved by the Food and Drug Administration (FDA), which receives roughly $100 million per year in "user fees" from drug companies for new drug applications. The pharmaceutical industry has over 1,200 registered lobbyists in Washington, D.C., and spent $900 million lobbying on legislation and $90 million in campaign contributions to politicians from 1998 to 2005 alone.[1] In 2003 the Bush administration passed Medicare Part D, which prohibits the federal government from negotiating prices with the pharmaceutical industry. This allows the drug companies to charge Medicare whatever prices they want. In addition, Medicare and private health insurers waste nearly $3 billion every year throwing away unused cancer medicines because many drug makers distribute the drugs in one-size-fits-all vials with a dose that is too large for most patients; the unused drugs get tossed in the trash.[2]

There are only three countries in the world that allow drug companies to advertise to consumers: the United States, New Zealand, and to a lesser extent, Canada. In the States, drug ads are everywhere: on TV, on billboards, in magazines, and online. How did this happen? Lobbying. Decades of lobbying have led to government legislation that funnels American tax dollars directly to the drug companies. Pharmaceutical companies create their own philanthropies, fund research to create and patent drugs with tax-exempt dollars, sell themselves the patents to the drugs, and then sell those drugs to the public.

We the taxpayers fund the research; then the drug companies make billions in profit selling the drugs back to us. The U.S. government spent $484 million developing the cancer drug Taxol and then licensed it to Bristol-Myers Squibb, which has made over $9 billion on the drug and only paid $35 million in royalties to the National Institutes of Health.[3]

The pharmaceutical industry has spent billions of dollars to convince Americans that patented drugs are the answer to all of our ailments, but in most cases of chronic disease drugs don't cure us. They only alleviate some of the symptoms of disease, enabling us to continue the behaviors that are making us sick. Drugs make our sickness tolerable so we are able to function while unwell, in a state of "vertical illness." And they create long-term dependence. They've made us addicts.

MEDICATION NATION

We the people are heavily medicated. Half of Americans are taking one prescription drug monthly, 21 percent are taking three or more, and 10 percent of us are taking more than five prescription drugs per month. And Americans now pay twice as much for prescription drugs on average than the citizens of any other developed country.[4]

Many prescription drugs have side effects that can cause new problems with long-term use, creating a vicious cycle in which patients are taking drugs for the side effects of drugs, and then more drugs for the side effects of those drugs. Some prescription drugs are highly addictive, while others help just enough to perpetuate continual use. It seems that the strategy of the drug marketers—and it has been remarkably successful—is to convince Americans that there are only two kinds of people: those with medical conditions that require drug treatment and those who don't know it yet.[5]

In the United States alone, the number of prescriptions written for painkillers nearly tripled from 1990 to 2010. There were 209.5 million painkiller prescriptions written in 2010 alone, enough to medicate every single American all day and night for an entire month. As a result, the number of unintentional overdoses has quadrupled.[6] Prescription drug reactions are the seventh leading cause of death in the United States, killing over 100,000 people every year. Opioid painkillers like methadone, oxycodone, and hydrocodone are killing more people than cocaine and heroin combined. As bad as the opioid epidemic is, surprisingly only about 15 percent of prescription drug deaths are from painkillers. Roughly 85,000 deaths per year are caused by all the other drugs we are taking. Those prescription meds with a "low risk of side effects" in your medicine cabinet may not be so low risk after all. Fun fact: Bayer used to sell heroin as cough medicine.

For the better part of the last century, the pharmaceutical industry has enjoyed a monopoly on medicine and the public trust. But in the last two decades, the rise of the internet and widespread access to information have led to a collective consciousness of the pitfalls and perils of conventional medicine and to a resurgence in the interest in and use of nutrition and natural, nontoxic therapies for healing and preventing disease. In response to the natural health movement, pharmaceutical-based medicine rebranded itself as "science-based medicine" and "evidence-based medicine," using the word "science" to imply truth and the word "evidence" to imply proof. Like all manufactured goods, it goes without saying that there is science involved. Of course drugs are science-based, and so are Pop-Tarts. When it comes to evidence-based medicine, however, in some cases, the more closely you look the less you find.

Pharmaceutical medicine is most accurately described as patent-based, profit-based medicine because drug companies are only interested in evidence that can lead to patented, highly profitable pharmaceutical drugs. Over 100,000 nutritional science studies are published each year and for the most part ignored by the medical and pharmaceutical industry, despite the fact that these studies continue to contribute to the mountain of evidence that many of the leading causes of premature death from chronic disease (such as heart disease, diabetes, cancer) can be prevented and reversed through simple, inexpensive diet and lifestyle changes. The pharmaceutical and medical industries ignore this information because it isn't profitable. They can't make billions of dollars prescribing diet and lifestyle interventions like nutrition, exercise, and stress reduction. So they only focus on evidence that can produce patentable drugs. The inherent implication of evidence-based medicine is that it must have strong scientific evidence behind it. But that's not always the case. A large-scale meta-analysis of published and unpublished antidepressant drug trials found that placebos worked as well as the drugs 82 percent of the time![7] In addition, 57 percent of the drug trials failed to show any benefit, but most of those trials were not published.

In March 2012 C. Glenn Begley, a former head of global cancer research at pharmaceutical giant Amgen, reported that during the 10 years he spent at Amgen, he and his team of 100 scientists discovered that 47 of 53 "landmark" cancer studies could not be replicated, in some cases after 50 attempts.[8] Amgen's intention was to verify the reliability of the 53 studies before spending millions of dollars to develop new drugs based on them. Here's what Begley had to say about their findings:

> It was shocking. . . . These are the studies the pharmaceutical industry relies on to identify new targets for drug development. But if you're going to place a $1 million, or $2 million, or $5 million bet on an observation, you need to be sure it's true. As we tried to reproduce these papers we became convinced you can't take anything at face value.[9]

Our favorite heroin cough syrup makers, Bayer AG, published a similar report entitled "Believe It or Not," in which they revealed that less than a fourth of 47 cancer projects undertaken in 2011 reproduced the findings of previously published research, despite the efforts of three or four scientists working full-time for up to a year. Those projects were dropped.[10]

The failed replication projects at Amgen and Bayer clearly indicate that many of the "landmark" scientific studies that have significantly influenced cancer drug development and treatment were either flukes or fakes. The incentives to publish nonreplicable drug studies can be traced to both the pharmaceutical companies and the researchers themselves. With increasing competition for academic jobs and research funding, getting published in a scientific journal can be a significant career booster, resulting in job security, bonuses, research grants, and job offers. Thus if a researcher conducted the same experiment ten times and only got a positive result once, he could ignore the nine times it didn't work and publish findings on the one time it did—the fluke. And no one is the wiser until an attempt is made to replicate the study. The fakes, in contrast, occur when researchers falsify or manipulate data to support their hypothesis or achieve a desired outcome, such as proving that a drug works.

In 2006 alone nearly one-third of 1,534 cancer research papers published in major journals disclosed that the study was either funded by the pharmaceutical industry or conducted by an industry employee. These studies were more likely to have positive findings, indicating that researchers were biased toward their industry connections.[11] Between 2001 and 2010, the number of published journal articles increased by about 44 percent but the number of scientific papers that had to be retracted increased by over 1,000 percent. A review of over 2,000 retracted papers found that only 21 percent were due to errors and 67 percent of retractions were due to fraud or suspected fraud and plagiarism.[12] Consider the opinions of the editors in chief of two the most prestigious and well-respected medical journals in the world.

> The case against science is straightforward: much of the scientific literature, perhaps half, may simply be untrue. Afflicted by studies with small sample sizes, tiny effects, invalid exploratory analyses, and flagrant conflicts

of interest, together with an obsession for pursuing fashionable trends of dubious importance, science has taken a turn towards darkness.[13]

— DR. RICHARD HORTON,
editor-in-chief of *The Lancet*

It is simply no longer possible to believe much of the clinical research that is published, or to rely on the judgment of trusted physicians or authoritative medical guidelines. I take no pleasure in this conclusion, which I reached slowly and reluctantly over my two decades as an editor of *The New England Journal of Medicine*."[14]

— DR. MARCIA ANGELL

In November 2013 it was reported that breast cancer patients taking paclitaxel, a 20-year-old generic drug, actually lived one to three months longer than patients taking "promising new drugs" Abraxane and Ixempra, which cost $4,000 to $5,000 per dose and had nearly $500 million in combined sales in 2012. The cheaper 20-year-old drug worked better. In this case, the word "better" is relative because the patients still died. The report also noted that patients taking any of those three drugs combined with Avastin typically had their cancer return or progress within seven to nine months.[15,16]

Inaccurate and incomplete scientific research leads to the development of drugs that don't work well, or at all. A 2017 study published in the *British Medical Journal* found that over half of the new cancer drugs approved in Europe between 2009 and 2013 showed no benefit. These expensive new drugs did not improve survival or even quality of life.[17,18] In some cases, hyped-up, evidence-less drugs rushed to market can cause serious damage and death.

One of the most egregious examples of the harm caused by "evidence-based" medicine used without actual evidence is Avastin. One of the world's top-selling cancer drugs at the time, Avastin was approved for use on metastatic breast cancer in 2008 under the FDA's accelerated approval program, which allows a drug to be fast-tracked even with insufficient data. After Avastin's approval, drug maker Genentech completed two clinical trials, only to find that the results could not back up their claims. In November 2011, the FDA revoked Avastin's approval for treatment of breast cancer after concluding that the drug was dangerous and didn't work. FDA commissioner Margaret Hamburg issued the following statement:

> After reviewing the available studies, it is clear that women who take Avastin for metastatic breast cancer risk potentially life-threatening side effects without proof that the use of Avastin will provide a benefit, in terms of delay in tumor growth, that would justify those risks. Nor is there evidence that use of Avastin will either help them live longer or improve their quality of life.[19]

For two and a half years, tens of thousands of women were prescribed Avastin for breast cancer and many of them suffered from its life-threatening effects, including severe high blood pressure, perforations in their stomach and intestines, internal bleeding, and hemorrhaging, as well as heart attacks, heart failure, and death.

In November 2014, the FDA approved Avastin for use in platinum-resistant recurrent ovarian cancer because Avastin was shown to reduce the risk of the disease worsening or death by 62 percent when used along with 60-year-old chemo drug paclitaxel, when compared to chemotherapy alone. According to Sandra Horning, M.D., head of Global Product Development for Genentech, "Avastin plus chemotherapy is the first new treatment option for women with this difficult-to-treat type of ovarian cancer in more than 15 years." An impressive claim, but the patients taking Avastin only lived about three and a half months longer on average.

Genentech brought in over $48 billion in net sales revenue between 2006 and 2014, largely from selling Avastin. The drug is still on the market today, approved for use for several other cancers and typically given to terminal cancer patients, hoping it might buy them a bit more time, at a cost of over $50,000 per year.

A recent study found that patients who took Avastin combined with chemotherapy had a 50 percent increased risk of dying from its complications versus those who received standard chemotherapy. Patients given Avastin along with platinum- or taxane-based chemotherapy agents, such as carboplatin or paclitaxel, had over triple the risk of dying.[20,21]

In 2016, Genentech and OSI Pharmaceuticals were ordered to pay a $67 million fine for giving promotional materials to oncologists that included misleading and overstated survival data about the effectiveness of Tarceva to treat non–small cell lung cancer. Oncologists were persuaded to prescribe Tarceva as a first-line therapy and were not informed that there was little evidence to show that the drug had any benefit unless the patient had never smoked or had a mutation in their epidermal growth factor receptor, which is a protein involved in the spread of cancer cells.[22,23]

THE 2 PERCENT STUDY

In 2004, my first year of cancer, a groundbreaking study was published in the *Journal of Clinical Oncology* examining the five-year survival rates of cancer patients in the U.S. and Australia. The study included over 154,000 Americans and 72,000 Australian adults with 22 types of cancer who were treated with chemotherapy.[24] The study's conclusion:

> The overall contribution of curative and adjuvant cytotoxic chemotherapy to 5-year survival in adults was estimated to be 2.3% in Australia and 2.1% in the USA. . . . As the 5-year relative survival rate in Australia is now over 60%, it is clear that cytotoxic chemotherapy only makes a minor contribution to cancer survival. To justify the continued funding and availability of drugs used in cytotoxic chemotherapy, a rigorous evaluation of the cost-effectiveness and impact on quality of life is urgently required.

In this study, only 3,306 of 154,971 American cancer patients had five-year survival that could be credited to chemotherapy. The study did not distinguish between the survivors who were NED (no evidence of disease) or AWD (alive with disease). The only thing we know is that 3,306 patients were still alive at the five-year mark. Patients in hospice and on life support are considered successfully treated five-year survivors as long as their hearts are beating at the five-year mark. It is likely that some of these five-year survivors still had cancer or had a recurrence in subsequent years and eventually died.

In fairness, averaging the five-year survival rates of 22 different cancers and claiming that "chemo only works 2 percent of the time" is misleading. This is not unlike when my first oncologist told me I had a 60 percent chance of living five years, which was the average survival of all cancer patients lumped together. According to this study, chemotherapy would have only contributed about 1 percent to my five-year survival for colon cancer, worse than the 2.1 percent average. To its credit, chemotherapy was found to increase five-year survival of testicular cancer by 40.3 percent and Hodgkin's disease by 37.7 percent. Chemotherapy also contributes to better five-year survival rates for childhood acute myeloid leukemia (85 percent), and rare cancers like Burkitt's lymphoma, which has a cure rate of over 90 percent. Those cancers were not included in this study.

A major factor impacting the conclusion of the 2 percent study was that the five-year survival benefit for many cancers after chemo treatment was zero. No survivors. The cancers for which chemo reportedly made no difference toward five-year survival were melanoma, multiple myeloma, and soft-tissue sarcoma, as well as pancreatic, uterine, prostate, bladder, and kidney cancers.

SIDE EFFECTS MAY INCLUDE . . .

Side effects of prescription drugs can sometimes be worse than the disease the drug is designed to treat and can increase your risk of cancer, and many other debilitating and life-threatening diseases, and death. All prescription drugs abnormally alter metabolic functions in your body and many cause additional health problems with extended use. For example, according to the disclaimer in a commercial for the arthritis drug Xeljanz, "Serious, sometimes fatal infections and cancers have happened in patients taking Xeljanz." The drug companies are telling us that their drugs can cause life-threatening infections and cancer, and we're taking them anyway.

Oral contraceptives (birth control pills) are classified as a Group 1 carcinogen, a special designation reserved for known cancer causers like cigarette smoking. In October 2006, the Mayo Clinic published a peer-reviewed meta-analysis that showed a 44 to 52 percent increased risk of premenopausal breast cancer in women who used oral contraceptives before their first full-term pregnancy. Women who used oral contraceptives for four or more years before their first full-term pregnancy had the highest risk.[25]

Sometimes pharmaceutical companies neglect to inform consumers of the potentially life-threatening side effects of their drugs and get in big trouble for it. In April 2014 a U.S. jury ordered Takeda Pharmaceutical Company Ltd and Eli Lilly and Company to pay a total of $9 billion in punitive damages for concealing the fact that their diabetes drug Actos increased cancer risk.

CANCER DRUGS CAN CAUSE CANCER

Many chemotherapy drugs are carcinogenic, which means they can cause new cancers in the body. Other chemo drugs, while not directly cancer causing, can severely damage your immune system, which can give existing cancers the opportunity to spread rapidly. Some of the chemotherapy drugs identified as carcinogenic by the U.S. National Toxicology Program are Adriamycin, chlorambucil, cisplatin, Cytoxan, dacarbazine, Leukeran, Mustargen, Myleran, nitrosourea agents (CCNU, BiCNU, Streptozotocin, STZ, Zanosar), melphalan, tamoxifen, and thiotepa.

Chemotherapy can also backfire and boost cancer growth. When healthy cells are damaged by chemotherapy, they can secrete a protein called WNT16B. This protein can feed existing tumors, helping them grow and making them resistant to further treatment, which is why approximately 90 percent of patients with solid metastatic cancers, including breast, prostate, lung, and colon cancer, develop resistance to chemotherapy.[26] Research published in 2017 found that when cancer cells are injured or killed by chemotherapy, targeted therapies, and radiotherapy, they trigger an inflammatory "cytokine storm" in the tumor microenvironment that sets the stage to promote new tumor growth.[27] Researchers in Israel had a similar finding. When they dripped the blood of patients treated with chemotherapy on cancer cells in the lab, it made those cancer cells more aggressive.[28] Despite these recent revelations, this is really not new information. Doctors and researchers have known that chemotherapy causes more aggressive cancers to spread throughout the body since chemotherapy was first introduced. One example is the cancer drug tamoxifen, which has been reported to reduce a woman's risk of a secondary estrogen receptor-positive breast cancer by 60 percent. But if the cancer returns, it is four times more likely to be a more aggressive, estrogen receptor-negative breast cancer.[29] Tamoxifen also increases a woman's risk for uterine cancer and potentially fatal blood clots.[30]

COLLATERAL DAMAGE

Chemotherapy drugs can cause damage throughout your body all the way down to your DNA. Many chemotherapy drugs carry an FDA "black box" warning because they can cause life-threatening side effects and death. Nurses who administer chemo drugs are required to wear protective gear to make sure they don't get these dangerous chemicals on their skin while they inject them into a patient's veins. If any chemo drugs spill on the floor, medical staff have to use a special kit to clean up the spill, which is at that point considered hazardous waste.

Most folks know that chemotherapy drugs can cause hair loss, but unfortunately for some cancer patients who took Taxotere (docetaxel), the drug caused permanent baldness. According to one lawsuit, drug maker Sanofi-Aventis allegedly knew that permanent hair loss was a potential side effect in 2005 but failed to disclose this to patients and doctors in the United States until 2016.[31]

One significant area of damage that chemo patients often suffer from is brain damage, which is known as "chemo brain" and marked by an inability to think clearly, organize thoughts, and concentrate. Chemo brain has been reported to affect as many as 70 percent of cancer patients, and severe symptoms include memory loss, mental and emotional instability, and even dementia. For years the industry claimed there was no such thing as chemo brain, until recent studies validated patients' claims.

Platinum-based chemo drugs like cisplatin and carboplatin are nephrotoxic, causing kidney damage, or ototoxic, causing temporary or permanent hearing loss. Drugs such as doxorubicin are cardiotoxic and can cause heart damage. Drugs like bleomycin and busulfan can cause pulmonary fibrosis, which is lung damage. Other chemo drugs such as methotrexate and 5-fluorouracil (5-FU) cause myelosuppression, which is bone marrow damage that decimates your immune system and in severe cases may require a bone marrow transplant.

Drugs in the vinca alkaloid family like vincristine and vinblastin can cause peripheral neuropathy, or nerve damage in your hands and feet, causing the loss of feeling and function. This can cripple you for life, and as a result some cancer patients are unable to feed, clothe, or bathe themselves.

Chemo drugs such as cyclophosphamide can cause hemorrhagic cystitis, resulting in bladder damage and permanent loss of bladder control. Chemo drugs can also induce early menopause in women and result in a significant loss in bone density in premenopausal women, increasing the risk of fractures. In severe cases, chemo drugs can cause potentially fatal blood clots or destroy your blood, requiring a blood transfusion. Chemo can also make both men and women sterile.

In early 2013, the FDA and Health Canada both issued warnings that in rare cases Avastin was linked to a life-threatening flesh-eating bacterial infection called necrotizing fasciitis.

WHAT ABOUT IMMUNOTHERAPY?

In recent years, immunotherapy drugs, which attempt to harness a patient's immune system to seek and destroy cancer cells, have been hailed as "a new hope," "a game changer," and "the biggest breakthrough since chemotherapy." Your immune system is vitally important in keeping you well and cancer free, and improving the immune system's ability to eliminate cancer is a step in the right direction for cancer therapy.

Immunotherapy is currently the hottest trend in the cancer treatment world, and as I write this, there are roughly 800 clinical trials under way using immunotherapy drugs, but the initial results do not justify the hype. Immunotherapy drugs only show a response rate in about 20 percent of patients for some cancers and have no effect on others. It's currently estimated that only 8 percent of cancer patients will get any benefit in terms of tumor shrinkage or delayed cancer progression from immunotherapy drugs.[32] And the risks with immunotherapy drugs can be just as severe and life threatening as chemo drugs. Patients in trials have died from reactions to immunotherapy drugs. Beyond that, the cost of these drugs is astronomical.

One example is a headline-making trial that reported that combining Yervoy and Opdivo to treat patients with melanoma increased median progression-free survival by 11.5 months, which was much better than either drug alone, but cost nearly $300,000 per patient. Coincidentally, only 11.5 percent of patients had complete remission during the trial. Sixty-five percent of the patients in the trial had to stop the therapy because of drug toxicity, disease progression, or death.[33]

Another trial on Opdivo for lung cancer reported that patients got an extra three months of life at a cost of $100,000. Based on that finding, Bristol-Meyers Squibb actually trademarked the slogan "A chance to live longer" for use in their Opdivo commercials, which also discloses that "Opdivo can cause your immune system to attack normal organs and tissues in any area of your body and can affect the way they work. These problems can sometimes become serious or life threatening and can lead to death." Another immunotherapy drug, Keytruda, is estimated to cost as much $1 million dollars per year, per patient, depending on the dose amount.[34] Merck and Bristol-Myers Squibb sold almost $9 billion worth of immunotherapy drugs between 2015 and 2017.[35]

RADIATION EXPLOSION

Radiation exposure in the U.S. population from diagnostic imaging has increased sixfold in the last 30 years, primarily due to the rapid increase in CT scans from 1 million per year to about 80 million per year. Ionizing radiation from CT scans is powerful enough to damage DNA, which can lead to cancer. But would you believe that one-third of the patients getting a CT scan didn't even know the test exposed their body to radiation? In a 2012 study, researchers found that 85 percent of patients underestimated the amount of radiation delivered by a CT scan and one-third of patients didn't know CT scans produced radiation at all.[36] On a personal level, I had no idea how much radiation was used in CT scans until I researched on my own. One CT of the abdomen and pelvis exposes you to as much radiation as 100 chest X-rays. A PET/CT combo is the equivalent of 250 chest X-rays.[37]

Radiation treatments are one of the top five causes of secondary cancers for cancer survivors. The most common radiation-related cancers are lung, breast, thyroid, stomach, and leukemia. Eight percent of secondary cancers are related to radiation therapy. The percentage is a bit higher for prostate cancer (11 percent), cervical cancer (18 percent), and testicular cancer (25 percent).

The radiation from a CT scan is considered to be twice as carcinogenic as the gamma rays from the atomic bombs dropped on Hiroshima and Nagasaki.[38] After only one CT scan, your risk of radiation-related cancer remains elevated throughout the rest of your life and your risk increases with every scan. It's estimated that diagnostic radiation causes 1 to 3 percent of all cancers and that the number of radiation-related cancers will triple in the coming years if diagnostic radiation use continues at current levels. A recent National Cancer Institute study estimates there will be about 29,000 future cancers as a result of scans done in 2007 alone.[39]

From 1995 to 2008, the use of CT scans on children at general hospitals increased by a factor of five. In children's hospitals, CT scan use increased by a factor of 13, from nearly 15,000 in 1995 to 200,000 in 2008.[40] Children are especially vulnerable to radiation damage. A 2012 study reported that a childhood CT scan (or scans) resulting in a cumulative exposure of 50 to 60 mGy (milligrays) of radiation before age 15 can nearly triple their risk of developing brain cancer and leukemia in the future.[41] The cancer risk from CT scans decreases significantly after age 25. Good evidence suggests that 20 to 50 percent of childhood CT scans could be replaced with another type of imaging or not done at all.

CT SCANS: RESULTS MAY VARY

In 2011 a team of researchers at Memorial Sloan Kettering Cancer Center took 30 patients with stage III or IV lung cancer and a minimum tumor size of 1 centimeter and gave them two CT scans 15 minutes apart. Three expert radiologists were on hand to read the scans and measure the tumors but were not told that the same patients were being scanned twice.

Nearly two-thirds of the patients had a measurable difference in tumor size of a millimeter or more, and a third of them had a difference of two millimeters. Some of the tumors shrunk by as much as 23 percent and some grew by as much as 31 percent.[42] Again, this was after only 15 minutes. So did the CT scan cause the cancers to shrink, or grow, or both?

None of the above. What this study demonstrated is that CT scans can be unreliable when measuring cancer progression. Measuring the diameter of a tumor perfectly in the center in scan #1, then measuring it slightly off center in scan #2, or vice versa, can lead to a discrepancy in size between the two scans. And a small discrepancy in a CT scan can have massive consequences.

For example, if a CT scan indicated that your tumor grew by 31 percent, you would assume that treatment is not working. In which case, your doctor might be prompted to recommend more aggressive treatment, which may be completely unnecessary and harmful. In reality, a scan showing up to a 30 percent change in tumor size may not mean anything at all. Even if your tumor did grow by 30 percent—although that sounds huge—this may only represent a change of a few millimeters. A 1 centimeter tumor that grew by 30 percent is still only 1.3 centimeters, which is tiny, and in many parts of the body would not be considered life threatening.

LITTLE-KNOWN RISKS OF RADIOTHERAPY

When radiotherapy shrinks a breast cancer tumor by 50 percent, everyone assumes that's a good thing, but researchers at UCLA discovered that the radiation often kills benign cells. It also makes the surviving breast cancer stem cells resistant to further treatment and up to 30 times more likely to form new tumors than the non-irradiated breast cancer cells.[43]

Another study found that ionizing radiation reprogrammed less-malignant breast cancer cells into breast cancer stem cells, creating treatment-resistant "super cells." Radiotherapy can not only make existing breast cancer stem cells stronger and more aggressive, but it can also create new breast cancer stem cells. Radiotherapy has also been found to increase cancer stem cells in the prostate, resulting in cancer recurrence and worsened prognosis.[44] Another commonly undisclosed side effect of chest radiotherapy, especially when treating breast cancer, is that it can cause significant damage to the heart and arteries, leading to heart disease.[45]

In 2004 a large randomized trial (CALGB 9343) found that women 70 and older with estrogen-positive and/or progesterone-positive stage I breast cancer had no increase in overall survival after radiation treatments. Five years after this study was published, nearly two-thirds of breast cancer patients over 70 were still being unnecessarily treated with radiation therapy.[46] According to study author Dr. Rachel Blitzblau, "We should consider omitting radiation for these women, because the small observed benefits might not be worth the side effects and costs."

WHAT ABOUT DENTAL X-RAYS?

All ionizing radiation is harmful, and small doses add up over time. Ionizing radiation from dental X-rays increases your risk for meningioma, the most common type of brain tumor. In a 2012 study of 1,433 cases, researchers reported that those who reported ever having a bitewing X-ray at any age had twice the risk of developing a brain tumor. Those who had a panoramic (panorex) full mouth X-ray before age 10 had nearly five times the risk.[47] In addition, there have been several studies linking dental X-rays to an increased risk of thyroid cancer. If you need to have a dental X-ray, make sure they use a neck shield. Also avoid the 3-D cone-beam CT, which uses about six times more radiation than traditional dental X-rays. The American Dental Association has acknowledged that routine dental X-rays are unnecessary, and that there is no need for dental X-rays on patients who are not having any pain or teeth problems.[48] In 2006, the *Journal of the American Dental Association* stated that "dentists should not prescribe routine X-rays at preset intervals for all patients." Yet many still do.

The conventional medical model is an approach that tends to treat symptoms of disease with drugs, surgery, radiation, or other procedures, rather than the causes of disease. These limited procedures are largely a one-size-fits-all approach to treatment, and doctors today have become highly specialized, treating only individual body parts rather than the whole body. Medical doctors do not have the freedom to practice medicine. Instead they have a strict set of guidelines they must follow. If they deviate from these guidelines, they risk losing their license to practice medicine and their livelihood.

The pharmaceutical industry is pulling the strings of the health-care industry. It is producing more drugs every year and spending millions of dollars to convince us that we need them. We are taking more drugs than ever before, but we aren't healthier. The evidence and effectiveness behind drug therapies can easily be manufactured, while the risks are downplayed. Many cancer patients are not told enough about the side effects of treatment and have no idea what they are in for when they agree to it. And the collateral damage can be lethal. The risk that chemotherapy and radiotherapy can make cancer more aggressive or cause more cancer in the body is rarely explained.

The tragedy is that even with the overwhelming evidence that conventional treatments don't cure most metastatic cancers, the pharmaceutical and medical industries have shown little interest in abandoning these destructive treatments. Instead they see it as an opportunity to create more drugs they can sell in conjunction with chemotherapy, in an attempt to make chemo work a little better or lessen its side effects. More drug therapies equal billions more in profits, regardless of curing the disease or saving the patient.

IT'S NOT LIKE I NEED YOUR BUSINESS

It is difficult to get a man to understand something when his salary depends upon his not understanding it.

— UPTON SINCLAIR

DURING WORLD WAR I autopsies revealed that soldiers exposed to the chemical warfare agent mustard gas had very low white blood cell counts and depleted lymph nodes because of the effect the poison had on their bone marrow. It was then theorized that a mustard gas derivative might slow down the growth of certain types of cancer cells. In 1943, pharmacologists Louis Goodman and Alfred Gilman, along with thoracic surgeon Gustaf Lindskog, injected nitrogen mustard into six terminal cancer patients. Two of the patients with lymphosarcoma had "significant" but temporary tumor shrinkage, which had never been seen before. The patients were not cured and eventually died. This led to another series of experiments on approximately 150 patients. Some of these patients with Hodgkin's disease, leukemia, and lymphosarcoma also had tumor shrinkage, but again none were cured.[1]

When the war was over, the results of these studies showing tumor shrinkage were published and the multibillion-dollar chemotherapy industry was born. Chemotherapy literally means "treating disease with chemicals." Nitrogen mustard was banned for use as a weapon under the 1993 Chemical Weapons Convention. It is still used today, however, decades later, in the form of several cancer drugs: cyclophosphamide, chlorambucil, ifosfamide, melphalan, and mechlorethamine, aka Mustargen. Here's what the manufacturer Merck has to say about Mustargen, as per the FDA website:

> Therapy with alkylating agents such as Mustargen may be associated with an increased incidence of a second malignant tumor, especially when such therapy is combined with other antineoplastic agents or radiation therapy.

CANCER IS BIG BUSINESS

Over $40 billion is spent every year on cancer drugs around the world. Cancer drugs are the second-largest category of pharmaceutical sales in the United States, after heart disease drugs, and are growing twice as fast as the rest of the market. Treating cancer is not a humanitarian pursuit; it is a billion-dollar business.

After eight years of undergrad and medical school, the average graduate ends up with about $150,000 in student loan debt. Their next step is three to five years of residency, which typically pays about $50,000 to $60,000 per year. After roughly 12 years of education and training, an oncologist can finally begin their career. It takes another five to ten years before they see firsthand that the cancer treatment methods they were taught in med school don't produce permanent remission for metastatic cancers, and that most of these patients do not survive. According to the 2017 Medscape Physician Compensation Report, oncologists make $330,000 per year on average yet only 57 percent of those surveyed felt "fairly compensated."

The oncology business model is different from other branches of medicine because you can't buy most chemotherapy drugs at your local pharmacy. Hospitals and oncology clinics buy cancer drugs at wholesale prices and then mark them up and sell them to you, charging you for the privilege of putting them in your body. Private practice oncologists make up to two-thirds of their income on the profit from chemo drugs.[2] This conflict of interest and legal profiting on drugs, known as a "buy and bill scheme," is unique to the cancer treatment world.

In 2003 in an attempt to reduce the financial incentives attached to drug therapies and clean up the seedy side of cancer treatment, Congress passed the Medicare Prescription Drug, Improvement, and Modernization Act, capping the markup on cancer drugs at 6 percent plus an administration fee. Consequently, oncologists began prescribing drugs with higher profit margins and increasing the number of treatments given to patients.[3] More expensive drugs plus more office visits equal more money.

The financial incentives aren't limited to drug therapies for cancer. As I mentioned in Chapter 4, the use of CT scans has increased from 1 million per year to about 80 million per year in the last 30 years. A 2013 study published in *The New England Journal of Medicine* found that urologists who owned their own radiotherapy equipment prescribed radiation three times as much as urologists who did not. The 10-year survival rate for all types of prostate cancer is about 98 percent because it's typically very slow growing, but doctors who own their own equipment were found to be treating 80-year-old men just as aggressively as young men.[4] According to Jean Mitchell, author of the report and professor at Georgetown University:

> It's crazy the way the system is set up. The patients are going to do what their physician tells them to do. The patient becomes almost like an ATM machine, with the doctor extracting as much revenue as they can.

In 2014 UnitedHealth Group published a study in which they paid oncologists in five medical groups a flat-rate payment per patient instead of paying them for each drug or service they provided. As a result the cost of cancer care in these groups fell by 34 percent over three years, saving patients $33 million.[5] When you remove the financial incentives, it changes the way oncologists treat patients.

INSIDE THE FDA

Nutrition and natural remedies have been used for centuries to support the body in healing, and many herbal medicinal formulas have been passed down from one generation to the next. Along the way, entrepreneurial types have bottled and sold all manner of tonics, lotions, and potions with curative claims. The FDA was established in 1902 to regulate the safety of ingredients in the food and drug industry and to limit the health claims that a manufacturer of medicine could make. Many popular "health tonics" sold before the FDA was established contained dangerous and highly addictive ingredients.

In the late 1800s, a small Atlanta company developed an elixir that they marketed as a "brain tonic" and pain reliever. The original formula contained cocaine from the coca leaf and caffeine from the African kola nut. It was sweet and fizzy and made you feel really, really good. In 1903, after 17 years of distribution, Coca-Cola removed the active cocaine from its formula and eventually stopped making health claims. Today the FDA requires extensive clinical trials before a drug or medicine is approved for medical use to treat a specific disease. The goal of the FDA approval process is to determine whether a drug is safe and effective, but a lot of inside money influences the approval of new drugs because of the enormous cost of drug development and clinical trials. One of those costs is the $2.1 million "user fee" that drug companies pay to the FDA each time they submit a new drug application for approval.

According to the Tufts Center for the Study of Drug Development, the average out-of-pocket cost to take a new drug from inception all the way to FDA approval is $1.3 billion. But that's only an average of the costs of the drugs that got FDA approval. It doesn't count all the money the drug companies spent researching and developing drugs that failed to get approval.

Forbes writer Matthew Herper totaled R & D spending from the 12 leading pharmaceutical companies from 1997 to 2011 and found that they had spent $802 billion to gain approval for 139 drugs, at an astounding average cost of $5.8 billion per drug.[6] Each new drug has the potential to make tens of billions of dollars in profit. With that much money at stake, it's not surprising that pharmaceutical companies try to influence the drug approval process in any way they can, including putting their own people on the FDA approval panels.

In October 2005 the renowned science journal *Nature* published an investigation of panels that write the clinical guidelines governing the diagnosis and treatment of patients with new drugs. They discovered that more than one-third of these authors declared financial links to relevant drug companies, with around 70 percent of panels being affected. In one case, every member of the panel had been paid by the company responsible for the drug that was ultimately recommended.[7]

Once the FDA approves new medications, drug company sales reps push them to doctors, who then prescribe them to you. If a significant number of patients die or suffer severe health problems caused by the drug, the FDA will eventually recall the dangerous medication. In most cases the manufacturer of the recalled drug has already made astronomical profits—enough to settle lawsuits for the permanent injuries and death that their drugs caused before they were recalled. Unless it's a vaccine. In that case, the U.S. government uses your tax dollars to settle the claims because the pharmaceutical industry has immunity from vaccine injury lawsuits. You can thank the National Childhood Vaccine Injury Act of 1986 for that.

Every drug medication available in the U.S. is a result of a cost-benefit analysis of its therapeutic value versus its harmful effects. Unfortunately, the behind-the-scenes process by which the FDA approves drugs, as well as the influence that pharmaceutical companies exert on the process, is not understood by the public. What may be the most surprising is that the FDA does not actually conduct its own independent drug safety testing. This research is done by the very companies who make the drugs. *PLoS Medicine* reported in 2013 that as many as half of all clinical trials are not published.[8]

Here are a few examples of "evidence-based," FDA-approved drugs that have been recalled in recent years. Painkiller Vioxx, taken by over 80 million people, was recalled for doubling heart attack risk if taken for 18 months or longer. In its promotional efforts, Merck created a fake scientific journal that contained ghost-written articles promoting Vioxx, which was marketed to doctors.[9] According to testimony in a Vioxx class action case in Australia, Merck also created a hit list to "destroy," "neutralize," or "discredit" doctors who spoke out against the irritable bowel syndrome drug Zelnorm, which was recalled due to eightfold increase in risk of heart attacks.[10] Diet drug Redux was recalled for a twenty-three-fold increase in the risk of primary pulmonary hypertension—abnormally high blood pressure in the arteries of the lungs that causes significant strain on the heart—after only three months on the drug.

CANCER CENTERS ARE COMPETING FOR YOUR BUSINESS

From 2005 to 2014, the amount of money spent on advertising by cancer treatment centers tripled. In 2014 alone 890 cancer centers spent $173 million on ads and over half of that was spent by Cancer Treatment Centers of America.[11] The majority of TV and magazine ads for U.S. cancer centers use emotional appeals rather than facts, leading to unrealistic expectations about treatment. A recent review of 409 television and magazine ads for 102 cancer centers found that 85 percent of ads used potentially misleading emotional appeals that seemed to equate treatment with cure.[12] Sixty-one percent of ads featured messages evoking hope for survival. Over half the ads included patient testimonials. Forty-one percent of ads described cancer treatment as a fight or battle, and a third of the ads were categorized by the study authors as "fear inducing."

Twenty-seven percent of cancer center ads promoted the benefits of cancer therapies, but none of the ads cited specific data to support their claims. Only 5 percent of ads mentioned costs and only 2 percent of ads gave objective information on treatment or talked about the typical results and risks such as physical suffering, financial hardship, cancer recurrence, and likelihood of eventual death.

Cancer center television ads often feature images of bald women and children accompanied by dramatic orchestral music, followed by witty taglines like "Fighters Wanted" or "Making Cancer History." The study authors suggested that cancer center ads that evoke emotions of fear and hope may mislead patients and their families to pursue treatments that are either unnecessary or unsupported by scientific evidence.

CANCER TREATMENTS DESTROY HEALTH AND WEALTH

One often unanticipated side effect of cancer treatment is its "financial toxicity." For most patients, the cancer treatment conveyor belt involves countless office visits, blood tests, CT and PET scans, surgical procedures, radiation therapy, chemotherapy, additional drugs for the side effects of treatments, emergency room visits, hospital stays, physical therapy, and cosmetic procedures like breast reconstruction, custom wigs, and nipple tattoos. It all adds up to a ton of money. In 2012, 11 of the 12 cancer drugs approved by the FDA were priced at over $100,000 per year. That same year physicians at Memorial Sloan Kettering Cancer Center took a stand and refused to prescribe colon cancer drug Zaltrap because it cost over $11,000 per month and was not shown to work any better than Avastin, which only cost $5,000 per month. As a result, the manufacturer of Zaltrap came down on the price. These conscientious doctors deserve kudos for standing up to Big Pharma, but unfortunately, since then, new drugs are more expensive than ever.

Cancer treatment can be financially devastating for someone who doesn't have insurance, but even those covered by insurance can end up bankrupt. The total cost of cancer treatment can range from several hundred thousand dollars to well over a million, and it's not uncommon for a cancer patient's medical debt to range from tens of thousands of dollars to over six figures. The financial problem is compounded when many cancer patients find themselves unable to work, often not because of the cancer but because of the brutal debilitating treatments they are told they must endure to increase their chances of survival, or to maybe live just a little longer.

A comprehensive study on cancer patients in Washington state diagnosed between 1995 and 2009 reported that they were two and half times more likely to go bankrupt than anyone else, and younger cancer patients were two to five times more likely to go bankrupt than patients over 65.[13] According to the 2004 Medical Expenditure Panel Survey, $130 million is spent out of pocket every year by cancer patients not on Medicare. Patients and their families are draining their life savings, mortgaging their houses, borrowing from friends, maxing out their credit cards, and begging for money from anyone who will give, with the hopes that another round of treatments might cure them or buy them more time. After suffering through months, even years of brutal therapies, many cancer patients find themselves dropped off at the end of the line, broke or bankrupt, with irreversible damage done to their bodies and little time left to live.

THE CATCH-22 OF CANCER TREATMENT

Both chemotherapy and radiation are capable of shrinking tumors and reducing cancer in the short term, but in many cases, the cancer comes back more aggressively than before and the patient is then subjected to more aggressive treatments. Thus begins the downward spiral. Endless rounds of chemo and radiation treatments may keep the cancer under control for a while but destroy the patient in the process. The unfortunate and all too common end result is that the cancer eventually becomes resistant to all treatments, at which point either hospice is suggested or, as a last-ditch effort, the patient is given the opportunity to be a guinea pig in an experimental clinical trial, a practice known inside the industry as "desperation oncology."

At this point, many cancer patients are devastated, discouraged, tired of suffering, and too broke to try anything else. Many are depressed and hopeless, and lose the will to live. The few who still have a strong desire to live after doctors have told them, "We've done everything we can" often begin looking into natural, nontoxic, and alternative therapies as a last-ditch effort. Despite having the odds stacked against them, I have met many terminal cancer patients who have healed themselves after doctors sent them home to die. There is always hope!

THE ELEPHANT
IN THE WAITING ROOM

Men occasionally stumble over the truth,
but most of them pick themselves up and hurry off
as if nothing ever happened.

— WINSTON CHURCHILL

I stood in line for an hour and fifteen minutes for the Dumbo ride.
After a minute I was like, I'm the Dumbo.

— JIM GAFFIGAN

TODAY IN THE UNITED STATES, 1 in 537 people die from cancer, with an annual death toll of over 580,000. Every day over 6,000 people are diagnosed with cancer and roughly 1,500 people die of the disease. More people are dying from cancer each year than in all of the U.S. wars combined, and cancer is now the number one killer in the world with an annual death toll of about 7.6 million people. Nearly half of American men and a third of American women are expected to get cancer in their lifetime.

At the turn of the 20th century, cancer was killing 1 in 1,500 Americans. By the 1950s, the cancer death rate had tripled and chemotherapy was introduced. Twenty years later, President Nixon declared "War on Cancer" with the passage of the National Cancer Act of 1971. Since then over $500 billion American tax dollars (adjusted for inflation) have been spent on research for promising new treatments. Undeterred by the "war," the cancer death rate continued to climb and peaked at 215 deaths per 100,000 people in 1991. It has declined since then, but the reason for this decline has very little to do with improvements in cancer treatment.

Brace yourself for the most shocking statistic in all of Cancerdom. Since the introduction of chemotherapy in the 1950s, the overall cancer death rate in the United States has only improved by 5 percent. And that includes an adjustment for age and population size. The death rate is the purest measure of progress and we've barely made any in 60 years. To give credit where it is due, the most notable progress has been made in curatively treating a handful of cancers like chronic myeloid leukemia, Hodgkin's and non-Hodgkin's lymphoma, testicular cancer, and childhood leukemia, many of which have an average 10-year survival rate between 80 and 90 percent. The cancer industry frequently highlights these exceptions, but treatments for epithelial cancers (solid tumor carcinomas), which make up about 80 percent of all cancers, have made little to no progress in lowering the death rate. So why is this lack of improvement so at odds with what we hear from the medical industry about our progress in the war on cancer?

In 2016 the American Cancer Society, which receives funding from drug companies including Merck, Pfizer, Eli Lilly, AstraZeneca, and Genentech, released a report celebrating the fact that the cancer death rate had dropped 23 percent from its peak in 1991 and claiming that 1.7 million deaths have been avoided. This blurb circled the globe and was lauded by the media as "significant progress in the war on cancer due to increased screening, early detection and better treatments." But that doesn't tell the whole story.

THE SMOKING GUN

The real cause for the 23 percent improvement in the overall cancer death rate since 1991 is largely attributed to the reduction in cigarette smoking, and to a lesser extent the reduction in hormone replacement therapy (HRT) for women. Smoking is the number one cause of cancer, and lung cancer is our number one cancer killer. Eighty-three percent of lung cancer patients die within five years of diagnosis. Conservative estimates indicate that the reduction in smoking is responsible for 40 percent of the decrease in male cancer deaths from 1991 to 2003.[1] This 40 percent drop in the death rate of our number one cancer killer had a huge impact on the overall cancer death rate, but somehow "early detection and innovations in cancer treatment" got most of the credit in the headlines.

Another factor that contributed to the drop in the overall cancer death rate is that women are taking fewer prescription drugs that cause cancer. In 2002 the Women's Health Initiative reported an increased risk of breast cancer, heart attacks, and strokes among women taking Prempro, an HRT that combined estrogen and progestin. In the following year, HRT prescriptions dropped sharply. In 2001 61 million HRT prescriptions were written. By 2004 the number of HRT prescriptions had dropped by two-thirds to 21 million. In that same period of time, new breast cancer diagnosis rates dropped by 8.6 percent.[2]

A 2015 analysis of 52 studies suggested an association between short-term use of HRT during menopause and a 40 percent increased relative risk of developing ovarian cancer. This risk declines after stopping treatment, but women who used HRT for 5 years or more were found to have increased risk even after 10 years.[3]

PHANTOM SURVIVORS

According to the National Cancer Institute's Surveillance, Epidemiology, and End Results (SEER) data, the overall five-year survival rate for all cancers combined has improved about 40 percent since 1975. This improvement in five-year survival, the standard by which the effectiveness of cancer treatment is measured, looks phenomenal on paper but often means very little in the real world of cancer patients.

Oftentimes five-year survival statistics do not distinguish between disease-free survival (DFS) and those who are alive with disease (AWD). If a woman is diagnosed with breast cancer and is alive five years later, she is counted as a successful five-year survivor. If she still has cancer, she is still a success. If she is an invalid, bedridden, unable to feed herself, or on life support, she is still a success. If she dies five years and one month after diagnosis, she is still a success. But if during those five years she dies from one of the various side effects of cancer treatment like a surgical complication, a hospital-acquired infection, a drug reaction, chemo toxicity, or organ failure, she may not be counted at all if she didn't technically die from "cancer."

Here's how misleading and biased five-year survival statistics can be. If 10 women are diagnosed with late-stage breast cancer at age 60 and all die by age 64, their five-year survival rate is 0 percent. If these same women are diagnosed with cancer earlier at age 58 and all die by 64, their five-year survival is now 100 percent. Increased screening and early detection made a remarkable improvement in their five-year survival, but they are all still dead at 64. That statistical phenomenon is known as lead-time bias. Surprisingly, your doctor may have no idea what lead-time bias is or how it has inflated survival statistics. In one study, 54 of 65 physicians surveyed did not understand lead-time bias. Of the 11 physicians who indicated they did, only two explained it correctly.[4]

Many cancer patients are not actually living longer due to improved cancer treatments; they are just finding out sooner that they have cancer, thanks to early detection. In addition, early stage cancers that are not life threatening and may spontaneously regress (heal) without treatment are also being counted and treated with lumpectomies, mastectomies, radiation, and chemo. One example is ductal carcinoma in situ (DCIS), also known as stage 0 breast cancer, which accounts for 20 to 30 percent of all breast cancer diagnoses and has a nearly 100 percent 10-year survival rate. A study of more than 100,000 women with DCIS found that their risk of dying of breast cancer was the same as women with no signs of breast cancer. Thanks to current guidelines, 20 to 30 out of every 100 breast cancer patients are being unnecessarily diagnosed and treated for something that isn't cancer.[5] Just like lead-time bias, overdiagnosis bias has made huge improvements on five-year survival rates and virtually no improvement on cancer death rates.

The elephant in the waiting room is that the cancer industry isn't curing most cancers. The fact that the overall cancer death rate has barely improved in 60 years, while the cancer industry continues to tout dubious 5-year survival rates and take credit for the reduction in cancer deaths from less smoking, is a powerful indictment against this institution. There's simply no other logical explanation for the spinning of statistics on such a grand scale. Meanwhile, the cancer industry continues the widespread practice of "finding and successfully treating" cancers that would never have been life threatening, while simultaneously failing to cure the cancers that are. If winning the war on cancer means curing the disease, the cancer industry is most definitely losing. In the meantime, the cancer industry is generating over $100 billion in revenue per year. Losing has never been more lucrative.

As frustrating as the overdiagnosis and overtreatment problem is, the tide is turning. The use of chemotherapy to treat early stage breast cancer is on the decline. A study of roughly 3,000 women with early stage breast cancer—and some 500 doctors who treated them—found that use of chemotherapy declined overall from 34.5 percent of cases in 2013 to 21.3 percent of cases in 2015.[6]

A significant advance occurred in August 2016 when the results of the MINDACT phase 3 clinical trial were published confirming that nearly half of early stage breast cancer patients have been receiving unnecessary treatments. The trial used a genetic test called MammaPrint to determine a patient's risk of breast cancer recurrence after surgery. Use of the test reduced chemotherapy treatment by 46 percent among the over 3,300 patients in the trial categorized as having a high risk of breast cancer recurrence based on current treatment criteria. The "high risk" patients with a low risk MammaPrint score who did not do chemo had a 95 percent five-year distant metastasis free survival rate.[7]

You now know vastly more about the cancer industry than I did when I decided to take control of my health and start my healing journey. Back in January 2004, I had one book with one cancer healing testimony and very little scientific evidence to substantiate the author's claims. Even so, the message of radical life change to get to the root cause of disease and restore health resonated with me, and in the absence of verifiable facts, I made my decision based on instincts, intuition, and faith.

Despite my critical view of the cancer industry, I am not anti-doctor or anti-chemo. I am pro-life, pro-health, and pro-healing. Any strategy or therapy that promotes health and healing is one worth pursuing. Any therapy that is destructive, threatens to do more harm than good, and has little evidence of long-term success is one that should be approached with caution and considered carefully.

Although I've highlighted many of the perils, pitfalls, and failures of the conventional cancer industry, my intention is not to talk you out of conventional treatment. Rather, it is to equip you with knowledge to make an informed decision, the best decision for you. And hopefully to spur you on to continue researching and educating yourself. In the following chapters I will show you what I did and what my radical life transformation looked like.

THE BEAT CANCER
MINDSET

Luck is not a factor.

Hope is not a strategy.

Fear is not an option.

— JAMES CAMERON

Whether you believe you can do a thing or not,

you are right.

— HENRY FORD

IN THE FIRST YEAR OF MY HEALING JOURNEY, one of the physical therapies I employed, along with chiropractic adjustments and acupuncture, was a form of therapeutic massage called structural integration, also known as "Rolfing." Three months after my diagnosis, I went to see a structural integration practitioner named Elinor. During our first meeting, she asked me a series of questions, the last of which was surprising and slightly terrifying. She said, "Before we get started, I need to know if you really want to live."

Like many cancer patients, I had mainly been focused on not dying. No one had ever asked me if I actually wanted to live. Isn't that a given? Doesn't everybody want to live?

Did I really want to live? For a brief moment, I feared that maybe deep down I didn't, that perhaps, subconsciously, I had a death wish. So I asked myself, *Do I want to live? Do I?* I searched my heart. At first I didn't know what the answer was. Despite my ambition and the confidence I outwardly projected, I had never really liked myself. I was afraid that secretly maybe I didn't want to live and that maybe my cancer was the manifestation of years of painful insecurity and mental and emotional self-sabotage. But in that moment, I realized that even if that was true, I could confront those thoughts and feelings and behavior. I could change.

"Yes. I want to live."

If you've been diagnosed with a terminal illness, this is the most powerful question you can ask yourself. So go ahead, ask yourself, "Do I want to live?" If your answer is yes, my next question for you is "Why?" Why do you want to live? If you are not sure, take a few minutes to think about what you have to live for. Your reasons to live might be people in your life who need you, people you want to love and serve. Your reason might be a purpose, a calling, a mission you haven't accomplished, a dream you haven't fulfilled, or it might be all of the above. Write down or type up the list of your reasons to live and put this list in places where you will see it every day. Tack the list on the wall. Write it in lipstick on your bathroom mirror. Make it the background on your computer screen. Take a picture and make it the lock screen on your phone. Keep your reasons to live in front of you and on your mind throughout the day every day.

I had several strong reasons to live. First and foremost I wanted to live for my wife and for my parents. At the time of my diagnosis, Micah and I had been together for eight years (dated for six, married for two). I couldn't bear the thought of leaving her a widow. Equally painful was the thought of my parents standing beside her at my graveside, burying me, their only child. Beyond that I had dreams and aspirations. I wanted to live a long, full life. I had an entrepreneurial spirit, and I wanted to build a successful business. I wanted to have children and grandchildren, and maybe even meet my great-grandchildren. I wanted to have adventures and travel the world. I wanted to serve the purpose of God in my generation.

Healing cancer starts in your mind and your heart, and with a choice. The choice to live.

Some cancer patients don't have a strong will to live. They may be satisfied with what they've accomplished in life and are ready to die. If this is you, that's okay! What I would like to encourage you to do is to help the people around you understand that you are ready to die so they won't continue to pressure you into doing things you don't want to do. If you don't want to do treatment, don't do it. This is your life and you should do what you want to do. You should make the most of the time you have left and live your life to the fullest. Spend time with people you love. Make your bucket list and start checking it off.

In January 2012 my cousin Jeff was diagnosed with stage IV colon cancer. He was told that he would only live for about six months without chemo but that he could live up to two years if he did treatment. He accepted his prognosis and agreed to the treatments that his doctors said would "buy him more time" but would not cure him. He set up a CaringBridge page and chronicled his journey through cancer treatment, which showed his inspiring strength and courage. In one e-mail to family, he mentioned that he hoped to be able run one more marathon between chemo treatments, but the tone of his e-mails suggested that he had accepted that he would not be cured. During this time his mother was strongly encouraging him to get a second opinion and to consider incorporating nutrition and nontoxic therapies as I did. She begged him to talk to me and I reached out to him via e-mail, but he did not respond. Later he told his mother in another e-mail that he and I were very different and that he didn't buy into fads or self-help books.

After surgery to remove the tumor in his colon, Jeff felt better and was in good spirits, but within a few weeks after starting chemo his health took a dramatic turn for the worse as the tumors grew rapidly in his abdomen and liver. He could not eat or even keep water down, and he told the doctors that if living meant continuing to be in the condition he was in—i.e., not being able to eat or drink—he did not want to live and would just let the cancer take him, and he hoped it would be quick. Jeff was gone in about three months after diagnosis, just after his 49th birthday.

THE BEAT CANCER MINDSET

As I've thought about my cousin's cancer experience and reflected on the path he chose, I've come to realize that he was right. He and I are different. Introspection does not come naturally to me, but as I began teaching others about health, nutrition, healing, and survival, I was often asked why I made the decisions I made, and I was forced to self-analyze. I realized what made me different; it was the mindset I adopted, which was born out of my determination to get well and to live. Since I started my journey, I've read about, met, and interviewed many people who have healed all types and stages of cancer, and I've seen that same mindset in every single one of them. I call it the Beat Cancer Mindset. This mindset is the single most important factor, the linchpin in every successful healing story.

The Beat Cancer Mindset has five components:

- ➤ Accept total responsibility for your health.
- ➤ Be willing to do whatever it takes.
- ➤ Take massive action.
- ➤ Make plans for the future.
- ➤ Enjoy your life and the process.

1) Accept total responsibility for your health.

The first question on a cancer patient's mind after diagnosis is "Why did this happen to me? How did I get cancer?" The revelation I had in January 2004 was that the way I was living was killing me. If you have cancer, I believe you should assume the same. My intention is not to blame you or shame you but to empower you to take control of your situation and change your life. Many of the cancer-causing factors in your life can be removed and your risk of getting a recurrence or dying from cancer can be greatly reduced, just by your choices. Your choices matter.

People who care about you are going to tell you the truth. Sometimes the truth stings a little, but the truth will set you free. Accepting responsibility for your health starts with considering the possibility that cancer may be your fault. Maybe some bad decisions, bad habits, or ignorance over the course of your life contributed to your cancer. I know mine did. There's no need to beat yourself up about it or wallow in guilt, self-pity, or regret. Instead now is the time to evaluate your life, accept whatever part you played, and learn from your mistakes. Now is the time to identify the cancer causers in your life, radically change, and move forward.

One of the most troubling things I've ever heard a cancer patient say is, "I'm not going to let cancer change me." On the surface, this proclamation of defiance to the disease gives the impression of strength, determination, and willpower and could easily serve as a rallying cry for cancer fighters, but tragically, it is denial and disempowerment in disguise. It was denial that she had contributed in any way to her situation, and it was an acknowledgment that she did not believe she had the power to affect her health and her future. She did not survive. And the gravity of her statement still haunts me. Denial is far more dangerous than blaming yourself. Accepting the blame is taking responsibility. Taking responsibility for your circumstance empowers you to take control of your life and to change for the better.

Every day in cancer clinics all over the world, patients are told that their cancer is probably the result of bad luck or bad genes. This turns patients into victims. The logic is simple: nothing you did caused or contributed to your disease; therefore, there is nothing you can do to reverse it. If you have family history, they may tell you it's genetic. If you don't have any family history, they may still tell you it's genetic. Heredity and genetics are easy scapegoats, but fewer than 5 percent of cancers are genetic, and not everyone with a "cancer gene" develops cancer. Genes may load the gun, but your diet, lifestyle, and environment pull the trigger. However, if you believe that you are powerless and that there is nothing you can do to positively affect your health and your future, your only hope is medical procedures and pharmaceutical drugs.

You are not powerless and you are not a victim. The health or disease you are experiencing today is largely the result of the diet and lifestyle decisions you've made in the past. If you abuse your body, it is going to break down sooner, but if you take care of your body it will work better and you will increase your odds of health, healing, and long life. Today's choices affect tomorrow's health. Your choices matter!

Cancer is not the cause of a sick body. It is the effect of a sick body. You aren't sick because you have cancer—you have cancer because you are sick. When you accept that you may have played a part in your body becoming vulnerable to developing cancer, you will also realize that you can play a part in healing it. If you broke it, maybe you can fix it. If you caused it, maybe you can cure it. If the way you were living resulted in disease, maybe changing the way you live will result in health. Early in my cancer journey, I realized that I had never really taken care of myself. Being thin I assumed I had a free pass to eat whatever I wanted, and for many years I was unknowingly poisoning and polluting my body. I was living on processed food, fast food, and junk food. I was well fed but nutrient deficient. I was stuffed but starving. I had a history of exposure to environmental toxins. And I had a lot of unhealthy stress and negative emotions in my life. Deep down I hated myself, and I was desperately seeking the attention and approval of others to combat my insecurity and unhappiness. All of these factors contributed to my disease. And they all had to do with my choices. I needed to change, and cancer was the divine tap on the shoulder, the catalyst for that change.

2) Be willing to do whatever it takes.

Once you have accepted responsibility for your health, the next step is being willing to do whatever it takes to get well, which means being willing to turn your life upside down, to change everything. If restoring my health meant getting as close to nature as possible by sleeping in the woods in a tent, I was willing to do it. If it meant trekking out into the wilderness for a 40-day water fast like Jesus, I was willing to do it. Fortunately I didn't have to resort to either of those two things, but they were on my radar. I became a detective, determined to identify and eliminate anything in my life that may have contributed to my disease. I stopped eating to satisfy my appetite and sensual cravings and began eating to feed my cells, restore my health, and save my life. I wasn't living to eat anymore; I was eating to live.

Most cancer patients have a strong will to live in the beginning, but unfortunately most of them have also been convinced that "doing whatever it takes," "living strong," and "fighting cancer" just mean suffering through brutal and destructive cancer treatments. Whether you do conventional treatments or not, the Beat Cancer Mindset means taking an active role in your health and healing, not solely relying on someone else to cure you. I radically changed my diet and lifestyle. I gave up all the unhealthy food I loved to eat. I did every natural, nontoxic therapy I could find and afford. I faced my fears, admitted my faults, changed the way I thought, reached out to God and asked for help, and forgave everyone who had hurt me. This was a lot more work than showing up for chemo and having my doctor's permission to eat burgers, ice cream, and pizza, and not changing my life, but I knew I had to do it.

The difference between successful people and unsuccessful people is not motivation. Motivation is unpredictable and unreliable. It is easy to be motivated when you've started something new and exciting, but when the excitement wears off so does the motivation, and lack of motivation becomes an excuse for inaction. What keeps people going when their motivation is low is determination. Determination is the force inside you that cannot be stopped, even when the storms of life come against you. Determination is doing what you know needs to be done, whether or not you feel like it at the time.

During this process I became acutely aware of the spirit-mind-body connection as it relates to health and realized that not only did I need to change my diet and lifestyle, but I also needed to change the way I was thinking.

My perspective on cancer is different from most. I don't see cancer as something to be fought or killed; I see it as something to be healed. There is a battle involved in healing cancer, but it's not so much a battle in the body as it is a battle in the mind. In order to heal your body, you must first win the battle in your mind. *Changing your thoughts will change your life.*

But first you have to stop lying to yourself. You have to stop making excuses and stop making bad decisions that sabotage your life and your health. And this starts with changing your thoughts.

Instead of dwelling on negativity, feeling sorry for myself, being jealous of everyone who didn't have cancer, worrying about my future, and allowing depression and discouragement to paralyze me, I took control of my thoughts and chose to think of myself the way I wanted to be. *I am healed. I am healthy. I am well. I am going to live.* That Beat Cancer Mindset prompted me to take massive action every day to promote health and healing in my body.

Did these thoughts come naturally? Absolutely not. I had to choose to think that way every single day. Worry was not an option. Failure (death) was not an option. I had to succeed, and I had to live. I realized that my mind was like a track on repeat, playing the same negative thoughts over and over again. I had to reprogram my mind. When I caught myself thinking negatively, I chose to think positively. I chose to speak life out of my mouth and not allow outside influences, fear, and doubt to sway me. When you think and speak this way, you empower your creative subconscious mind to assist you in the process, and you find supernatural strength to do things you never thought you could.

Your conscious mind and subconscious mind are powerful. Your beliefs are powerful. Patients who believe treatment will help them often respond better than those who don't. The placebo effect is real. In my experience patients who go through the motions of treatment and therapies to appease those around them but don't believe they can get well rarely do. They subliminally sabotage the process and often make impulsive, irrational, emotion-based decisions that are not conducive to healing.

When a doctor tells a patient they are going to die in a matter of months, it can become a self-fulfilling prophecy. They often lose all hope and stop trying to live. They believe they are going to die and they usually do, as predicted. This is eerily not unlike a hex or a curse. No doctor has the authority to dictate the end of your life unless you give it to them. They do not know when you will die. They are just lumping you into a statistical group based on your age, cancer type, stage, and other factors. Your thoughts and beliefs create your life, your health, and your future. And when faced with a terminal prognosis, you have a choice of how to process that information. You can choose to believe it, or you can choose to reject it and become determined to prove your doctor wrong. It's okay to accept a diagnosis, assuming it has been validated by several sources, but you don't have to accept a prognosis that you're going to die in a certain amount of time because a doctor or a statistic said so. Defy the odds and be the exception. That's the Beat Cancer Mindset.

3) Take massive action.

The third characteristic of successful survivors is massive action. Minimal action typically produces minimal results, but massive action produces massive results. Massive Action is radical action. It's going against the grain. It's swimming upstream when everyone else is floating downstream. It's action that draws jealousy and criticism from others. Humans by nature are resistant to change and tend to have a "crab mentality." If you put crabs in a bucket and one tries to escape, the other crabs will pull it back down. In the same way, people often pull each other down out of envy, spite, or competitiveness. Massive Action may appear crazy to people around you and they may try to talk you out of it, like they did me, but don't let them.

Massive Action is facing your flaws, faults, and fears, changing your whole life, getting rid of everything that might be keeping you sick, and replacing disease promoters with health promoters. Sometimes small changes can produce big results. I love when that happens. But if that's what you're hoping for, your hope is in the wrong place because your hope is for a quick fix. That's not the Beat Cancer Mindset. That's the Magic Bullet Mindset. And the conventional and alternative cancer industries are both full of people ready to take advantage of anyone looking for a shortcut. You didn't get cancer overnight and you aren't going to get rid of it overnight. There is no miracle cure or magic bullet. Long-term healing requires massive action and a total life change. *Point your ship toward Healthy Island and stay the course.*

I've seen many cancer patients experience dramatic turnarounds in their health and have tumors shrink and even disappear in as little as 30 to 90 days using nutrition and nontoxic therapies, but I've also seen some of them become lazy and complacent and slide back into their old unhealthy habits. Then the cancer comes back. The first two years after a cancer diagnosis are the most critical. This is when cancer is most likely to return or spread. Two years of hard-core healthy living is an ideal short-term target, and beyond that, in order to stay healthy long term, you have to make your health a priority for life. Every day of your life is a page in your story. Your thoughts, decisions, and actions each day write your story. Take massive action to change your life and be 100 percent committed to the process. 100 percent is easy. 99 percent is hard.

4) Make plans for the future.

Document every detail of your cancer journey. Journal. Do a video diary. Plan on being well and document what you're doing so you can use what you've learned to help other people once you are well. You need a future goal to work toward, and making plans for the future is very important. The spirit-mind-body connection is a mystery, but something powerful happens when you plan for the future. You're planning to live. You're sending signals of life to your body. Don't be afraid to make plans for the future. I know the default response is, "Well, I don't know if I'll be here in a year or two years . . ." Instead of thinking that way, plan on living a long life. Sketch out your life goals, write down the things you want to accomplish, and keep those goals in front of you and start working toward them.

Making plans for the future is so important. When I was diagnosed, I didn't have children and I really wanted to have a family. I wanted to be a dad. The decision to start a family three months after being diagnosed was a huge risk, but it took my focus off cancer, strengthened my will to live, and brought a new dimension of purpose into my life. If Micah and I had agreed not to have children for fear of an unknown future, we would not have our two beautiful daughters, the greatest joys in our life.

5) Enjoy your life and the process.

Don't let fear and worry steal your joy. Make a decision to live in the present and to enjoy your life right now. Depression suppresses your immune system. If you're depressed, fearful, anxious, or worried, it makes you more vulnerable to cancer. Instead focus on things that bring you hope, optimism, encouragement, and joy. Start living your life, really living. There's an organization for young adult cancer patients called Stupid Cancer and I love their slogan, which is "Get Busy Living."

Now is the time to live. There are a thousand different ways you could die besides cancer. You could die in a car wreck. You could trip and hit your head on the pavement. You could choke on a peppermint. There's no point in letting cancer paralyze you into depression and inaction. Start doing things you've always wanted to do. Get out there. Live your life. Do fun stuff. Do some skydiving, mountain climbing, and bull riding like it says in the Tim McGraw song "Live Like You Were Dying." Make a commitment to enjoy your life and to enjoy the process. And Get Busy Living!

Even if some of these changes are difficult for you, like quitting smoking, giving up your favorite unhealthy foods, or eating vegetables you've never liked, you've got to keep your perspective because there are way worse things than vegetables. And when you get well, you can look back and know it was all worth it. This is a new chapter, a new season in life, a new adventure that should be dominated by gratitude. *Gratitude is the secret to happiness.*

Count your blessings every day. Don't focus on what you don't have. Focus on what you *do* have. Don't focus on what you can't do. Focus on what you *can* do. Cancer cut a dividing line in your life. If you're focused on the past, longing for the days before cancer and wishing things were the way they used to be, you will only make yourself more miserable. *What you focus on expands.*

Focus on joy, happiness, love, and gratitude and they will increase in your life. Focus on the present and on the things you can do today to improve your health and make your life better. In 2004 I was struggling to build a real estate business, barely making ends meet, and living in a tiny house, and I had cancer. I had every reason to be negative, bitter, and angry. But I learned how to exercise gratitude, how to be thankful, how to focus on all the good things in my life instead of the bad, and how to be happy in my most difficult season of life. And although I would rather not go through cancer again, I know with absolute certainty that what it taught me changed me for the better. The worst thing that ever happened to me has made my life more fulfilling than I could ever have imagined.

In the following chapters, I'm going to show you how to transform your life and how to take Massive Action to promote health and healing, which includes eliminating cancer causers, eating an evidence-based anti-cancer diet, and replacing your health-destroying habits with health-promoting ones. Finally, and most importantly, we'll talk about how to heal mentally, emotionally, and spiritually.

PLANTS VERSUS ZOMBIES

How Nutrition Fights Cancer

OVER 100,000 NUTRITIONAL SCIENCE STUDIES are published every year that demonstrate how naturally occurring compounds in plants can assist the body in preventing and reversing chronic disease. But because the pharmaceutical industry can't figure out how to extract most of the beneficial compounds in fruits, vegetables, herbs, and spices, synthesize them, and patent them for profit, this valuable research is largely ignored by the medical industry.

We've spent a lot of time talking about what you shouldn't put in your body and about how our Western diet promotes cancer. Now, as we begin to build your Massive Action Plan, we're going to talk about what you should put on your fork and into your body. In this chapter, we go deeper into the foods that fight cancer.

EATING TO BEAT CANCER

There are many different ways cancer can be stopped. Some compounds cause DNA damage, killing the cancer cell directly. Others cause apoptosis, which is programmed cell death, aka cancer cell suicide. Some are anti-proliferative; they stop cancer cells from spreading. Some compounds disrupt cancer cell metabolism. And others are anti-angiogenic. (Bet you can't say that last one five times fast.) We all have microscopic cancer cells in our bodies, but they can't grow into tumors any bigger than about 2 millimeters without first forming new blood vessels. This process is called angiogenesis, and blocking tumors from forming new blood vessels—a process known as anti-angiogenesis—is a very good thing. Avastin was the first anti-angiogenic drug approved by the FDA for cancer treatment but it is not a cure, has deadly side effects, and lost FDA approval for use in breast cancer. Fortunately there is a natural, nontoxic alternative: fruits and vegetables! Many phytonutrients in plant foods, such as apigenin and luteolin in parsley and celery, as well as fisetin in onions and strawberries, also have the ability to block the formation of new tumor blood vessels through anti-angiogenesis.

According to the research of Dr. William Li, president, medical director, and cofounder of the Angiogenesis Foundation, some of the most potent anti-angiogenic foods are green tea, ginseng, strawberries, blackberries, blueberries, raspberries, oranges, grapefruit, lemons, apples, pineapples, cherries, red grapes, kale, maitake mushrooms, turmeric, nutmeg, lavender, artichokes, pumpkins, parsley, garlic, tomatoes, olive oil, and even red wine and dark chocolate.[1] However, if you have cancer, I think it's a good idea to avoid alcohol until you are several years in the clear, as alcohol consumption can increase cancer risk. Dr. Li gave an excellent TED talk highlighting his discoveries in the field of nutrition and anti-angiogenesis called "Can We Eat to Starve Cancer?" And many of the foods I just listed aren't just anti-angiogenic. Like most plant foods, they contain compounds that cause cancer cell death, stop cancer from spreading, and disrupt cancer cell metabolism.

FRUIT VERSUS CANCER

Researchers at Cornell University conducted a study in which they dripped the freshly extracted juice of 11 common fruits on human liver cancer cells to see what would happen. Pineapples, pears, oranges, and peaches had very little effect on the liver cancer cells directly, but bananas and grapefruit cut the cancer cell growth by about 40 percent. Red grapes, strawberries, and apples were twice as potent as the bananas and grapefruit, but the tart fruits—cranberries and lemons—were the most powerful. Cranberries had the highest anti-cancer phenolic and antioxidant activity and cut liver cancer cell growth by 85 percent with only a third of the dose of apples and strawberries.[2] Lemons came in a close second. Researchers also noted that the higher the dose used, the more effective they were.

Cranberries have been shown to have anti-cancer effects on 17 different cancers in vitro and on 9 different cancers in animal studies, including cancers of the colon, bladder, esophagus, stomach, and prostate as well as lymphoma and glioblastoma.[3] In one study cranberries were fractionated in an attempt to isolate the active cancer-fighting compounds, but the isolated compounds did not work nearly as well as the whole fruit extract.[4] This is because the nutrients in whole foods are perfectly designed to work together synergistically to promote health in the body. The whole is greater than the sum of its parts, which is why many natural compounds don't translate to patented pharmaceutical medicine. In many cases they just don't work when isolated or altered in the lab. Anti-cancer nutrients are typically most potent when eaten in whole-food form, and the pharmaceutical and medical industries can't make any money selling lemons and cranberries to cancer patients.

Berries are the most potent anti-cancer fruits, partly due to their ability to protect and repair damage from oxidative stress and inflammation. Blueberries contain immune-boosting and anti-cancer compounds like ellagic acid, anthocyanins, and caffeic acid. One study reported that athletes who ate about two cups of blueberries per day for six weeks nearly doubled the amount of cancer-destroying natural killer cells in their blood from about 2 billion to 4 billion cells.[5] When eaten immediately before exercise, blueberries were also found to reduce oxidative stress and inflammation.

Raspberries, strawberries, and blackberries also contain ellagic acid and other compounds with anti-mutagenic effects that can protect your cells from free radicals and DNA damage, as well as slow down or stop cancer cell growth for many types of cancer. One laboratory study of berries versus cancer cells found that raspberry extract blocked cervical cancer cell growth by 50 percent. Strawberries blocked it by 75 percent.[6] Another study found organic strawberry extracts to be more potent and effective against colon and breast cancer cells than conventional strawberries.[7] In a 2011 randomized phase II clinical trial, researchers gave patients with precancerous esophageal lesions 60 grams of powdered freeze-dried strawberries every day for six months. At the end of six months, half the patients were disease free. The precancerous lesions were gone, and their tumor markers dropped dramatically, with just strawberries.[8] Another study found that black raspberries could stop the growth of precancerous oral lesions and even reverse cancer completely when patients applied black raspberries topically, simply spreading a black raspberry paste on the cancerous lesions in their mouth for six weeks.[9]

Lemons are everywhere and they're super cheap. Blueberries, blackberries, raspberries, and strawberries are also not hard to find, but cranberries present a few challenges. Fresh cranberries are not easy to find and even harder to eat because they are so tart. Store-bought cranberry juice is not an option because it's pasteurized, filtered, and often has sugar added. Dried cranberries, aka "craisins," are tasty, but they almost always have added processed sugar and oil, which could negate some of their beneficial effects. The best options are buying frozen organic cranberries at your local grocery store to blend into smoothies. You can also buy organic freeze-dried cranberry powder online and add it to juice or smoothies.

SUPERFOOD SPOTLIGHT: INDIAN GOOSEBERRY

Used for centuries in Indian ayurvedic medicine to treat nearly every condition known to man, and currently the top contender for the most incredible berry on earth, is amla, aka amalaki, the Indian gooseberry. Amla berries look like a cross between a green grape and a Ping-Pong ball and have the highest antioxidant content of any food known to man, with 200 times the antioxidant content of blueberries. Alma also has the second-highest concentration of vitamin C next to camu camu fruit. To put it in perspective, the average American meal has 25 to 100 units of antioxidants. One teaspoon of amla powder has nearly 800 units of antioxidants.

In a 2010 study, amla fruit extract was tested against six human cancer cell lines: lung, liver, cervical, breast, ovarian, and colon cancer. Amla not only stopped the cancer growth completely but also killed the existing cancer cells, reducing their population by over 50 percent, and significantly blocked the cancers' ability to spread.[10] Another study showed that just ¾ teaspoon per day of dried amla powder worked better at lowering high blood sugar into a normal range than the diabetes medication glyburide. In addition to regulating blood sugar, the study also found that the equivalent of one gooseberry per day cut bad cholesterol and triglycerides in half and boosted good cholesterol after only three weeks of supplementing daily.[11] Food trumps pharmaceuticals!

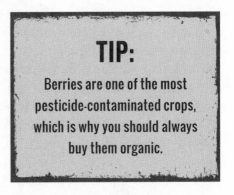

TIP:

Berries are one of the most pesticide-contaminated crops, which is why you should always buy them organic.

One small problem with amla, though, is that it tastes terrible. It is bitter, sour, pithy, and just plain awful. The first way I ever had amla was in an herbal fruit paste from India called Dabur Chyawanprash, which is a thick brown paste that's sweet and spicy.

But years later, when I first tried an amla berry whole . . . wow, was it gross. The easiest way to get amla in your body is by adding organic dried amla powder to water, juice, or a smoothie. You can get organic amla/amalaki powder online.

I'm often asked, "If sugar feeds cancer, what about the sugar in fruit?" The naturally occurring sugars in fruits and vegetables provide energy to every cell in your body, and the antioxidants and phytonutrients provide a wide range of anti-inflammatory and anti-cancer benefits in the body. Fruit is a wonderful health-promoting food, and nearly every fruit on earth has been found to contain anti-cancer compounds. I don't worry about the naturally occurring sugars in whole fruit. If there's one thing I'm sure of, I didn't get cancer from eating too much fruit.

THE TOP 10 ANTI-CANCER VEGETABLES

In January 2009 researchers published a study in the journal *Food Chemistry* comparing the anti-cancer effects of 34 vegetable extracts on eight different tumor cell lines. Researchers basically just ran vegetables through a juicer and then dripped the juice on different cancer cells to see what would happen. Many of the vegetables had significant anti-cancer effects, but the most powerful anti-cancer vegetable was garlic.

Garlic stopped cancer growth completely against the following tumor cell lines: breast cancer, brain cancer, lung cancer, pancreatic cancer, prostate cancer, childhood brain cancer, and stomach cancer. Leeks ran a close second and were number one against kidney cancer. But garlic and leeks weren't the only superstars: almost every vegetable from the allium and cruciferous families completely stopped growth in the various cancers tested. The allium family vegetables tested were garlic, leeks, yellow onions, and green onions. The cruciferous family veggies tested were broccoli, Brussels sprouts, cauliflower, kale, red cabbage, and curly cabbage. Spinach and beet root also scored in the top 10 against many of the cancers tested. Honorable mentions include asparagus, green beans, radishes, and rutabaga. Here is an excerpt from the study:

> The extracts from cruciferous vegetables as well as those from vegetables of the genus *Allium* inhibited the proliferation of all tested cancer cell lines whereas extracts from vegetables most commonly consumed in Western countries were much less effective. The antiproliferative effect of vegetables was specific to cells of cancerous origin and was found to be largely independent of their antioxidant properties. These results thus indicate that vegetables have very different inhibitory activities towards cancer cells and that the inclusion of cruciferous and *Allium* vegetables in the diet is essential for effective dietary-based chemopreventive strategies.[12]

The most powerful anti-cancer veggies in this study, including dark leafy greens, cruciferous veggies, and garlic, account for less than 1 percent of our Western diet. Something else worth noting in this study is that radishes were shown to stop tumor growth by 95 to 100 percent for breast and stomach cancer but had no effect and may have even increased tumor growth in pancreatic, brain, lung, and kidney cancer.

Researchers at Cornell conducted a similar study in 2002 in which they dripped the extracts of 11 common vegetables on human liver cancer cells. Spinach showed the highest liver cancer stopping power, followed by cabbage, red pepper, onion, and broccoli.[13] Garlic and leeks were not included in their study. Most of the top anti-cancer vegetables identified in both studies are the same vegetables I ate twice per day every day in a giant salad. The only veggies I did not eat were leeks, radishes, and rutabaga because I had no idea they were so great.

Brocc-Out and Crucify Cancer Cells

High intake of cruciferous vegetables including broccoli and cauliflower has been associated with reduced risk of several cancers such as breast cancer and aggressive prostate cancer.[14,15] Here are a few clues as to why. Your immune system begins in your intestines, and your body's first line of defense against pathogens, bacteria, viruses, parasites, and cancer-causing toxins are immune cells called intraepithelial lymphocytes. These cells are covered in aryl hydrocarbon receptors. Broccoli and other cruciferous veggies contain an anti-cancer compound called indole-3-carbinol, which activates the aryl hydrocarbon receptors on your intraepithelial lymphocytes, supercharging your intestinal immune cells. Broccoli also contains a compound called sulforaphane, which is created by a chemical reaction that happens when you chop or chew raw broccoli and is the most potent phase 2 liver detoxification enzyme known. If you plan to cook cruciferous veggies, chop them 30 to 40 minutes before cooking to allow the sulforaphane reaction to take place.

Broccoli sprouts contain roughly 25 times more sulforaphane and 100 times more indole-3-carbinol than mature broccoli, and they can be found in the refrigerated produce section of most grocery stores right next to the alfalfa sprouts. You can also purchase broccoli seeds and sprout them in three to four days at home, which makes them the cheapest and most powerful immune-boosting and detoxifying medicinal food on earth. Broccoli sprouts should be eaten raw and are great on salads. I should note that it is possible to get too much of a good thing. Too much sulforaphane could be toxic and make you feel sick, so it's recommended that you do not eat more than four cups of broccoli sprouts per day. Two to three cups per day should keep you on the safe side.

Medicinal Mushrooms

Mushrooms are a powerful immune-boosting, health-promoting food, and daily intake of mushrooms may have significant anti-cancer properties for many cancers, including breast cancer. Estrogen-positive (ER+) breast cancers need estrogen to grow, but simply eliminating estrogen from the diet may not be enough because many breast cancer tumors can synthesize their own estrogen by converting testosterone to estrogen with an enzyme called aromatase.

In one study, white button mushrooms were shown to suppress aromatase by 60 percent, which was better than any other vegetable and mushroom tested.[16] Mushrooms also boost your immune system and reduce inflammation in your body. Eating one cup of cooked white button mushrooms per day is shown to accelerate the salivary secretion of an immune system antibody called immunoglobulin A by 50 percent.[17] That's a very good thing.

Some of the powerful anti-cancer compounds found in mushrooms, oats, barley, and nutritional yeast are polysaccharides called beta-glucans. They are known as "biological response modifiers" because of their ability to activate the immune system.[18] Simply put, they make your immune system work better. Beta-glucan supplementation has even been tested on endurance athletes like cyclists and marathon runners. It's not uncommon for endurance athletes to get sick after a long race because extreme exercise causes immune suppression, but in one study, a control group taking beta-glucans cut their post-race infection rate in half.[19]

The rate of breast cancer in American women is six times higher than in Asian women. Two protective dietary factors that have been identified are green tea and mushrooms. In 2009 researchers found that Chinese women who ate an average of only 15 mushrooms per month along with drinking 15 cups of green tea per month had an astounding 90 percent reduced risk of developing breast cancer when compared to Chinese women who didn't consume green tea or mushrooms regularly.[20]

Drinking green tea and eating mushrooms daily could have a significant impact on your health. I ate raw mushrooms daily in my giant salads, but recent studies indicate that it might be better to eat mushrooms cooked because cooking destroys a toxin found in raw mushrooms called agaritine. If you really don't like the taste of mushrooms or you just want to maximize your immune benefit from mushrooms, you can also take them as supplements from a reputable company like Host Defense or Mushroom Wisdom.

Turmeric

The turmeric plant is a relative of ginger and has been used for thousands of years in Indian ayurvedic medicine as an antiseptic and antibacterial agent to heal wounds and treat infection, inflammation, digestive issues, and more. Indians eat a mostly plant-based diet with some of highest spice consumption in the world, and have significantly lower cancer rates than Western countries.[21] Indians have roughly 9 times less melanoma, endometrial cancer, and kidney cancer, 5 times less breast cancer, 10 times less colorectal cancer, 7 times less lung cancer, and 23 times less prostate cancer.[22]

Turmeric is one of the most powerful cancer-fighting spices known because it contains the anti-inflammatory antioxidant polyphenol curcumin, which has been shown to inhibit growth of many types of cancer cells.

Curry powder, a spice mix commonly found in Indian, Middle Eastern, Thai, and Malaysian cuisine, typically includes turmeric, coriander, cumin, chili peppers, and fenugreek and may also include clove, cinnamon, cardamom, fennel, and ginger. I love turmeric and curry powder, and I put them on nearly everything I eat. I even put a teaspoon of turmeric in oatmeal and a tablespoon in fruit smoothies.

Most cancer drugs target only one cancer pathway. For example, 5-FU targets DNA and methotrexate targets folic acid reductase. Curcumin, the active anti-cancer compound in turmeric, targets at least 80 cancer-linked cell-signaling pathways like p53, tumor necrosis factor, interleukin-6, NF-kB and mTOR.[23] Curcumin has the ability to block every stage of cancer development, from cancer formation to tumor growth to metastasis. It can also kill many different types of cancer cells by triggering apoptosis (programmed cell death) without harming normal cells.

Multiple clinical studies have found that doses of 8 grams per day of curcumin had no toxic effects in humans.[24] One study on Curcumin C3 Complex reported no toxic effects in humans taking 12 grams per day.[25] To date, a maximum daily dose has not been identified. Curcumin reaches peak blood concentrations in one to two hours. Taking it three times per day keeps therapeutic levels fairly consistent. A number of studies have shown that high-dose curcumin supplementation (8 grams per day) can enhance the effectiveness of chemotherapy drugs.[26] But in some cases, high-dose curcumin could cause adverse effects, depending on which drugs it is combined with. *Exercise extreme caution.* Dr. Bharat Aggarwal, curcumin researcher and author of more than 600 scientific papers, recommends dosing gradually starting with 1 gram per day for the first week and doubling the daily dose each week. By week 4 you will be taking 8 grams per day. In 2017 the *British Medical Journal* published the first ever case report of a woman who reversed her late-stage myeloma by taking 8 grams of Curcumin C3 Complex with BioPerine per day.[27] BioPerine is a patented formulation of piperine, an extract of black pepper or long pepper, which has been found to increase the absorption of curcumin by 2000 percent.[28]

Oregano

Oregano is an antibacterial, anti-inflammatory, and anti-cancer spice with high levels of antioxidants and antimicrobial compounds. Oregano ranks as one of the top ten highest antioxidant spices on earth, and one teaspoon of oregano has the same antioxidant power (oxygen radical absorbance capacity, or ORAC) of two cups of red grapes. It contains the flavonoid quercetin, which is known to slow cancer growth and promote apoptosis. It is also a good source of vitamin K and iron. Laboratory studies have found oregano extracts to cause cancer cell death in colon cancer, breast cancer, and prostate cancer.[29, 30,31]

Garlic

Garlic is one of the most powerful anti-cancer vegetables. Numerous studies have shown it to lower the risk of developing all types of cancers, especially colon, stomach, intestinal, and prostate cancer. It has strong antibacterial properties as well as the ability to block formation and halt activation of cancer-causing substances. It can also enhance DNA repair, slow down cancer cell reproduction, and, like turmeric and oregano, induce apoptosis. The World Health Organization even recommends that adults eat one clove of fresh garlic per day.[32] I consumed several cloves per day during my most intensive cancer healing season. I often chopped the cloves up into tiny bits and downed them with a swig of water or juice.

Black garlic is a super potent form of garlic that involves aging garlic for 40 days in 140 to 170 degrees Fahrenheit with 85 to 95 percent humidity, which produces sweet, chewy cloves that are less pungent and easier to eat. As powerful as garlic is against cancer, black garlic has been found to have even higher antioxidant, anti-inflammatory, and anti-cancer activity.[33]

Cayenne Pepper

Cayenne pepper, like most hot peppers, contains capsaicin, the active compound that sets your lips, tongue, and everything else on fire. Capsaicin has been shown to alter the expression of several genes involved in cancer cell survival, growth, angiogenesis, and metastasis. Like curcumin in turmeric, capsaicin has been found to target multiple signaling pathways, oncogenes, and tumor-suppressor genes in various types of cancer models.[34] And the hotter the better. Cayenne will spice up your salad quickly, so go easy on it the first time. If you can handle the heat, habanero peppers contain four to six times more capsaicin than cayenne, with a Scoville rating of 200,000 units.

TEA UP

Another key component of an anti-cancer diet is drinking copious amounts of herbal teas, specifically the ones reported to have immune-boosting, detoxification, and anti-cancer properties. Here are a few of the teas known to be the least friendly to cancer.

Essiac Tea

This herbal tea made from burdock root, sheep sorrel, rhubarb root, and slippery elm bark was discovered by Canadian nurse Rene Caisse in 1922. (*Rene* is like Irene without the "I". *Essiac* is Caisse spelled backward.) As the story goes, Rene obtained the formula from a woman who had been given the formula by an Ojibwan Indian medicine man and used it to cure her own breast cancer 20 years prior. Two years later Caisse used the tea to cure her aunt of terminal stomach and liver cancer and her mother of liver cancer. Caisse opened a clinic and treated cancer patients with the herbal formula for 18 years until Canadian government pressure and litigation forced her to close it down. Despite numerous offers, Caisse was very protective of the formula and refused to sell it for profit.

In 1959 she partnered with Dr. Charles Brusch to continue research on the formula. Dr. Brusch expanded the formula adding watercress, blessed thistle, red clover, and kelp and used it to treat cancer patients in his clinic. He even used it to cure his own bowel cancer.

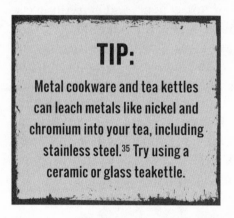

TIP:

Metal cookware and tea kettles can leach metals like nickel and chromium into your tea, including stainless steel.[35] Try using a ceramic or glass teakettle.

In laboratory studies, Essiac tea has been shown to have five times the antioxidant power of green tea and has significant anti-cancer effects by inhibiting tumor growth and stimulating immune response for various cancers.[36] Two reputable brands are Essiac Tea made by Essiac Canada International and Flor-Essence made by Flora. Essiac tea only requires a small dose of 1 to 3 ounces, two to four times per day. You can also make your own, as the formula is now widely known. I recommend the Essiac tea instructional videos by Mali Klein on YouTube.

Jason Winters Tea

In 1977 Jason Winters was diagnosed with terminal cancer and given three months to live. With nothing to lose, he decided to travel the world in search of a cure. He discovered medicinal herbs used for centuries on three different continents to promote healing in the body: red clover, chaparral, and a Chinese herbal tonic known as Herbalene, which contains astragalus and *Ligustrum*. The individual herbal remedies had little effect when consumed separately, and his condition worsened. As a last-ditch effort, he combined them all together in a tea and proceeded to drink about a gallon per day, and the large tumor on his neck began to shrink and was gone in three weeks. After his recovery, he began selling this blend, now known as Jason Winters Tea. In the last 30 years, research has shown that the herbs in Jason Winters Tea appear to have blood purification and immune supporting properties.[37,38] Chaparral has anti-cancer activities.[39] Astragalus has antioxidant, anti-inflammatory, immunostimulant, anti-cancer, and anti-viral activities.[40] Red clover has antioxidant activity and is also an aromatase inhibitor.[41,42]

Jason Winters wrote a book documenting his experience called *Killing Cancer*. He dedicated the rest his life to health education and won numerous awards around the world, including being knighted in Malta in 1985. Jason Winters Tea is delicious and naturally caffeine free. Our kids call it "Jason tea," and we love to drink it iced at our house.

Dandelion Root Tea

This pesky weed that pops up in your yard every spring is a powerful anti-cancer plant. Dandelion root tea has been shown to kill various types of cancer cells in the lab and in animals, including those for colon cancer, breast cancer, leukemia, melanoma, and even pancreatic cancer without harming healthy cells.[43,44,45,46,47]

Making dandelion root tea is simple. Dig up a dandelion that hasn't been sprayed with weed killer, cut off the root, and chop it or grind it up. Put ½ teaspoon to a teaspoon in a tea bag, steep it in boiling water for 20 minutes, and drink two or more cups per day. Dandelion root tea and dandelion root extract can be found at health food stores and ordered online. Don't throw away the dandelion greens. They are also highly nutritious and can be added to a salad or blended up in a smoothie. Don't eat the puffball.

Green Tea

The practice of drinking green tea dates back over 1,000 years to the Tang dynasty in China. Green tea contains known anti-cancer phytonutrients called catechins (epigallocatechin gallate, or EGCG) and about 13 times more antioxidants than blueberries and pomegranates. Regular consumption of green tea has been associated with a lower risk of death from cardiovascular disease and death from all causes.[48] It has also been shown to reduce the risk of certain cancers including breast cancer, prostate cancer, and colon cancer.[49] Matcha green tea is considered to be the most nutritious form of green tea. The matcha process involves grinding young green tea leaves into a fine powder that dissolves in water. (You don't have to grind it up; it comes that way.) And unlike steeping tea in a tea bag, you're consuming the entire tea leaf so you get all the nutrients. Green tea is wonderful and matcha green tea may be even better. You can drink matcha green tea hot or cold or add it to juice or smoothies.

Hibiscus Tea

Recent research has shown that hibiscus tea has an even higher antioxidant content than green tea. It is also rich in phenolic acids, flavonoids, and anthocyanins. Hibiscus extracts have been shown to inhibit the growth of cancer cells in the lab and have beneficial effects on inflammation, atherosclerosis, liver disease, diabetes, and other metabolic syndromes, which are all good reasons to drink it. Celestial Seasonings organic Zinger teas are all hibiscus-based teas.[50] You can also buy dried organic hibiscus in bulk, brew it yourself, or blend it into your smoothies, water, or juice.

FOOD FOUNDATIONS

Healing cancer does not require a secret formula, an exotic Amazonian plant, or a therapy costing tens of thousands of dollars. Cancer patients don't have to climb remote mountaintops to access a hidden cure. Nor do they have to fork over every dollar they have to access expensive treatments only available to a select few. Fruits, vegetables, mushrooms, spices, nuts, seeds, and herbal teas are the foundational ingredients of the anti-cancer diet. The truth is simple: whole foods from the earth give your body vital nutrients that enable it to repair, regenerate, detoxify, and heal.

Whether you have cancer or you want to prevent it, hopefully now you have a sense of how important your dietary choices are. The food on the end of your fork has the power to promote health or promote disease. Choose wisely.

HEROIC DOSES

The Anti-Cancer Diet

If man made it, don't eat it.

— JACK LALANNE

IN THE OLD TESTAMENT OF THE BIBLE, the Book of Daniel records a period of time when the Jewish people were living as captives of their conquerors in Babylon. The Babylonian king Nebuchadnezzar ordered young men from the Israelites' royal family to be trained to serve in his palace for three years. Daniel was one of those men.

The king ordered that the young men be fed the food from his table, but Daniel, in order to not violate his religious tradition, asked the chief official for permission not to eat the king's food. The official refused. Daniel then said, "Please test your servants for ten days: Give us nothing but pulse to eat and water to drink.

Then compare our appearance to the rest of the men who eat the royal food, and see what happens."

The word "pulse" refers to plant food like whole grains, beans, peas, fruits, vegetables, nuts, and seeds—whatever was available in that region at the time. Daniel was given permission to do the test, and after just 10 days he and his friends who chose to eat humble plant food from the earth appeared remarkably healthier and more nourished than the young men who ate the king's finest fare. Was their improved health a miracle or was it the diet?

Twenty-seven hundred years later and two blocks from my house, researchers at the University of Memphis put 43 relatively healthy participants on a 21-day "Daniel fast," eating a strict plant-based (vegan) diet of fruits, vegetables, nuts, and seeds with no animal food as well as no processed food, additives, preservatives, white flour, sweeteners, caffeine, or alcohol. At the end of 21 days, the participants had significant increases in antioxidant capacity and nitric oxide in their blood—both very good things. They also had reductions in oxidative stress, blood pressure, cholesterol, insulin levels, insulin resistance, and C-reactive protein, a marker of inflammation in the body.[1] In just 21 days, eating a whole-food, plant-based diet significantly improved their risk factors for metabolic and cardiovascular disease. Just like Daniel and his mates, they got healthier. A king's diet is not a healthy diet. It is a diet of excess. The king's diet in Daniel's day sounds a lot like the diet most of us eat today—a diet rich in meats, cheeses, sweets, and alcohol.

THE ANTI-CANCER DIET IS A PLANT-BASED DIET

The first phase of my Massive Action Plan to heal cancer was essentially an amped up 90-day Daniel Fast. I was determined to live and to change my internal terrain in order to make my body an environment where cancer could not thrive. Step one in this process was eliminating all processed man-made food and animal products in favor of an organic, whole-foods, plant-based diet.

In 2005, medical doctor and clinical researcher Dean Ornish at the University of California San Francisco, along with colleagues from UCLA and Memorial Sloan Kettering Cancer Center, conducted a study which proved that the progression of early stage prostate cancer can be reversed with intensive diet and lifestyle changes, specifically a low-fat, whole-foods, plant-based diet, exercise, and stress reduction. The 44 patients in the study who adopted a plant-based diet and incorporated daily exercise and stress management techniques instead of conventional therapy had a 4 percent drop in their PSA cancer-marker counts on average after one year. A 4 percent drop may not sound like much, but it indicates that their cancer had stopped spreading and that their bodies were healing. The patients with the strictest compliance to the diet and lifestyle program had the best improvement.

Meanwhile, the 49 patients in the control group, who didn't make any diet and lifestyle changes, had an average 6 percent increase in their PSA counts after one year, indicating disease progression. Researchers took the blood of the patients put on a plant-based diet for one year, dripped it directly onto cancer cells, and found that it had eight times the cancer stopping power. The plant-based patient blood slowed down the growth of prostate cancer cells in the lab by 70 percent. The blood of the control group eating the standard American diet (SAD) only slowed cancer growth by 9 percent.[2]

Another study took ten men with advanced prostate cancer whose PSAs were rising after having their prostates removed and put them on a similar program, which included a low-fat, whole-foods, plant-based diet and stress management. After four months, five of the ten patients had significantly slower PSA growth and three of the patients had lower PSAs than when they started, indicating disease reversal. Only two patients did not show improvement.[3] Just as in the Ornish study, those who committed to the program and followed it as directed had the best results.

In 2006 some of the same researchers from the Ornish study conducted a similar study on breast cancer cells. They took blood from overweight and obese postmenopausal women eating a standard American diet and dripped it on three different types of breast cancer cells. The SAD blood had only a small effect in suppressing the growth of the breast cancer cells. Then they put the women on a low-fat, whole-foods, plant-based diet and had them take an exercise class every day. Twelve days later they took more blood samples from the same women and dripped their blood on the breast cancer cells again. After just 12 days on a whole-foods, plant-based diet with daily exercise, the women's blood stopped the cancer cell growth between 6 and 18 percent and increased apoptosis (programmed cell death) between 20 and 30 percent.[4]

In 2015 after reviewing 800 scientific studies, the World Health Organization's International Agency for Research on Cancer (IARC) classified processed meats including bacon, sausage, ham, corned beef, canned meat, and jerky as Group 1 carcinogens. That means these foods directly cause cancer. They reported that eating 50 grams or 1.75 ounces of processed meat per day—that's only about two strips of bacon—increases your risk of colorectal cancer by 18 percent.[5] The IARC also classified red meat as a Group 2A carcinogen, which means there is limited evidence indicating that it probably causes cancer. The highest risk is for colorectal cancer, but links between red meat and processed meat consumption and pancreatic cancer and prostate cancer were also reported. Another meta-analysis associated increased consumption of red meat and processed meat with colorectal, esophageal, liver, lung, and pancreatic cancers.[6]

Will eliminating processed meat and red meat from your diet cut your cancer risk? Absolutely. But that's just one part of the equation. Eating animal products can also promote the growth of cancers in a number of ways.

One significant anti-cancer effect of a whole-foods, plant-based diet appears to be its ability to reduce insulin-like growth factor-1 (IGF-1) in the body. IGF-1, a growth hormone directly linked to uncontrolled cancer growth, increases in your body when you eat a diet high in animal protein and/or refined sugar. After just two weeks on a whole-foods, plant-based diet, the blood of breast cancer patients was found to have significantly lower levels of IGF-1 and increased cancer stopping power.[7]

Many human cancer cells, including colorectal, breast, ovarian, melanoma, and even leukemia, are dependent on an amino acid called methionine.[8,9] Without it, they die. Methionine is one of nine essential amino acids that cannot be made by the body. It must come from food. And guess which food group has the highest levels of methionine: animal foods! One way to deprive cancer cells of methionine and control cancer growth is to stop eating animal foods. Overall, fruits contain little to no methionine. Vegetables, nuts, and whole grains have small amounts of methionine. The highest source of methionine in the plant kingdom is beans, but animal foods have more. Milk, eggs, and red meat have more than twice as much methionine as beans, and chicken and fish have five to seven times more.

Beans, split peas, chickpeas, and lentils contain a valuable anti-cancer compound called inositol hexaphosphate, also known as IP6 or phytic acid. IP6 has been found to reduce cell proliferation and contribute to tumor cell destruction. It's even been shown to enhance the anti-cancer effects of chemotherapy, control cancer metastases, and improve quality of life.[10]

A 2014 study found that middle-aged Americans ages 50 to 65 who reported eating a high-protein diet with more than 20 percent of calories coming from animal protein were four times more likely to die of cancer or diabetes and twice as likely to die of any other cause in the next 18 years. But those who ate a plant-based diet did not have any increase in risk.[11] A diet high in animal protein is typically also high in saturated fat. A diet high in saturated fat has been found to increase your risk of lung, colorectal, stomach, and esophageal cancer.[12,13,14] It also increases your risk of breast cancer if you're a woman and prostate cancer if you're a man.[15,16]

Another cancer promoter found in animal food is heme iron, a highly absorbable form of iron found in meat—especially red meat, organ meat, and shellfish—but not in plant food. In small amounts, iron is good for the body and necessary for the formation of healthy blood cells, but in excess iron causes oxidative stress and DNA damage and can catalyze endogenous formation of N-nitroso compounds, which are potent carcinogens. Excess dietary iron has been linked to an increased risk of esophageal and stomach cancer as well as colorectal cancer.[17,18] Excess iron that is not used in blood cell formation accumulates in your liver, heart, and pancreas and can contribute to iron overload because your body has no way of ridding itself of iron except by bleeding. In addition, research published in 2018 concluded that two common forms of iron used in iron supplements, ferric citrate and ferric EDTA, might be carcinogenic as they increase the formation of amphiregulin in colon cancer cells, a known cancer biomarker most often associated with long-term cancer with poor prognosis.[19] Another form of iron, ferrous sulphate did not have this effect. A little-known benefit of menstruation is that women naturally shed excess iron every month until menopause. A 2008 VA Hospital study found that intentional blood iron reduction every six months in patients with cardiovascular disease resulted in a 37 percent drop in their cancer incidence and that those who developed cancer had a much lower risk of death.[20]

Non-heme iron is abundant in plant foods, especially in legumes, sesame seeds, pumpkin seeds, spinach, Swiss chard, quinoa, and dried apricots.

When you stop eating animal products and replace them with whole plant foods from the earth, you stop eating animal-derived protein and saturated fat; reduce the levels of cancer promoters like growth hormone IGF-1, methionine, and heme iron in your body; and increase the levels of thousands of anti-cancer phytonutrients found only in plant food.

PLANT POWER

For many years, the Centers for Disease Control and the National Cancer Institute have recommended that we eat at least 5 servings of fruits and veggies per day to protect against cancer, but a 2017 study concluded that eating 10 servings is even better. Eating 10 servings of fruits and vegetables per day (800 grams) was associated with a 24 percent reduced risk of heart disease, a 33 percent reduced risk of stroke, a 28 percent reduced risk of cardiovascular disease, a 13 percent reduced risk of all cancers, and a 31 percent reduction in premature deaths![21,22] Fewer than one-third of Americans eat the recommended five servings of fruits and vegetables per day. In addition, the fruits and vegetables most commonly consumed by Americans have the smallest amount of cancer-fighting nutrients. Our modern diet, loaded with animal products and processed food and deficient in fruits and vegetables, is not only polluting our bodies, but is also depriving us of essential anti-cancer compounds.

My anti-cancer dietary strategy was to "overdose on nutrition." I wanted to saturate my body with the vital nutrients in fruits and vegetables in order to give it all the fuel and firepower it needed to repair, regenerate, and detoxify, and I went way beyond the recommended daily allowances. I went from eating a typical American diet that might include 1 to 2 servings of fruits and vegetables on a good day to eating between 15 and 20 servings *every single day*.

The first book I read about healing cancer with nutrition recommended taking the plant-based diet a step further and eating like Adam and Eve in the Garden of Eden—all raw and all organic. Like most of the world in January 2004, I had never heard of the raw-food diet, and I was fascinated by it. There were no raw-food social media superstars back then, and I didn't have anyone to follow other than a handful of fringe health and wellness authors. But something about it made sense. I was fascinated by the idea of only eating organic fruits and vegetables straight from the earth. I loved the simplicity and purity of the raw diet, and I was excited to see what effect it would have on my body.

My anti-cancer diet had two major objectives. First, eliminate all foods that might be a burden to my body and promote cancer growth, like processed food and animal food. Second, "overdose" on nutrient-dense foods from the earth. I wanted to saturate my body with vitamins, minerals, enzymes, antioxidants, and the thousands of phytonutrients and anti-cancer compounds found in plant food. You can't accomplish this by taking a handful of supplements. This approach required massive action and my Massive Action Plan consisted of three main elements, aka the Super Health Triad:

1. Juices
2. The Giant Cancer-Fighting Salad
3. The Anti-Cancer Fruit Smoothie

JUICING

In order to understand the value of juicing, you need to understand what happens when you eat. When you chew food, you are essentially juicing it in your mouth. You are breaking it down into liquid form and splitting open the cell walls. Your saliva contains enzymes that begin the digestive process and enable nutrients to be absorbed by your body. The food particles that cannot be broken down by your digestive system, such as fiber, pass through and head out the back door. Chewing separates the fruit and vegetable nutrients from the insoluble fiber. The better you chew before you swallow, the more nutrients you will absorb from your meal. Juicing is a great way to extract massive amounts of nutrients from fruits and vegetables without having to sit down and chew through 20 pounds of vegetables per day. Juicing releases approximately 90 percent of the nutrients in food, which is about three times better than you can do with your teeth.

Another key factor is absorption. If your digestive tract is inflamed and overrun with bad bacteria, you may only be absorbing a small amount of the nutrients in the food you eat. Fresh juice is alive, nutrient rich, and easy for your body to absorb and use. Breaking down and digesting whole foods require a lot of energy, which is why eating a big meal will often make you sleepy. Sick people usually have an energy problem. They need nutrients and energy from food, but the energy required to digest food robs energy from the healing processes in the body. As a result, many late-stage cancer patients have difficulty absorbing nutrients from food. But when you drink freshly extracted juice, the vitamins, minerals, enzymes, and phytonutrients are quickly absorbed into your bloodstream, where they are carried to all the cells in your body with almost no digestive energy required.

In the beginning, I drank 64 ounces per day of straight carrot juice, broken up into roughly eight 8-ounce servings throughout the day. Then, as I did some research, I began adding more ingredients to it. There are a thousand different combinations of veggie juice, but I kept it simple and typically either drank straight carrot juice or one of the following combinations.

MY BASIC JUICE FORMULA

(ONE SERVING)

  5 small carrots
  1 to 2 celery stalks
  ½ beet root (and a few beet greens)
  1 knuckle gingerroot

MY ADVANCED JUICE FORMULA

(TWO SERVINGS)

  5 small carrots

  1 to 2 celery stalks

  ½ beet root (and a few beet greens)

  1 knuckle-sized piece of gingerroot (or as much as you
  can stand)

  1 to 2 knuckles turmeric root (or as much as you can
  stand)

  ¼ to ½ lemon or lime, unpeeled

  1 whole green apple, unpeeled

  1 clove garlic (or as much as you can stand)

NOTE: A knuckle is the length from your fingertip to your first knuckle.

Juice all the ingredients together and determine how many
ounces of juice your juicer yields. Then multiply the ingredients to the get the desired amount of juice you want to
make each day.

These additional ingredients may be added after the fact to amp up the nutritional value:

1 scoop greens powder
¼ to 1 teaspoon amla powder
¼ to 1 teaspoon moringa powder
¼ teaspoon matcha green tea powder
2 to 6 ounces aloe vera gel

CARROTS

Carrots are rich in cancer-fighting nutrients. Carrot juice has more naturally occurring vitamin A, alpha carotene, and beta carotene than anything else on earth. One 8-ounce cup of raw carrot juice has over 45,000 IU of vitamin A, which promotes liver detoxification and is healthy, unlike the isolated synthesized vitamin A found in most supplements. Carrots are rich in vitamin B-6 and also contain vitamins E and K; minerals including sodium, potassium, calcium, magnesium, and iron; flavonoids and carotenoids such as lycopene; and lutein. All of these nutrients work together to feed your cells, support your body's ability to inhibit the growth of many different cancers, and stimulate the activity of your immune system. Carotenoids and vitamin A have shown a strong ability to inhibit cancer induction, not only by viruses, but from chemicals and radiation as well. At least part of this effect is from these nutrients acting directly on your genes.[23] Another powerful anti-cancer compound in carrots is falcarinol, a fatty alcohol (which sounds terrible, but isn't), and is also found in *Panax* ginseng. Falcarinol has been demonstrated to have antibacterial, anti-fungal, anti-inflammatory, immune-boosting, and anti-cancer properties in laboratory studies, specifically against leukemia and colon cancer.[24]

BEETS

Beets are one of the highest antioxidant vegetables, and, like carrots, they are also rich in carotenoids, lycopene, and vitamin A, with strong anti-cancer and anti-mutagenic activity. Beets contain a potent anti-cancer phytonutrient called proanthocyanidin, which gives them their color. They contain betaine (a natural anti-inflammatory compound), vitamin C, folate, manganese, and potassium. Beets have also been shown to help lower high blood pressure and increase athletic endurance. Make sure to juice both the beetroot and the greens.

CELERY

Like carrots, celery contains the anti-cancer compound falcarinol, along with vitamins A, C, and K; minerals like potassium, calcium, and magnesium; and many other phytonutrients, including polysaccharides, antioxidants, phenolic acids, and flavonoids. Two noteworthy anti-cancer flavonoids in celery are apigenin and luteolin. In May 2013 researchers at Ohio State University demonstrated that apigenin could stop breast cancer cells from inhibiting their own death.[25] In other words, it made the cancer cells mortal again, like normal cells. Apigenin blocks aromatase, an enzyme in the body that helps promote the cancer growth hormone estrogen, and inhibits breast and prostate cancer cells.[26] Apigenin has even been found to make cancer cells more sensitive to chemotherapy by activating a tumor-suppressor gene called p53.[27] Luteolin helps protect cells from DNA damage, and both apigenin and luteolin have been shown to be anti-angiogenenic.[28,29] Another good source of luteolin is artichokes, while parsley and chamomile tea have high concentrations of apigenin.

GINGER

Ginger is a powerhouse root that contains antioxidant, anti-inflammatory, and anti-cancer compounds.[30,31] Multiple studies have shown that ginger can inhibit tumor cell growth, slow down metastasis, induce cancer cell death, protect healthy cells from radiotherapy damage, and enhance the effectiveness of chemotherapy.[32,33,34] Fresh gingerroot is spicy, and a small slice or knuckle goes a long way. Go easy on it the first time you add it to your juice.

JUICING TIPS

First and foremost, it's important to buy organic produce for your juice. In the United States, most commercial nonorganic produce contains traces of toxic pesticides, fungicides, and herbicides. Having said that, if you do not have access to or cannot afford organic produce, don't let that stop you. The benefits still outweigh the risks; just juice what you can get.

Don't get too hung up on the juice formula or ratio. The type of juicer you use will determine how much produce you'll need, and you'll figure it out in no time. There are a thousand possible juice combinations, so have fun experimenting. Vegetable juice is wonderful for you. Just get it in your body. You can also dilute the juice with purified water if the taste is too strong.

I didn't juice leafy green vegetables because they didn't produce as much juice as fruits and root vegetables, and I always felt like I was wasting them. In addition, some leafy greens, such as spinach and kale, contain high levels of oxalic acid, which can be problematic for some people. I prefer to eat leafy greens whole in a salad or blend them up in a smoothie.

I often supercharge my juice with an organic greens powder. There are many brands on the market today, and they typically have a variety of ingredients like barley grass, wheat grass, chlorella, and spirulina, along with lots of sprouts and veggies. Greens powders are rich in chlorophyll, trace minerals, antioxidants, and enzymes. Some brands also sell them in individual serving packets, which are great for travel and green juice on the go.

When juicing large batches, the best practice is to store the juice in the fridge in airtight glass mason jars or recycled glass bottles. Fill the bottles all the way to the top, leaving as little air as possible. This will slow down oxidation and help keep your juice fresh and potent throughout the day. I recommend drinking juice in the early morning, mid-morning, lunchtime, afternoon, dinnertime, and finish what's left before bed.

If you're serious about juicing large amounts of produce every day, you will need a good juicer. Cheap ones tend to jam up or don't produce much juice, and can frustrate you to the point where you won't juice at all. I bought a $300 Champion Juicer with a commercial motor in 2004, and it served me well for over a decade before I replaced any parts on it. Omega, Green Star, and Breville are also high-quality brands.

To get the maximum amount of juice out of your produce, you can use a Champion Juicer as a grinder and then press the juice out with a Welles or Peoples hydraulic juice press, which will yield about 50 percent more juice. This two-step process can produce as much as 2 ounces more juice per pound of carrots than the Rolls Royce of juicers, the $2,400 Norwalk, at only a third of the cost.

If money is tight, look for a used juicer on eBay or Craigslist, or ask your friends on social media. Chances are, someone you know has a juicer collecting dust that they will give to you for free or lend to you indefinitely. Don't let your circumstances stop you. Ask for help. The most important thing is that you get on the juice!

I'm often contacted by people who are concerned that carrot or beet juice contains too much sugar and "sugar feeds cancer." While it is true that cancer cells feed primarily on glucose, so does every other cell in your body. All fruits, vegetables, grains, and animal protein are converted to glucose to feed your cells. Carrots and beets contain anti-cancer nutrients that can turn off cancer genes, interfere with cancer cell reproduction, block metastasis, and cause cancer cell suicide. In my opinion, the positive benefits of the phytonutrients and anti-cancer compounds in carrots, beets, and fruit far outweigh any potential negative related to their sugar content. We aren't getting cancer from eating too much fruit, carrots, or beets. Carrot juice and beet juice are staples in the legendary anti-cancer nutritional protocols from Dr. Max Gerson and Dr. Rudolph Breuss, and I've known many cancer survivors whose healing protocols included lots of carrot and beet juice. I never worried about the sugar content in carrots and beets, and I don't think you should either.

What about fruit juice? Some of the literature I read back in 2004 claimed that even freshly juiced fruit juice had too much concentrated sugar for cancer patients, so I avoided fruit juice and only ate fruit whole or blended up in smoothies. Since then my attitude toward fresh fruit juice has changed. There are some powerful anti-cancer compounds in fruit juices, especially green apple and lemon juice. The Gerson Therapy for cancer includes one serving of fresh orange juice every morning and several 50/50 green apple and carrot juices throughout the day. If you are concerned about the sugar in fruit juice, you can eat apples and oranges whole instead, but definitely don't skip the lemon juice.

MY DAILY JUICE ROUTINE

Store-bought fruit and vegetable juices are not recommended because they are often not fresh and has been processed, pasteurized, and preserved. Fresh, organic juice is the best strategy. Some health experts recommend drinking fresh juice immediately in order to get the most nutritional value, but fresh juice has been found to retain its enzyme and nutritional content for several days. Back in 2004 I didn't have the luxury of making a fresh glass of juice eight times per day, so I had to devise a system that was simple and sustainable. My number one priority was getting large amounts of juice in my body every day. So first thing every morning, I made one big batch of juice to last me throughout the day. I started with 5 pounds of organic carrots, which yield approximately 40 ounces of juice, and then I added gingerroot, beet root, celery, and other ingredients to get me to 64 ounces, which I drank throughout the day. Ideally 64 ounces of juice should be consumed as eight 8-ounce servings, every hour or so. Many holistic cancer clinics have their patients drink between 1 and 3 quarts of juice per day. On the Gerson Therapy, cancer patients drink 13 juices per day, once every hour. Think of juice as medicinal food. Hourly dosing is the best way to maintain high levels of nutrients in your blood throughout the day.

OVERDOSING ON NUTRITION

I wanted to ensure that my body was getting all the nutrition it needed to repair, regenerate, and detoxify, and as a result I ended up drinking so much carrot juice that I turned orange. Overdosing on carotenoids temporarily turns your skin yellowish orange; it's common in babies when they eat too much carrot or sweet potato mush. This phenomenon is called carotenemia, but one nurse thought I was jaundiced, a symptom of a sick liver. The major difference between jaundice and carotenemia is that jaundice turns your eyes yellow. If your skin starts to turn yellow/orange, don't worry; it will eventually go away after you cut back on carrot juice. It's not uncommon for cancer patients who have turned orange from carrot juice to be warned by their doctor that too much vitamin A can be harmful and damaging to the liver. This opinion is based on studies using isolated vitamin A supplements, not carrot juice.

THE GIANT CANCER-FIGHTING SALAD

The second component in my anti-cancer diet was eating the biggest, baddest salad on the planet. The reason behind this salad was simple. I wanted to put as many anti-cancer vegetables into my body as possible every day. When I first started the raw-food diet, I bought several raw-food recipe books, but many of the recipes were complicated and time consuming and didn't contain the large variety of foods I wanted to be eating daily, so the giant salad ended up being my staple meal for lunch and dinner. I didn't mind eating the same thing every day because it was quick to prepare and delicious. Plus, I didn't have to put any time into planning my meals; I knew exactly what to buy at the grocery store every week and I ate everything I bought. No waste! There's really no secret formula, but I did follow some guidelines: No meat, cheese, or store-bought salad dressing. Use organic produce if you can get it and afford it to reduce your exposure to toxic chemical pesticides, herbicides, and fungicides.

THE GIANT CANCER-FIGHTING SALAD

Leafy greens: for example, kale, spinach, Swiss chard, watercress, arugula

Broccoli or broccoli sprouts

Cauliflower

Purple cabbage

Slice of red, yellow, or green onion

Leeks

Red, yellow, or green peppers (I know these are technically fruits)

½ or whole avocado (and so is this)

Sunflower seeds

Almonds or walnuts (unsalted, raw, or roasted)

Sprouted garbanzo beans

Sprouted black lentils

Sprouted mung beans

All vegetables are wonderful. Feel free to add any others you like. Availability and pricing will vary based on the season. Also, soaking and sprouting unlock enzymes and nutrition in nuts and seeds and may make them easier to digest, but it is not mandatory. Unsprouted nuts and seeds are wonderful healthy foods as well. Legumes should be soaked and sprouted if consumed raw. Otherwise, cook them.

Fun with Fermented Food

Health starts in the gut, and it's not uncommon for sick people to have digestive problems and unhealthy guts. The causes: eating a diet rich in meat, dairy, and processed food; eating conventionally grown produce sprayed with glyphosate; and taking antibiotics, all of which can either directly damage the gut or promote the abundance of inflammatory, disease-promoting bacteria. A critical part of the health restoration process is healing your gut and rebuilding your digestive tract. The first step is eating tons of plant food, which is rich in starch and fiber (these are prebiotics) and serves as food for probiotics, the good gut bacteria. The second step is eating a small amount of fermented foods daily, which contains live cultures of probiotic bacteria. Fermented foods help repopulate your intestinal flora with good bacteria, which displace bad bacteria and can improve your digestion and immune function. Pickled vegetables like sauerkraut, kimchi, and pickles, as well as apple cider vinegar, are my preferred fermented foods.

Traditional sauerkraut is made with only three ingredients: cabbage, water, and salt. Kimchi is a spicy Korean version of sauerkraut typically consisting of fermented cabbage, onions, garlic, and pepper. Recognized as one of the top five "World's Healthiest Foods" by *Health* magazine, kimchi has high concentrations of vitamin C and carotene in addition to vitamins A, B1, B2, calcium, iron, and beneficial bacteria.

As the old saying goes, "The dose determines the poison." Fermented foods may end up being unhealthy if you consume too much. Asian cultures with the highest intake of pickled vegetables also have the highest incidence of stomach cancer. A meta-analysis of observational studies conducted in Korea and Japan found that a high intake of pickled vegetables was associated with a 28 percent increased risk of gastric cancer. Kimchi accounts for approximately 20 percent of sodium intake in the Korean diet, and the high amounts of sodium used in pickled foods may be the real culprit.[35] Knowing what I know now, I still don't see any problem with adding a small amount (¼ cup) of either sauerkraut or kimchi to my salads every day. Look for organic sauerkraut, kimchi, and pickles in the refrigerated section of your local grocer or health food store. When comparing brands, look for the one with the lowest amount of sodium.

MY ANTI-CANCER SALAD DRESSING

Apple cider vinegar (I love Bragg)

Extra virgin olive oil and/or extra virgin flax oil (I recommend Bragg and Barlean's)

Organic oregano

Organic garlic powder

Organic turmeric or curry powder

Organic cayenne pepper

Organic black pepper

Bragg organic sprinkle (a blend of 24 herbs and spices)

Nutritional yeast (I recommend Bragg, again!)

Lightly drizzle olive oil or flax seed oil and organic apple cider vinegar to taste. If you don't like the taste of apple cider vinegar, lemon juice is a great addition or substitute for ACV. Sprinkle on the spices to taste.

NOTE: Some people who switch to a raw-food diet may experience gas and indigestion. That's normal at first. If your body isn't used to eating lots of plant food, it may take a few days or weeks to adapt. Chewing your food really well, eating fermented foods daily, and taking a high-quality digestive enzyme with meals can help your body adjust. If digestion is difficult or painful, try the Giant Cancer-Fighting Salad blended up as a smoothie or blended and cooked as a soup.

Oleocanthal, a compound in olive oil, has been found to kill cancer cells in the lab in less than an hour.[36]

THE GREEN SMOOTHIE

Another way to get all of these anti-cancer veggies into your body is to put all (or most of) the ingredients of the giant salad into a blender with 1 to 2 cups of purified water, liquefy it, and drink it. This is especially good if you cannot eat solid food, want to consume it on the go, or want to give your jaws a break from all the chewing. Liquefying in a blender also increases the amount of absorbable nutrients. A liquefied salad is going to taste a bit unusual, kind of like a cold, bland vegetable soup. Not very appetizing sounding, I know, but keep in mind that this is medicinal food. You aren't drinking it for the taste. Even if you have to hold your nose, do it. Just get it in your body. Another option with this blended-up salad concoction is to warm it up on the stove. If you want to keep it raw, just warm it up to around 100 degrees, spice accordingly, and eat it like soup. If you have a hard time digesting raw food (such as having painful cramps or bloating), it can also be fully cooked and consumed warm or cooled.

APPLE CIDER VINEGAR

Apple cider vinegar (ACV) is a staple in my salad dressing. If you've never had it, it's exactly what it sounds like—vinegar made from apple juice. It tastes like vinegar, but with an apple-y twist, and it is celebrated in the natural health world for its many uses. ACV is a fermented food rich in probiotics, enzymes, potassium, and polyphenols, which are antimicrobial and antibacterial.[37] Apple cider vinegar contains acetic acid, which can help increase nutrient absorption in your body. Anecdotally, it has also been reported to assist in healing allergies, infections, candida, acid reflux, arthritis, and gout, and to support detoxification and immune function. Whether all these claims are true, I can't say. All I know for sure is that it is, at the very least, healthy, and I love it.

Bragg organic apple cider vinegar is the best of the best. It's raw and unfiltered, leaving all the vital nutrients and enzymes intact, unlike most vinegars, which are pasteurized, filtered, processed, and nutritionally dead. Paul Bragg was a lifelong health crusader and mentor to Jack LaLanne. He literally wrote the book on apple cider vinegar and numerous other books on diet, exercise, and fasting, and was a true pioneer in the world of health and wellness. My mom had many of his books in her library until I absconded with them. You can find Bragg ACV at most grocery and health food stores. I also recommend Bragg organic extra virgin olive oil.

NUTRITIONAL YEAST

Nutritional yeast contains a type of fiber called beta-glucan, an immunomodulatory compound that enhances your body's defenses against infections and cancer.[38] Beta-glucans have been shown to increase immune function, specifically monocyte and natural killer cell activity against cancer.[39] In one study, breast cancer patients who were given a small amount of beta-glucan daily—the equivalent of 1/16 of a teaspoon of nutritional yeast—had a 50 percent increase in monocytes in their bloodstream after just two weeks.[40] Beta-glucan supplementation has also been found to accelerate wound healing after mastectomy.[41] There have been over 20 studies in Japan showing beta-glucans can enhance the effects of chemo and radiotherapy treatment and improve survival and quality of life.[42] Nutritional yeast has a mild cheesy, nutty flavor and can be added to oatmeal, smoothies, salads, and pretty much anything you eat. Bragg is my brand of choice, and I also take beta-glucans in supplement form.

YOU'RE GONNA NEED A BIGGER BOWL

When I first started making the Giant Cancer-Fighting Salad, I quickly realized that our little soup and side salad bowls were not going to cut it, so I bought some giant bowls that hold over 6 cups. That's 6 servings of vegetables in one meal. Remember: 10 servings per day of fruits and vegetables are considered ideal for cancer prevention; cancer healing may require more. I ate two giant salads per day and drank eight glasses of vegetable juice, plus a fruit smoothie. I was giving my body an abundance of nutrition with 15 to 20 servings of fruits and vegetables per day, every day. Like I said before, massive action produces massive results. And that, my friend, is what massive action looks like.

Note: The salad really doesn't have to be "giant." I made big ones because that's what it took to fill me up. Obviously, not everyone needs to eat as much as I did. Just make your salads big enough to satisfy your appetite and not leave you hungry an hour later.

MY ANTI-CANCER FRUIT SMOOTHIE

Berries are the most potent anti-cancer fruits, but it can be difficult to get organically grown berries, and they tend to be expensive and often get moldy within a few days. The most practical way to consume berries is to buy them frozen and blend them up in smoothies. I buy large bags of frozen organic berries at Costco, which are typically a mix of blueberries, blackberries, raspberries, strawberries, cherries, and sometimes even cranberries.

Depending on the size of the smoothie I want, I use:

1 to 4 cups of frozen organic berries
A handful of leafy greens like spinach or kale
A handful of almonds or walnuts, or both
1 banana or 3 to 5 pitted dates

I also like to add the juice and meat of a young Thai coconut. Fresh coconut is a delicious addition to the smoothie, but it tends to be expensive and it is difficult both to find and to open. And it is not essential.

Blend all ingredients in a blender with 1 cup of purified water. Add more water gradually if it's too thick. Note: If the smoothie is too thin, it may run through you.

If you want to amp your smoothies up even more, consider adding any of the following: 1 to 8 ounces Stockton aloe vera gel; 1 teaspoon to 1 tablespoon turmeric powder; 1 teaspoon amla powder; 1 teaspoon moringa powder; ½ to 1 teaspoon matcha green tea powder; pineapple; papaya; goji berries; acai berries; mangosteen; cauliflower . . . you get the idea. If it's a fruit or a vegetable, throw it in there.

If you need to gain weight, add more nuts and seeds, such as hemp hearts or pepitas.

GO NUTS

A 7-year study found that stage III colon cancer survivors who ate at least 2 ounces (57 grams) of tree nuts per week—roughly 48 almonds or walnuts (that's only about 7 per day)—were 42 percent less likely to have their cancer return and 57 percent less likely to die from their cancer than those who did not eat nuts.[43] This benefit applied only to those eating tree nuts (almonds, walnuts, Brazil nuts, pistachios, and cashews) but not peanuts. The study did not differentiate between raw or roasted nuts, so it's safe to assume that the study participants ate a variety of both. Roasting almonds doubles the antioxidant activity and phenolic compounds in almond skins.[44] However, nuts aren't just good for colon cancer. Eating a handful of nuts and seeds every day cuts your risk of several types of cancer (including breast cancer and pancreatic cancer), as well as cardiovascular disease, neurodegenerative disease, and diabetes.[45]

MY DAILY ANTI-CANCER ROUTINE

Here's what a typical day looked like for me while I was healing cancer, and even now. One of my intentions was to live as closely to nature as possible, to sleep in total darkness, and to let the sun wake me up naturally instead of being jarred awake by the radio or an alarm buzzer.

Once I'm up the first thing I do every morning is hydrate. I drink 20 ounces of purified water and/or tea cold-steeped overnight and take supplements that should be taken first thing in the morning. An additional benefit of drinking several cups of water first thing in the morning is that it gets your bowels moving. Next is 10 to 20 minutes of aerobic exercise such as jogging, cycling, or rebounding (jumping on a mini-trampoline) to wake me up, get my heart pumping and my blood circulating, and get me sweaty. Aerobic exercise not only has anti-cancer benefits in the body, but it also makes you feel good and promotes detoxification via sweating. Afterward I take a quick shower and spend a few minutes to get my mind on track for the day by reading a devotional passage, praying and/or meditating, journaling, and making or reviewing my to-do list. Next I make all my juice for the day, roughly 64 ounces. This process takes the better part of an hour. I recommend making it fun. Play some music you love or listen to a podcast while you're running the juicer.

In the first 90 days of my healing journey, I skipped breakfast and drank juice throughout the morning until lunch; some days I snacked mid-morning on fruit such as a grapefruit or a green apple. If you need to gain or maintain weight, oatmeal or the fruit smoothie is a great breakfast option. Lunch and dinner every day was the Giant Cancer-Fighting Salad. Some days I snacked on nuts or fruit mid-afternoon. Most days before lunch and dinner, I bounced on the rebounder for 10 minutes to incorporate more exercise into my day and get my lymphatic system moving. When the weather was nice, we often walked the dog after dinner. After dinner and before bed, I finished any remaining juice, sometimes drank herbal tea, and tried to get into bed within a few hours after sundown.

BUILDING
A NEW BODY

Tell me what you eat, and I will tell you what you are.

— JEAN ANTHELME BRILLAT-SAVARIN

YOUR BODY IS MADE UP OF TRILLIONS OF CELLS, almost all of which are dying and being replaced continually throughout your life. Your intestines are regenerated every two to three days, your taste buds take ten days, your skin and lungs take two to four weeks, your red blood cells take four months, your nails take six to ten months, and your bones take about ten years. About every hundred days, most of your soft tissue has been replaced. Your body is a perpetual construction site. And your body is built with the food you eat. That's it. You built your body. You are what you ate.

The ability of the human body to adapt to and use so many different types of fuel to repair, regenerate, and sustain life is an amazing testament to the intelligent design of our Creator. No matter what we put in it, it manages to keep working, which is why it's so easy for us take our bodies and health for granted. But you can only do that for so long, because if your nutritional requirements are consistently not met, and you replace vital, life-sustaining food from the earth with artificial, man-made factory food and high amounts of animal products, your health will decline. It's only a matter of time. Healthy cells and tissues are replaced with weaker ones as they regenerate, nutrient reserves are depleted, and the body becomes vulnerable to disease. Progressively, after many years, critical systems begin to break down, like your cardiovascular system, your central nervous system, your endocrine system, your digestive system, your reproductive system, or your immune system. All of these systems are connected, and when one system becomes dysfunctional it affects the others. And that's about the time when you begin to develop chronic pain, acid reflux, high blood pressure, irritable bowel syndrome, and high blood sugar, warning signs of diseases such as diabetes, heart disease, or cancer.

It takes multiple generations of cell degradation to produce a sick body but, thankfully, not nearly as many to heal it. When you stop polluting your body and give it the highest-quality raw materials (whole foods from the earth), it will reward you by rebuilding a healthier body. This is why many people experience a significant, even dramatic improvement in health in as little as three months after a radical diet and lifestyle change.

As encouraging as that is, I must emphasize that restoring health is not a quick fix. The experience of many practitioners and patients who have healed cancer shows that it can take several years to fully heal, and from there you must maintain a healthy diet and lifestyle for life. Every time you sit down to eat, remind yourself that you are building a new body. Before that first bite, ask yourself, *Is this food going to promote health or disease in my body?* In this chapter, I will highlight some time-tested, scientifically validated dietary principles for maintaining lifelong health.

In January 2004 I began working with a clinical nutritionist who took a holistic approach. Instead of treating symptoms, his focus was on supporting my body's ability to heal itself by identifying and correcting functional deficiencies and toxicities such as heavy metals. Along with blood work, he had me send samples of my urine, saliva, hair, and stool to various labs across the country for evaluation. When all of these tests came back, we had a detailed picture of what was happening in my body. From there he recommended individualized nutraceutical and herbal supplements to support various functions in my body.

After 90 days on a raw diet, he suggested I add some cooked food. At that point I had accepted that I would be on a raw diet indefinitely, maybe for the rest of my life, but at the same time I was open to doing whatever it took to get well. My nutritionist was the only person besides my parents who believed I was doing the right thing, so I trusted his advice.

When you are sick, there's no place for dietary dogmatism. It is easy to become convinced that one diet is the best diet for everyone, especially if you initially have good results with it yourself, but it's important that you stay open to refining your approach in order to give your body the optimal diet that it needs to thrive. The raw diet can be a powerful detoxification and healing diet in the short term, but it may not be sustainable for some people long term, depending on body type and metabolism. I'm an ectomorph (skinny frame) with a high metabolism. At that point, I was super skinny at six-feet-two, 130 pounds, and although I was eating tons of food and felt good on a raw diet, I was having trouble gaining weight and looked like Jack Skellington from *The Nightmare Before Christmas*.

I was clinically underweight, and it was clear that I needed more calories than juicing and giant salads could provide, so I started eating some cooked vegetables at night along with my giant salad. Contrary to what I'd been led to believe by raw foodists, cooking does not destroy the nutritional value of food; it actually breaks down cell walls and makes certain nutrients in food easier to absorb. Cooking can reduce the amount of water-soluble vitamins by about 15 percent, but it also reduces the volume of the food so you end up eating more of it, so there's no net loss. If you've ever cooked spinach, you've seen how drastically the volume is reduced after cooking—a giant bag cooks down to a bowlful. This is why cooked vegetables are considered to have about twice the calories as raw vegetables.

After the first 90 days, I modified my diet from 100 percent raw vegan to about 80 percent raw and not vegan. At the recommendation of my nutritionist, I added some starches, including sweet potatoes, lentils, brown rice, and quinoa, and a few servings of clean animal protein per week. He suggested wild-caught Alaskan salmon or organic lamb. I had no desire to eat cooked food or meat at the time, but this modification did help me get back to my normal weight in a few months.

Over the years, I have experimented with increasing the amount of animal food in my diet, including eating more servings of wild-caught fish or organically-raised chicken, beef, eggs, and even raw dairy to see how these foods affected my body. But I found no additional benefit. In hindsight, adding a few servings of animal protein per week back to my diet clearly wasn't enough to hurt me, but if I knew then what I know now, like how elevated levels of IGF-1, methionine, saturated fat, and heme iron from eating animal protein can promote cancer growth, I would not have added it back to my diet so soon. I think the safest approach is to stay off all animal products for the first phase of your healing journey, at least 90 days and maybe for several years. Cancer doesn't develop overnight and doesn't heal overnight. Healing can take several years, with ups and downs along the way. It's important to be in it for the long haul, committed to the process and to a total life change, which is what is often required for healing.

THE CANCER PATIENT WHO FORGOT TO DIE

Diagnosed with terminal lung cancer in 1976, 66-year-old Stamatis Moraitis left the U.S. and moved back to Ikaria, a Greek island, to be close to his family and enjoy his last nine months on earth. He planted a garden and a vineyard, got lots of fresh air and sunshine, ate homegrown local food, slept late, took naps, ate and drank with friends at night, and started going to church. This was a radical change compared to his former life back in the United States, and as a result something unexpected happened. Or rather, something expected didn't happen. He didn't die. Thirty years later, he celebrated his 96th birthday a cancer-free man without any help from doctors or drugs. Not even any alternative therapies or juicing. Stamatis slowed down, simplified his life, adopted a whole-foods diet, and reconnected with God, old friends, and family, and his body healed.

Stamatis Moraitis is not an anomaly. The island of Ikaria is classified as one of five Blue Zones documented by National Geographic fellow Dan Buettner. The Blue Zones are unique areas around the world where the healthiest, longest-living people live. Ikarians live on average 8 to 10 years longer than Americans and are four times as likely to reach age 90 in better health with less depression and dementia. Here's what makes life on Ikaria unique: The pace of life is slow. People wake up naturally. No alarm clocks. No stressful morning rush. They eat fresh local food that they produce themselves. They get exercise working in their gardens and walking up and down the hilly terrain. They eat lots of plant foods like garlic, potatoes, and wild greens and six times as many beans per day than Americans, including garbanzo beans, black-eyed peas, and lentils. They also eat breads from stone-ground whole wheat.

Ikarians are not vegetarians or vegans, but they eat a lot less meat than we do, only about three to four times per week. Typically, it's fresh-caught fish about twice a week and other meats about five times a month. They drink fresh goat's milk and eat honey. They drink lots of herbal teas with wild marjoram, sage, mint, rosemary, artemisia, and dandelion. They eat very little processed food and consume 75 percent less refined sugar than Americans. They spend a lot of time socializing and sharing meals with each other, and often stay up late drinking and dancing. Sounds pretty nice, right?

Speaking of drinking, they drink on average two to three cups of coffee and two to four glasses of wine per day. Multiple servings of coffee and wine per day are not a good strategy for anyone trying to transform their health, but it appears that the overwhelming healthiness of the Ikarian diet and lifestyle counteracts any negative effects of those indulgences. It is also worth noting that Ikaria is not a rich place. In fact, it's the opposite. Unemployment is around 40 percent, but almost everyone has access to a family garden and livestock, and they share what they have with each other. *The Blue Zones: Lessons for Living Longer from the People Who've Lived the Longest* by Dan Buettner is one of my favorite books on health and longevity. I've interviewed Dan on my blog as well.

LESSONS FROM RURAL AFRICANS

Dr. Denis Burkitt was a world-renowned Irish surgeon and devout Christian who spent many decades working as a medical missionary in Africa. Burkitt has been immortalized in Cancerdom for his 1958 discovery of Burkitt's lymphoma, a children's cancer caused by the Epstein-Barr virus, but what he did after that made him a legend in epidemiology. After many years spent working in African hospitals, Burkitt became discontent with simply treating the effects of chronic Western diseases and more interested in identifying the causes in order to prevent them. He surveyed hundreds of doctors at hospitals across Africa and discovered that many chronic diseases common to industrialized nations simply didn't exist in rural Africa. Rural Africans weren't getting our most common cancers, heart disease, diabetes, Crohn's disease, hemorrhoids, hernias, ulcers, gall stones, appendicitis, or autoimmune diseases. And if they made it through the infectious disease gauntlet of childhood, they were likely to live to be over 100 and simply die of old age.

One of Burkitt's first conclusions was that the absence of chronic Western diseases in rural Africa had nothing to do with genetics. Black Africans living in major cities eating the same diet as white Africans suffered from the same chronic diseases as they did. When Burkitt investigated the diets of rural Africans, he noted that they ate a high-fiber, plant-based diet that consisted of starchy vegetables such as potatoes, yams, cassava, peas, and beans; whole grains such as corn, millet, sorghum, teff, and wheat; and fruits like bananas and plantains, when available and in season. Unlike the Western diet, there was very little white flour and white sugar and very little meat and dairy. Rural Africans were eating a naturally high-carbohydrate, high-fiber, low-fat diet. The chief reason behind this diet was poverty and availability. There weren't any supermarkets in the African bush. The food they ate was the food they grew. Meat was scarce, a luxury eaten only on rare and special occasions. Burkitt also found that in any region where a Western diet rich in meat, dairy, and refined foods was adopted, chronic disease rates skyrocketed within a few decades.

Now let's talk about poop. One aspect of Burkitt's research involved measuring the stool size and bowel transit times of people all over the world, and his findings were revelatory. According to Burkitt, rural Africans were a model of healthy bowel function in comparison to American and British people, but in order to understand why, we must first discuss the liver.

The liver is responsible for as many as 500 functions in the body, one of which is detoxification. Along with the kidneys, it filters your blood, collecting, processing, and eliminating toxins and metabolic waste products from your body. One of the ways it does this is by excreting bile, your body's toxic waste, into your intestinal tract to be carried out by your stool. The longer that food and liver bile remain in the bowel, the more potential they have to putrefy and release toxic by-products and create fecal mutagens that cause irritation, inflammation, and ulceration in your intestinal walls, leading to bowel diseases like diverticulitis, colitis, Crohn's disease, and colorectal cancer. Some of the toxins in your poop can be reabsorbed into your bloodstream, causing a vicious cycle of autointoxication—poisoning and polluting your body and creating perpetual work for your liver. Meat, dairy, and eggs contain no fiber; move through your digestive tract very slowly, causing constipation; and putrefy in your colon, leading to the problems described above. Starch and fiber from plant food move through your digestive system quickly, absorbing toxic liver bile and carrying it out before it can cause any harm.

In his research Burkitt noted that rural Africans typically pooped twice per day and when they did, a lot more came out.

They expelled four times more poop per day by weight than Americans, Europeans, and Australians. Compared to the small, hard, dark poops of Western diet eaters, the Africans' poop was much larger, softer, and lighter in color, with no straining required. And the Africans' average bowel transit time—the time it takes a meal to go from mouth to anus—was about a day and a half, while Western diet eaters typically took three to five days. Perhaps most alarming was Burkitt's discovery that elderly Western diet eaters could take two weeks or more to pass a meal.

> To measure your bowel transit time, eat beets with a meal and then track the number of hours before you have beet-red poop.

Burkitt was adamant that the number of doctors, medical technology, and health care available had very little bearing on the overall health of a nation. And he was right. The U.S. has the highest health spending of any industrialized nation in the world per capita and some of the shortest life spans. We spend twice as much as the Japanese on health care, and they live three and a half years longer on average. Burkitt also famously stated that the overall health of a nation could easily be measured by evaluating its people's stools. By 1973 Burkitt had written 28 medical journal articles on the connection between nutrition and disease, and he believed a high-fiber diet was the key to health and Western disease prevention.

Burkitt's work is monumental but he made one mistake: reductionism—trying to pinpoint Western disease on a singular dietary factor, namely fiber. His work was largely responsible for the dietary fiber craze of the '70s and '80s that prompted food manufacturers to produce and promote "high-fiber" breakfast cereals like All-Bran and supplements like Metamucil, convincing the public that simply adding more fiber to our diets would make us healthier. At the time of Burkitt's research, rural Africans consumed four to six times more fiber per day than Western diet eaters, but we now know that the high amount of fiber wasn't the reason they avoided chronic Western diseases. Several decades after Burkitt's work was published, researchers reexamined the native African diet. They found that today it consists primarily of highly processed corn grits and provides only half the U.S. recommended daily allowance of fiber, but surprisingly, the rates of colorectal cancer in Africa were still 50 times lower than the United States. The researchers concluded that the low rate of colorectal cancer among Africans could not be due to "protective" dietary factors like vitamins, minerals, and fiber because the modern African diet was actually found to be deficient in many of those nutrients. They credited the extraordinarily low rates of colon cancer to an absence of "aggressive" dietary factors—namely, excess animal protein and fat—and to beneficial by-products produced by Africans' colon bacteria, which are also influenced by diet.[1] Less meat equals more health.

CLEAN MEAT

After my nutritionist recommended I add some clean (organic pasture-raised or wild-caught) animal protein back into my diet, I was inspired to revisit the dietary laws that God gave to the Israelites, which are detailed in the Book of Leviticus of the Bible. These were laws pertaining to which animals they were allowed to eat and which animals were "unclean" and forbidden to eat. I've read these dietary laws many times in my life, and I never really understood them. But after closer examination and research, I discovered why God put these laws in place.

God told the Israelites they could only eat land animals with split hooves that chew their cud, which includes cows, goats, sheep, and deer but excludes dogs, cats, rodents, rabbits, pigs, horses, and snakes. They were also allowed to eat any water animal with fins and scales, which includes most fish but excludes reptiles, shellfish, dolphins, seals, and whales. Birds including chicken, turkey, duck, and pheasant were allowed, but birds of prey and scavengers such as eagles, ravens, hawks, and vultures were not allowed. There's a common thread here. The land animals and birds they were allowed to eat were mainly herbivores that ate plants and insects but didn't kill and eat other animals.

God, in His infinite wisdom, forbade the Israelites from eating most carnivorous predatory animals and scavengers. The Israelites were also not allowed to eat or drink blood from *any* animal. What we know now, thanks to science, is that these guidelines actually make a lot of sense. Carnivorous animal flesh and all animal blood can contain high amounts of viruses, bacteria, parasites, pathogens, and heme iron. Making these foods off-limits was much simpler than trying to teach the complexities of biology and anatomy.

SCAVENGERS

Scavengers are animals that eat the remains of other dead animals and include birds of prey like vultures, as well as swine and shellfish. Even though they are smart and can make great pets, pigs are nature's garbage collectors, and they will eat anything, including decaying dead animals and their own poop. Pigs don't sweat, and they store the majority of toxins they collect in their fat. Barbecue is especially bad because of the carcinogenic compounds created in the smoking process.

Shellfish also clean up their environment. They absorb the toxins and pollution in our rivers, lakes, and oceans. Polonium, a by-product of uranium, has polluted the world's oceans as a result of nuclear weapons testing, sunken nuclear subs, satellites, isotope batteries, and waste dumping from nuclear power plants.[2] The majority of our exposure to radioactive polonium comes from eating fish and shellfish because radioactive waste bioaccumulates in fish tissue. The higher up the food chain a fish is, the more toxic it becomes. Researchers found that just one meal of mussels caused a 300 percent spike in polonium levels in human semen.[3]

A catastrophic amount of radioactive fallout from the Fukushima meltdown in Japan ended up in the Pacific Ocean. Within several days of the meltdown, low levels of radioactive iodine and cesium were detected in rain and drinking water, as well as in grass and milk samples all across the United States. Milk samples in San Francisco were found to have 10 times the legal limit of radioactive iodine, and the highest levels of radioactive iodine in rainwater were found in Boise, Idaho. Tokyo Electric Power Company admitted in August 2013 that around 300 tons of highly radioactive water had leaked out of storage tanks, but some research scientists believe it may have been a lot more. Researchers at Stanford reported that Pacific bluefin tuna are transporting radioactive waste from Fukushima across the entire North Pacific Ocean as they migrate from Japan to California.[4] Testing revealed that Pacific tuna meat contained 10 times more radioactive nuclides after Fukushima, along with already high levels of mercury. Other scavengers to avoid are catfish, crawfish, shrimp, crab, lobster, mussels, squid, and octopus.

The Israelites had specific dietary laws as to which animals they could eat and how the meat should be prepared. Meat prepared according to these ancient laws is called kosher. In order to be considered kosher, the animal must be free from disease or injury and slaughtered in a way that, if done properly, is instantaneous and painless. After all the blood is drained out and the internal fat is removed, the meat is soaked in clean water for 30 minutes and drips dry. Afterward, it is salted for about an hour to draw out more blood. Then it's washed three times in cold, clean water to remove the salt. Then it is dried, cut up, and packaged.

The cleanest, healthiest, most humane meat you can eat is either wild caught or killed and prepared in a kosher manner or organic pasture-raised kosher meat. If you do include a small amount of animal protein in your diet, this is the best way to limit your exposure to potentially harmful toxins and heme iron in meat.

PATHOGENS, VIRUSES, AND BACTERIA, OH MY!

What's grosser than gross? In 2013 *Consumer Reports* found fecal bacteria in over half of the packaged raw ground turkey meat and patties they tested. Some samples harbored other germs, including salmonella and *Staphylococcus aureus*. Ninety percent of the samples had one or more of the five harmful bacteria they tested for. Sixty percent of the samples had *E. coli*. Surprisingly, the organic ground turkey was just as contaminated with bacteria as the conventional varieties. And almost all the disease-causing organisms they found were antibiotic resistant, except for those found in organically raised or antibiotic-free turkey.[5]

But it's not just turkey. The Retail Meat Report published by the FDA in February 2013 found that 81 percent of turkey, 69 percent of pork chops, 55 percent of raw ground beef, and 39 percent of chicken parts in supermarkets were infected with an antibiotic-resistant superbug called *Enterococcus*, a bacteria that is also the third leading cause of hospital infections. The FDA report also found that 74 percent of poultry contained antibiotic-resistant salmonella.[6]

In recent years there has been a growing concern about the increase in antibiotic-resistant bacterial infections in humans. This problem is largely caused by the rampant overuse of antibiotics in the meat and poultry industry. They are overdosing livestock with antibiotics to keep them from getting sick while living in the unsanitary conditions of factory farms. Nearly 80 percent of the antibiotics sold are used on food-producing animals. Roughly 30 million pounds of antibiotics are used on animals every year, which is four times more than the amount of antibiotics used on humans.[7] The simple and obvious way to protect yourself from unnecessary antibiotic exposure is to stop buying and eating factory-farmed meat.

As far as bacterial content goes, ground meat is the worst. Hamburger meat can contain as much as 100 million bacteria per quarter-pound patty. This is why it is strongly recommended that burgers be cooked well done. But even if the meat is completely cooked, the dead bacteria still release endotoxins into your bloodstream and cause an immediate inflammation response throughout the body, which causes stiffening of your arterial walls and lung inflammation.[8,9] This reaction typically lasts about five to six hours, and eating animal products three times per day keeps the body in a state of endotoxemia, or chronic, low-grade inflammation that can eventually lead to a host of diseases, including Crohn's disease, heart disease, diabetes, and cancer.

COOKED MEAT IS SAFER . . . AND MORE DANGEROUS

As if all those bacterial endotoxins weren't bad enough, cooking meat releases mutagenic compounds called heterocyclic amines (HCAs) and polycyclic aromatic hydrocarbons (PAHs). These are cancer-causing chemicals formed when muscle meat such as beef, pork, fish, or chicken is cooked at high temperatures, as in barbecuing, baking, pan frying, or grilling over an open flame. HCAs and PAHs are linked to various cancers, including kidney, colorectal, lung, prostate, and pancreatic cancer.[10,11,12,13,14] One large study found that the people with the highest consumption of meat cooked at high temperatures had a 70 percent greater risk of developing pancreatic cancer compared with those with the lowest consumption of well-done meats.[15] Fried bacon and fried fish have the highest concentrations of these mutagens, about five times more than beef and chicken. Chicken cooked without the skin has been found to have twice the levels of mutagens as chicken cooked with the skin on.

Meat cooked medium-rare has two-thirds less cancer-causing compounds than meat cooked well done,[16] but when you eat undercooked meat you risk the exposure to live bacteria like salmonella and *E. coli*. Boiling meat, as in stews and soups, is the safest cooking method because it kills bacteria without causing carcinogens. In recent years, there have been some fascinating discoveries in the world of nutrition science with regard to safely cooking meat.

HERBS AND SPICES TO THE RESCUE

In multiple studies, researchers have found that marinating meat with various herbs and spices before cooking blocks the formation of heterocyclic amines and polycyclic aromatic hydrocarbons. One study found that a marinade blend containing garlic, ginger, thyme, rosemary, and chili pepper reduced HCA production by 90 percent in pan-fried beef.[17] Another study comparing different marinades on grilled beef steaks found that a Southwest marinade with paprika, red pepper, oregano, thyme, black pepper, garlic, and onion reduced HCAs by 57 percent. An herbal marinade with oregano, basil, garlic, onion, jalapeño, parsley, and red pepper reduced HCAs by 72 percent. A Caribbean marinade containing thyme, red pepper, black pepper, allspice, rosemary, and chives reduced HCAs by 88 percent.[18] A third study in *Food Control* found that a simple lemon juice marinade could reduce the PAH content by as much as 70 percent.[19] Thus, always marinate your meat before cooking.

FIGHT FREE RADICALS WITH HERBS AND SPICES

Free radicals are caused by oxidative stress from external factors like radiation or pollutants and are also the toxic by-products of normal cell metabolism, kind of like your car exhaust. Free radicals damage cells, proteins, and DNA and are associated with causing disease including cancer, Alzheimer's, and Parkinson's disease. Your body is constantly neutralizing free radicals with the antioxidants that it makes, such as glutathione and super oxide dismutase, and with the antioxidants you eat. The more antioxidants you can get from food each day, the better. Plant food is rich in antioxidants, but herbs and spices have some of the highest concentrations of all, and are an easy way to supercharge the health benefits of any meal. The "Magnificent Seven" spices with the highest antioxidant content are cloves, peppermint, lemon balm, allspice, marjoram, cinnamon, and oregano.

Sweet Potato Tips and Tricks

> ➤ Sprinkle a little cinnamon and allspice on a sweet potato for more antioxidant power than nearly a week's worth of Western-diet meals.

> ➤ Sweet potatoes are delicious raw—just slice them up and dip them in some hummus.

> ➤ Raw sweet potatoes have higher antioxidant content than cooked, and boiled sweet potatoes have more than baked.

> ➤ Always eat the potato skin. It has about 10 times more antioxidant content than starch.

DOES MEAT CAUSE CANCER?

One of the largest prospective studies on diet and cancer found that the incidence of all cancers combined is lower among vegetarians than among meat eaters.[20] Processed meats like bacon, sausage, ham, and hot dogs are classified as Group 1 human carcinogens, which means there is strong evidence that processed meats cause cancer, specifically colorectal cancer. Red meat, including beef, lamb, and pork, is classified as a "probable" cause of cancer and has been linked to prostate and pancreatic cancer. There are many studies associating the consumption of animal protein and fat with an increased risk of certain cancers.

But haven't humans been eating meat for thousands of years? Yes, but our dietary habits and food systems are very different from those of our ancestors. Americans are eating twice as much meat as our great-grandparents, and even they were eating more meat than many of the populations with the lowest cancer rates today. In addition, the processed and factory-farmed meat we are eating contains higher levels of fat, growth hormones, and contaminants. Considering the fact that half of men and one-third of American women are predicted to get cancer in their lifetime, it makes sense to imitate the diets of the people with the lowest cancer rates and to reduce our exposure to as many cancer-promoters as possible.

Our bodies are bombarded with toxins every day from three sources: our environment, our food, and the products we use. We have limited control over our exposure to environmental toxins, many of which are undetectable, but we have complete control over what we put in and on our bodies. The goal is to reduce your toxic load. I believe giving up all animal products is essential for anyone who is trying to reverse a chronic disease like cancer.

Even if you don't have cancer, cutting out processed foods and eating less meat and more plant food can have a significant impact on your health in both the short and long term. Financial guru Dave Ramsey is famous for saying, "Live like no one else now, so later you can *live* like no one else." The same wisdom applies to your health. If you live and eat the way everyone else does, you can expect to get the same chronic diseases everyone is getting.

It is human nature to look for the quick fix, the one thing we can consume to be healthy, but there is no single cause of health or chronic disease. Scientists have studied populations all over the globe and consistently found that the people with the lowest incidence of chronic disease and the longest life spans eat a traditional whole-food, plant-based diet naturally rich in starchy vegetables and containing an abundance of vitamins, minerals, enzymes, antioxidants, and phytonutrients. Most traditional/ancestral diets are low in animal products and contain no processed food. And we know from the National Geographic Society's Blue Zones project that the longest-living populations around the world on every continent eat diets that are on average about 95 percent plant based. That equates to eating animal products somewhere between a few times per week and a few times per month. If you live and eat the way the healthy longest-living people live and eat, you can expect to enjoy health and long life free from most chronic diseases everyone else gets.

TAKE OUT
THE TRASH

Garbage in, garbage out.

— ANONYMOUS

YOUR LIVER IS YOUR BODY'S DETOXIFICATION ENGINE and a critical component of your immune system. It processes nearly every toxin that enters your body. An overburdened, sick liver can lead to a toxic body, weakened immune system, and an environment where cancer cells can thrive. So it makes sense to reduce the workload on your liver and the rest of your body by reducing or eliminating your exposure to unnecessary toxins. The overwhelming awareness of how much potentially toxic stuff is around you may induce some anxiety and paranoia at first, but don't let fear take over and paralyze you; just make a to-do list and start cleaning up your life. The goal is to reduce your toxic load, and every little bit helps.

First, you must understand that your body is always detoxifying. Your body detoxifies when you pee, poop, and sweat and every time you exhale. And your body is able to detoxify much faster when you stop polluting it. Cigarettes are the number one cause of cancer. If you smoke, stop smoking. Although e-cigarettes, aka "vaping," are less toxic than tobacco, they still increase your risk of cancer.[1] Flex your determination muscle and break your nicotine addiction. You're better off without it.

If you're eating a Western diet, you're eating a lot of toxic stuff. Artificial additives, preservatives, flavors, colors, sweeteners, and trans fats are all man-made chemicals that you were never meant to ingest. Eliminating processed food and switching to an organic whole-foods, plant-based diet are critical steps in reducing your toxic load and restoring your health. If you are eating conventionally grown produce, you are ingesting trace amounts of toxic pesticides, herbicides, and fungicides that are sprayed on crops. Switching to an all-organic diet (as much as possible) is the first way you can reduce your body's toxic load. The less work your liver has to do to detoxify avoidable toxins, the more bandwidth it has to detoxify the unavoidable ones.

In 2013, researchers at MIT published a study demonstrating that Monsanto's Roundup—the most popular herbicide in the world, sprayed on genetically modified and conventionally grown (non-organic) crops—leaves glyphosate residue, especially on sugar, corn, soy, and wheat. According to their findings, glyphosate interferes with cytochrome P450 enzymes that help your body detoxify. Inhibited detoxification can enhance the damaging effects of other food-borne chemicals and environmental toxins, leading to diabetes, heart disease, autism, cancer, infertility, and more.[2] Glyphosate is also a xenoestrogen, an endocrine disrupter found to promote hormone-dependent breast cancer growth.[3] Internal FDA emails obtained by *The Guardian* through the Freedom of Information Act revealed that one researcher found traces of glyphosate in all the food he brought from home to test except for broccoli, which included wheat crackers, granola, and cornmeal.[4] Glyphosate has also been found in a variety of cereals, chips, crackers, cookies, and even wine and orange juice. This chemical is so widely used that it has polluted our rainwater, groundwater, and drinking water.

Each year the Environmental Working Group publishes a report of the most pesticide-contaminated produce. The rankings are based on the pesticide levels in washed produce reported by the FDA and the USDA Pesticide Testing Program. According to its findings, you can lower your pesticide exposure by nearly 80 percent simply by avoiding the top 12 most contaminated fruits and vegetables, known as the Dirty Dozen.

A study published in the *Journal of Environmental Research* found that after just seven days on an organic diet, dialkyl phosphate pesticide (DAP) levels in adults dropped by 89 percent in urinary excretion. DAPs make up 70 to 80 percent of organophosphate pesticides.[5] In a similar study, researchers also reported a dramatic drop in the levels of insecticides and herbicide in children's urine after only five days on an organic diet.[6]

Produce you should buy organic:

Apples, celery, cherry tomatoes, cucumbers, grapes, hot peppers, nectarines, peaches, potatoes, spinach, strawberries, sweet bell peppers, kale, collard greens, summer squash, corn, and berries.

Produce that isn't critical to buy organic:

Asparagus, avocados, cabbage, cantaloupe, eggplant, grapefruit, honeydew, kiwi, mangoes, mushrooms, onions, papayas (avoid Hawaiian papayas; they are genetically modified), pineapples, sweet peas, sweet potatoes, and watermelons.

The most effective fruit and vegetable wash for pesticide removal appears to be a 10 percent solution of salt water, 1 part salt to 9 parts water.[7]

CHECK THE LABEL

Conventional produce has a four-digit SKU on the sticker starting with a 3 or 4. Organic produce will have a five-digit SKU starting with the number 9. Genetically modified produce typically has a five-digit SKU starting with the number 8, but since it is not required by law, some GMO producers have dropped the 8 and shortened their SKUs to four digits.

If you can't afford or don't have access to organic produce, you should still eat tons of fruits and vegetables. The benefits of the abundance of vitamins, minerals, antioxidants, enzymes, and phytonutrients in a diet rich in fruits and vegetables outweigh any risk.

THE SOLUTION TO POLLUTION IS DILUTION

Our bodies are roughly 60 percent water. Water is the most critical element in your body. Depending on your metabolism and how much body fat you have, you can go anywhere from many weeks to many months without food, but you can only live a week or two without water. Water (hydrogen and oxygen) is essential to life and every system in the body, especially for flushing out toxins.

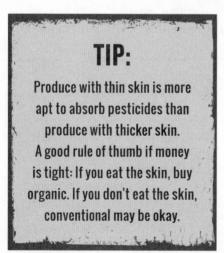

TIP:

Produce with thin skin is more apt to absorb pesticides than produce with thicker skin. A good rule of thumb if money is tight: If you eat the skin, buy organic. If you don't eat the skin, conventional may be okay.

This is why it is vitally important to put clean water in your body. And lots of it. Half a gallon of purified water per day is ideal (juice counts toward this). Although tap water is relatively clean, and is certainly an improvement over drinking sugary drinks, it still can contain hundreds of contaminants, including lead, copper, bacteria, industrial waste chemicals, and sewage. And even if your tap water is 100 percent contaminant free, it still likely contains chlorine bleach and fluoride. Chlorine bleach is added to kill bacteria, which is good. But then you end up drinking the bleach, which is bad. Fluoride is added to our drinking water for our teeth, but the fluoride used is not naturally sourced or pharmaceutical grade.

Cities with fluoridated water have higher cavity rates and higher cancer death rates than cities with non-fluoridated water. Ninety-eight percent of Western Europe now has rejected water fluoridation, and their children's teeth are just as healthy as children's teeth in the United States. Since 1997, the FDA has required all fluoride toothpaste sold in the United States to carry this poison warning:

> Keep out of reach of children under 6 years of age. If you accidentally swallow more than used for brushing, seek professional help or call a poison control center immediately.

This is because a tube of toothpaste contains enough fluoride to kill a small child, and it's not uncommon for young children to swallow some toothpaste while brushing. But even if you don't swallow your toothpaste, fluoride is still absorbed directly into your bloodstream through the capillaries under your tongue.

Roughly 66 percent of U.S. water supplies are currently fluoridated and 90 percent of these municipalities use hydrofluorosilicic acid,[8] a waste product from phosphate fertilizer manufacturing that is often contaminated with arsenic, heavy metals, and radionuclides. Since 1999, over 60 U.S. communities have rejected fluoridation.

Fluoride is an ingredient in some prescription drugs, including Paxil, Prozac, Flonase, and Flovent. Most commercial crops are watered with fluoridated water and absorb it. Fruit juices from concentrate are reconstituted with fluoridated water. And bottled water, even if it's filtered, usually has fluoride in it, unless it's true spring water. Bottled water companies are not required to disclose what type of filtration they use, if any. And don't believe the "natural mountain spring" hype; many companies are simply selling tap water that may be further contaminated by hormone-disrupting chemicals leached from the plastic bottle. A 2018 study found that 93 percent of bottled water brands tested were contaminated with as much as 10,000 plastic microparticles per liter. Nestlé Pure Life bottled water had the highest levels.[9]

Cooking with tap water is also problematic because it concentrates the fluoride and other pollutants, some of which bind to the vegetables you're about to eat. Steaming is the best way to preserve nutrients in vegetables, but if you're going to boil veggies, make sure you use purified water and save the broth for soup stock.

MEET THE HALIDES: UNINVITED GUESTS IN YOUR BODY

Many people have thyroid problems today due to fluoride, chlorine, and bromine. These three toxic halides all displace iodine in the thyroid, essentially polluting it and eventually impairing its ability to function properly. The thyroid regulates your endocrine system, directly affecting breast, ovarian, uterine, and prostate health. Fluoride and chlorine are in our drinking and bathing water and most beverages sold today. Bromine is a flame retardant used to treat furniture, mattresses, and carpet to help keep them from catching fire. Bromine is also used in processed foods in the form of brominated vegetable oil and potassium bromate, as well as in prescription medications.

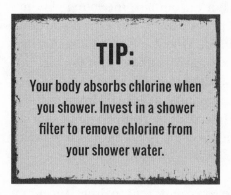

TIP:

Your body absorbs chlorine when you shower. Invest in a shower filter to remove chlorine from your shower water.

Brominated vegetable oil (BVO) is banned in over 100 countries (but not the U.S.) and is most commonly found in soft drinks and sports drinks like Gatorade, Powerade, Mountain Dew, Squirt, and Fresca. BVO has been linked to major organ system damage, hormone disruption, thyroid dysfunction, birth defects, brain development and growth problems in children, schizophrenia, hearing loss, and cancers of the breast, thyroid, stomach, ovaries, uterus, and prostate. In early 2013, due to public pressure, Pepsi agreed to remove BVO from Gatorade.

Potassium bromate (bromated flour) is used in many baked goods to speed up the baking process. It bleaches the dough and makes it unnaturally white and fluffy—think Wonder Bread. In the early 1980s, Japanese researchers began publishing studies showing that potassium bromate caused thyroid, kidney, and other cancers in rodents. Many countries other than the U.S., including the E.U., China, and Brazil, took these studies seriously and banned potassium bromate in food. The state of California requires a disclosure on food labels that contain it, which says, "Potassium bromate is an unnecessary and potentially harmful food additive, and should be avoided."

TOXIC MEAT AND DAIRY

Meat and dairy can harbor viruses, bacteria, and parasites, and factory-farmed animals are often injected with antibiotics and hormones and are fed unnatural GMO feed to fatten them up. Many wild fish are polluted with mercury, especially the fish at the top of the food chain, including tuna, tilefish, swordfish, shark, and king mackerel. On the other hand, farm-raised fish have been found to have some of the highest levels of PCBs, a toxic by-product of the manufacturing industry. Dairy, eggs, and meat also have been found to concentrate environmental toxins and pesticide residues in their fatty tissues.[10]

Aluminum is a potent neurotoxin linked to Alzheimer's.[11] You might be surprised to know that the highest source of dietary aluminum is cheese. Many cheese manufacturers use an additive called sodium aluminum phosphate, which is a form of salt that enhances flavor and texture. But you won't see sodium aluminum phosphate listed as an ingredient on the label because cheese makers are allowed to simply call it "salt." Other forms of aluminum, such as aluminum sulfate, are often used in baking powders, pickles, relishes, flour, and canned meat. The half-life of mercury in the body is estimated to be about two months. The same goes for aluminum. Your body can remove these heavy metals, but you have to stop putting them in.

The most important steps in detoxification are to stop putting toxins in your mouth via drinking, smoking, and eating man-made processed food and animal products, as well as prescription drugs (consult your doctor before stopping them).

TOXIC BEAUTY

Your skin absorbs what you put on it. Chemicals from creams, lotions, potions, oils, makeup, nail polish, deodorants, and other body care products are absorbed into your bloodstream through your skin, and these chemicals circulate throughout your entire body. Unlike the food industry, the skin care industry is largely unregulated. Mascara has traces of mercury. Lipstick has traces of lead. Talcum powder has been associated with ovarian cancer. According to a study conducted by the Organic Consumers Association, traces of suspected carcinogen 1,4-dioxane were found in almost half of personal care products tested, even though it is typically not listed on the label.[12] This included bath products, shower gels, lotions, and hand soaps. Aluminum salts in antiperspirants, which interfere with estrogen receptors, have been implicated as a potential contributor to breast cancer, as there is a disproportionately large number of breast cancers that occur in the upper outer quadrant of the breast tissue closest to the armpit.[13]

The Environmental Working Group website (ewg.org) has a large database of body care products rated by toxicity. It's a great place to research the brands you're using to see if they are potentially toxic and to find top-rated, clean brands.

Toxic Body Care Chemicals to Avoid

Here is a selected list of toxic chemicals commonly used in personal care products that you should steer clear of, courtesy of the Environmental Working Group.

1. **BHA** (butylated hydroxyanisole) is a suspected human carcinogen found in food, food packaging, and personal care products sold in the U.S. In animal studies, BHA produces liver damage and causes stomach cancers (such as papillomas and carcinomas) and interferes with reproductive system development and thyroid function (hormone levels). The European Union considers it unsafe in fragrance.

2. **Coal tar** and other coal tar ingredients (aminophenol, diaminobenzene, phenylenediamine) are used in hair dyes and specialty products such as dandruff and psoriasis shampoos. Coal tar is a known human carcinogen. Hair stylists and other professionals are exposed to these chemicals in hair dye almost daily and have a higher risk of cancer than many other professions. Europe has banned the use of many of these coal tar ingredients in hair dyes.

3. **Formaldehyde and formaldehyde releasers** (bronopol, DMDM hydantoin, diazolidinyl urea, imidzaolidinyl urea, and quaternium-15). Formaldehyde is a preservative and a known human carcinogen as well as an asthmagen, neurotoxicant, and developmental toxicant. It is used in hair straighteners and as a preservative in cosmetics. Formaldehyde releasers are widely used in U.S. products. Not surprisingly, more Americans develop contact allergies to these ingredients than Europeans. Also, the artificial sweetener aspartame breaks down into formaldehyde in the body.

4. **Fragrances** is the generic catch-all term used to avoid disclosing secret ingredients to competitors, but it's also

a way to hide potentially toxic ingredients. Federal law doesn't require companies to list any of the chemicals in their fragrance mixture on their product labels. Recent research from EWG and the Campaign for Safe Cosmetics found an average of 14 chemicals in 17 name-brand fragrance products, none of them listed on the label. Fragrances can contain hormone disruptors and are among the top five allergens in the world. I recommend buying fragrance free or from companies that provide full label disclosure.

5. **Parabens** (specifically propyl-, isopropyl-, butyl-, and isobutyl-parabens) are estrogen-mimicking preservatives used widely in cosmetics and body care products like shampoos and conditioners. Parabens may disrupt the endocrine system and cause reproductive and developmental disorders.

6. **Polyethylene glycol (PEGs) and other polyethylene compounds** are a family of conditioning and cleaning agents that go by many names. These synthetic chemicals are frequently contaminated with 1,4-dioxane, which the U.S. government considers a probable human carcinogen and which readily penetrates the skin.

7. **Petroleum distillates** are petroleum-extracted cosmetics ingredients, commonly found in mascara. They may cause contact dermatitis and are often contaminated with cancer-causing impurities. They are produced in oil refineries at the same time as automobile fuel, heating oil, and chemical feedstocks.

8. **Phthalates** are found in color cosmetics, fragranced lotions, body washes, hair care products, nail polish, and more. They can cause endocrine disruption, developmental and reproductive toxicity, organ system toxicity, and bioaccumulation of toxic substances. Pregnant women and breast-feeding mothers are especially vulnerable. Phthalates are banned from cosmetics sold in the E.U. but not in the U.S. Look for phthalate-free brands and avoid products with "fragrance," which may contain phthalates.

9. **Resorcinol** is a common ingredient in hair color and bleaching products. It is a skin irritant, toxic to the immune system, and a frequent cause of hair dye allergy. In animal studies resorcinol has been shown to disrupt normal thyroid function.

10. **Triclosan and triclocarban** are antimicrobial pesticides found in antibacterial soaps. Triclosan disrupts thyroid function and reproductive hormones. Overuse may promote the development of bacterial resistance. These chemicals are highly toxic to the aquatic environment. Colgate made national headlines in 2014 when it was discovered that Colgate Total toothpaste contained triclosan.

11. **Vitamin A compounds** (retinol, retinyl palmitate, retinyl acetate) are widely used in sunscreens, skin lotions, lip products, and makeup. Sunlight breaks down vitamin A to produce toxic free radicals that can damage DNA and hasten skin lesions and tumors in lab animals.

A CANCER CAUSE RIGHT UNDER YOUR NOSE

If you have cancer, the cause could literally be right under your nose, in your mouth, specifically from silver fillings. Silver amalgam fillings are 50 percent mercury, the most toxic nonradioactive metal on earth. Silver fillings release mercury vapor every time you agitate your teeth with chewing, brushing, eating acidic foods, and drinking hot liquids. Your body absorbs 80 percent of the mercury vapor you breathe in. Each amalgam in your mouth can release as much as 1 microgram of mercury per day, and the release of mercury vapor never stops, no matter how old the fillings are. Tests have found that people with silver fillings have mercury circulating in their blood, brain, liver, kidneys, and even amniotic fluid and breast milk. Because of the excessive use of mercury fillings, it is estimated that over 120 million Americans have mercury exposure that exceeds the safety limit set by the

California Environmental Protection Agency.[14] If you have two or more mercury fillings, you are probably in that group. (For more information, visit the International Academy of Oral Medicine and Toxicology at iaomt.org.)

The American Dental Association's official position is that mercury amalgams are safe. Mercury amalgams were first introduced into dentistry in the early 1800s, long before safety regulations were enacted. Today the EPA and OSHA classify mercury filings as hazardous waste, requiring strict disposal procedures to prevent further release of mercury into the environment after fillings are removed from dental patients' mouths.

If you decide to have your mercury fillings replaced, avoid bisphenol-A based epoxy resin composites. The New England Children's Amalgam Trial linked these types of resins to a greater risk of impaired physiological function in children, including learning impairment and behavioral issues. Make sure your dentist uses a non–BPA-based composite resin for your fillings.

The half-life of mercury in the body is estimated to be about two months.[15] If mercury exposure from sources like fish and silver fillings is stopped, it is estimated that the body can almost completely detoxify mercury within a year. Oral DMSA (dimercaptosuccinic acid) therapy is a mercury and lead detoxification protocol that may accelerate the process. This should only be done under the supervision of a qualified practitioner.

MERCURY IN OUR FOOD

Mercury has made its way into our food supply. Almost all fish and shellfish contain trace amounts of mercury in their bodies, trapped in their fatty tissue. Like polonium, mercury works its way up the food chain in a process called biomagnification. The bigger the fish and the longer it lives, the more toxic mercury it absorbs, and when you eat that fish you absorb it all and it accumulates in your tissues. The human body can detoxify mercury but it can take many months, and consistent mercury exposure over time can lead to a toxic buildup and eventual tipping point when your body's ability to repair, regenerate, and detoxify properly is compromised, its functions break down, and health problems begin.

Mercury consumption from fish has been linked to brain and nervous system damage in unborn babies and young children, which is why the FDA and EPA strongly advise that women who are pregnant, may become pregnant, breast-feeding mothers, and young children abstain from fish known to have high levels of mercury, such as tuna, tilefish, king mackerel, marlin, orange roughy, shark, and swordfish. Mercury poisons adults too. In 1969 the FDA determined that 0.5 ppm was the maximum allowable limit for mercury in fish, but mercury levels in fish kept rising. So in 1979 they raised the limit to 1 ppm. In 1984 they stopped measuring total mercury and decided to only check for methylmercury. In 1998 the FDA stopped widely testing for mercury in fish. To put it in perspective, eating mercury-containing fish like tuna just once per week may exceed the EPA safety level and expose you to more mercury than six thimerosal-containing vaccines.

MY MERCURY EXPOSURE

When I was in fourth grade, I got a fever and stayed home sick from school. While playing with the dog in the living room with a thermometer in my mouth, I hit my chin on the coffee table, biting the glass thermometer in half. This was a fairly common problem with kids and glass thermometers, which is why they don't sell them anymore. Years later when I was a junior in high school, I thought it would be cool to "accidentally" break a huge thermometer on the lab table in chemistry class. I poured some of the mercury into the palm of my hand and let it roll around for a few seconds. I remember one of the other kids saying, "I don't think you're supposed to touch that stuff." At which point I let it roll off my hand back onto the table. Holding mercury in my hand was strange because it was surprisingly heavy, like a liquid marble. When I was diagnosed with colon cancer, my doctor estimated it had been growing in my body for about 10 years.

FRESH AIR IS UNDERRATED

An important step to reduce your toxic load is to eliminate as many potential toxins as possible from the two places where you spend most of your time: home and work. A 2018 study published in *Science* found that volatile organic compounds from paint, varnishes, cleaning products, and personal care products including shampoo, hairspray, deodorant, perfume, air fresheners, and hand sanitizers contribute to more outdoor air pollution than automobile exhaust.[16] And we spend 90 percent of our time indoors! According to the EPA, indoor air can be as much as five times more polluted than outside air. Common indoor air pollutants also include radon gas, smoke, mold spores, and volatile organic compounds from chemicals used in furniture foam and fabrics. Radon gas is the second leading cause of lung cancer after smoking.[17] You can get a radon gas test kit for $15 at your local hardware store. While you're there, pick up a mold test kit. Toxic mold can lead to chronic infection and suppressed immunity, which can keep you perpetually sick and vulnerable to cancer. Scented candles, incense, and air fresheners can produce toxic chemical vapors and smoke. Look for 100 percent soy or beeswax candles with paper or cotton wicks scented with essential oils. Diffusing essential oils is also a safer option, but certain oils can be toxic to pets.

Air purifiers can help clean up the air in your home and so can houseplants. Multiple studies have found that houseplants remove common indoor air pollutants, such as benzene, trichloroethylene, formaldehyde, and ammonia. Some of the best performers are peace lily, Boston fern, bamboo palm, lady palm, Barberton daisy, mass cane, Janet Craig, and warneckei. For optimal air filtering, NASA recommends one plant for every 100 square feet of indoor space.[18,19] Note: Before you bring new plants into the house, make sure they aren't toxic to pets.

CLEAN UP YOUR CLEANING SUPPLIES

Many household cleaning products contain noxious and toxic ingredients than can be absorbed through your skin and when you inhale the fumes. An eight-year study following over 55,000 American nurses reported that nurses who used disinfectants to clean surfaces at least once a week had a 24 to 32 percent increased risk of developing chronic obstructive pulmonary disease, emphysema, bronchitis, and asthma when compared to nurses who used disinfectants less frequently.[20] The main cleaning chemicals linked to lung damage in the study were glutaraldehyde, a disinfectant used on medical instruments, as well as bleach, hydrogen peroxide, alcohol, and ammonia-based compounds, which are commonly found in household cleaners.

A 2018 study out of Norway found that women who reported using cleaning products at least once per week in their home or cleaned professionally for 20 years had substantial lung damage, equivalent to smoking 20 cigarettes per day, compared to women who didn't clean their own homes.[21] Women who cleaned for a living had the most damage and the highest decline in lung function. To prevent lung damage from harsh cleaning chemicals, the scientists who conducted the research advise using microfiber cloths and water instead of harsh chemical cleaning products.

Even laundry detergents and dryer sheets can be polluting your home. An analysis of gases produced by household laundry machines found more than 25 volatile organic compounds, including seven hazardous air pollutants, such as known carcinogens acetaldehyde and benzene.[22]

I recommend replacing standard chemical household cleaners, laundry detergent, and especially dish detergent with natural, nontoxic, biodegradable, organic cleaning products. Dr. Bronner's Pure Castile Soap is one of our favorites. You can use it in the shower. You can do your dishes with it. You can clean your house with it. You can even brush your teeth with it.

IS YOUR JOB TOXIC?

In 2009 an occupational study of cancer risk for 15 million people from Denmark, Finland, Iceland, Norway, and Sweden found the highest risk of cancer in beverage and tobacco workers, plumbers, seamen, mechanics, engine operators, miners, chimney sweeps, and some factory workers. These professions involve working around smoke, soot, dust, or chemical fumes. Hair stylists and salon workers also have elevated risk due to their exposure to chemical agents in hair care products like straighteners, bleaches, dyes, perfumes, and nail polish. Restaurant servers have an elevated risk of lung cancer from tobacco use and exposure, as well as liver cancer from alcohol use.[23] According to the study, the occupations with the lowest risk for cancer are farmers, gardeners, and teachers. But it's a different story for livestock producers. Multiple studies have linked American poultry, cattle, and pig farmers to elevated risk of blood cancers.[24,25]

Detoxifying your workplace can be tricky. Unless you're the boss, you may not be able to improve the air quality at work. Adding several small plants, or even a desktop air purifier, in your office or cubicle can help. If you are surrounded by toxic fumes at work, it might be a good time to start looking for another job.

ELECTROPOLLUTION

Your body is an electrically powered organic machine, and your cells communicate with each other through electrical impulses. Your brain tells your heart to beat. Your stomach tells your brain you are hungry. Your skin sends information to your brain about the texture, temperature, and weight of objects you touch, and so much more.

Your central nervous system is kind of like the internet. It is the conduit for trillions of messages to be sent back and forth between your cells, organs, and brain to keep your body functioning properly. When you cut yourself, distress signals are sent out by the wounded area and your body responds with reinforcements to clot the blood, fight infection, seal off the area, and rebuild the damaged tissue.

When electrical current flows through an object, it creates an electromagnetic field (EMF), and just like electrical wiring and electronic equipment, our bodies have an electromagnetic field surrounding them. We conduct electricity and radio frequencies, which is why getting close to or touching the TV antenna can affect the picture. Our bodies run on electricity, but not all electricity is good for us.

Electropollution is a term coined to describe our increasing exposure to harmful invisible electronic frequencies harnessed by man in our modern world. Electronic frequency can be divided into these basic groups:

➤ **Extremely low frequency (ELF):** power lines

➤ **Radio frequency (RF):** radio and TV signals, microwaves, and wireless devices

➤ **Intermediate frequencies:** emitted by appliances and electric circuits

➤ **High frequency:** ionizing radiation, X-rays, CT scans, and PET scans

➤ **Dirty electricity:** the harmful combination of distorted frequencies from various electronic sources in our homes, offices, schools, and elsewhere

According to the research and hypothesis of Samuel Milham, M.D., M.P.H., the widespread adoption of electricity in our homes, which was completed in 1959, is correlated to the rise in cancer, cardiovascular disease, diabetes, and even suicide in the United States. The incidence of these diseases was much lower in rural areas before they were electrified, and there was a distinct increase in the years following electrification.[26] In 1979 a study by Leeper and Wertheimer was published showing a correlation between living in close proximity to strong magnetic fields emitted by residential power lines and risk of childhood cancer.[27] Since then additional studies have also shown an increase in cancer risk while others have shown no increase in risk. Two pooled studies and a meta-analysis found a 1.4 to 2-fold increase in risk of leukemia in children exposed to electromagnetic fields at home measuring 0.3 μT or higher. However, according to the National Cancer Institute, the number of children exposed to this level of electromagnetic fields in the combined studies is considered to be too small to be statistically significant. Given the lack of conclusive evidence either way, I think it makes sense to follow the precautionary principle and take steps to reduce your exposure to potentially harmful electromagnetic frequencies. Not living next to power lines is a good start.

The microwave frequencies produced by 2.4 GHz Wi-Fi devices have been identified as an important threat to human health. Numerous repeated studies have linked Wi-Fi radiation to oxidative stress, DNA damage, hormone dysregulation, melatonin lowering and sleep disruption, infant brain development, calcium overload, and male infertility.[28]

If you're living near an industrial area, you could be exposed to higher levels of air and water pollution. And there may be significant pollution nearby that you aren't aware of. I suggest researching to see if there are any EPA superfund sites in your area. These are known toxic-waste hazard sites across the United States (https://www.epa.gov/superfund). Also check to see if you live in a cancer cluster, which is an area known to have higher than average rates of cancer. Deaths from all cancers in 2014 were highest along the Mississippi River, near the Kentucky/West Virginia border, in western Alaska, and in the South in general. Cancer deaths were lowest in western states like Utah and Colorado.[29] If you live in an area with high rates of cancer, if multiple neighbors are getting cancer, or if more than one person in your house is diagnosed with cancer, you may need to get the heck out of there.

How to Reduce Harmful EMF Exposure in Your Home

➤ Just like light, EMFs can also interfere with your body's production of melatonin. Don't charge your cell phone on the nightstand beside your bed.

➤ Turn off your Wi-Fi at night or when you aren't using it. Newer wireless routers have on/off switches for the Wi-Fi signal and some can even be controlled with your smartphone. If your wireless router doesn't have an on/off switch, a cheap hack is to plug it into a light timer programmed to shut off automatically at a certain time each night.

➤ Fluorescent bulbs generate more EMFs than standard bulbs, produce harmful blue light, and are filled with toxic mercury vapor. LED light bulbs generate less EMFs but also produce blue light, which you should avoid at night. Incandescent bulbs are best.

➤ If you would like to measure the EMF fields in your home or at work, you can use a gauss meter to measure EMF "hot spots" in your home or work environment so you can take steps to reduce your exposure.

Your cells are constantly sending and receiving messages via electrochemical pathways in your nervous system, but external electromagnetic frequencies can disrupt normal communication between cells. They can overload and confuse cells with false messages or messages they don't understand, like when too many people try to talk at the same time. This interference can disrupt cellular function in every part of your body. When you are exposed to harmful EMFs, they can disturb your nervous system and raise your stress hormones, which can lead to sleep disorders, depressed immunity, cardiovascular disease, premature aging, autoimmune disorders, and even neurological problems like depression. Harmful EMFs can rupture cell membranes and create free radicals, resulting in DNA damage. They can disrupt normal cell division, handicap your immune system, and create precancerous cells. If you have health problems, electropollution is not likely to be something your doctor is going to consider but it could be aggravating or even causing your condition.

WHAT ABOUT CELL PHONE RADIATION?

If cell phone radiation causes brain cancer, then it stands to reason that the widespread adoption of cell phones starting in the early 1990s should have caused a measurable increase in the number of new brain cancers diagnosed each year. However, data from the National Cancer Institute's SEER Program shows no increase in the incidence of brain or other central nervous system cancers between 1992 and 2015, despite the dramatic increase in cell phone use in the United States during this time.[30]

But these stats don't tell the whole story. According to a 2018 UK study, the rates of several types of brain cancers have fallen, but the overall annual incidence of glioblastoma multiforme, the most aggressive type of brain cancer, has doubled since 1995.[31] The authors of the study speculate that this could be due to increased exposure to factors such as medical X-rays and CT scans, pollution, or cell phone radiation.

The World Health Organization's International Agency for Research on Cancer has classified cell phone use as "possibly carcinogenic to humans," but along with the American Cancer Society, the National Institute of Environmental Health Sciences, as well as the FDA, CDC, and FCC, the IARC also states that there is not enough evidence to conclusively link cell phone use to brain tumors.

Given the lack of conclusive evidence concerning cell phones and cancer risk, I still think it makes sense to take precautions. I rarely if ever put my phone up to my head. I always try to use the speaker phone or earbuds, and I keep my phone away from my body whenever possible. I put my phone on my desk when

I'm working, on the table at restaurants, or in the console when I'm driving. I also put my phone on airplane mode for hours at a time, especially if it's in my pocket for long periods of time. When using your phone, be aware that the weaker your phone's signal, the more radiation it emits.

FASTING

Fasting was a regular part of life for many of our ancestors for religious reasons and during times of food scarcity. And it is a powerful detoxification method and regeneration therapy for your body. I fasted often during my cancer healing journey and did several extended-day juice fasts, drinking only vegetable juice for up to 10 days as well as taking shorter water fasts.

Fasting gives your body a break from digestion, which allows it to pay attention to things that have been overlooked. Around day two or three of a water fast, your body switches from burning glucose for energy to burning body fat. This process is called ketosis. When you enter a natural state of ketosis through fasting, which is technically controlled starvation, your body switches from normal daily operations to survival and protection mode and your cells begin a process of internal housecleaning. Realizing there is a shortage of glucose for fuel, healthy cells stop trying to grow and instead begin to break down and use old and damaged parts for fuel. The scientific term for this is autophagy, which is derived from Greek and means "self-eating." During this process, healthy cells "hunker down" and reinforce their defenses to protect themselves and survive, but cancer cells are mutated cells stuck in growth mode and have difficulty adapting. During a period of fasting or starvation, many types of cancer cells keep trying to grow without fuel and become weaker and die.

Sometimes cells live too long and become old and ineffective. These are not the kinds of cells you want in your body, especially when it comes to your immune cells. During a three- to five-day water fast, old and damaged immune cells in your body die off and regenerative stem cells are activated. Then when you start eating again, these activated stem cells ramp up production of brand-new immune cells to replace the old ones that died off.[32] Fasting essentially reboots and recharges your immune system and reduces levels of IGF-1, insulin, and glucose in your body.

Researchers have even found that short-term fasting protects healthy cells and sensitizes cancer cells to chemo and radiotherapy treatment in mice, extending their survival.[33] Fasting for 72 hours around cancer treatment—48 hours before and 24 hours after—has been determined to be safe for cancer patients and to reduce the side effects of platinum combination chemotherapy while protecting healthy cells.[34]

The guidelines for fasting are simple. Drink water throughout the day; somewhere between half and one gallon is sufficient. You can squeeze lemon into your water and drink non-caffeinated herbal teas like rooibos or hibiscus. Taking supplements may be okay too. There aren't enough calories in lemon juice, teas, or supplements to interfere with the process. Most people can handle a three- to five-day water fast without any problems, but under certain conditions—like if you are taking drugs that lower blood pressure or blood sugar—fasting could be dangerous. If you are taking pharmaceutical drugs or have any serious health conditions or concerns, you should check with your doctor before attempting a water fast.

An alternative to water fasting is the ProLon Fasting Mimicking Diet developed by Dr. Valter Longo, director of the Longevity Institute at the University of Southern California. The Fasting Mimicking Diet is a five-day, plant-based, calorie-restricted meal plan that has been proven in human clinical trials to produce the same powerful benefits in the body as a water fast, including autophagy and stem cell activation and regeneration.[35] My wife and I have done the ProLon Diet. It is easier than a water fast because you don't have to stop eating completely, and it may be safer for individuals with serious health conditions. For maximum physiological benefit, Dr. Longo recommends doing this diet once per month for three months in a row, and then once per quarter or every six months. He and his team are currently conducting clinical trials examining the extent to which a fasting mimicking diet protects healthy cells and enhances conventional cancer treatments.

It's normal to feel lousy during the first few days of a fast. This is known as the Herxheimer Reaction, or the "healing crisis." You may even experience this just by converting from a Western diet to a raw-food or plant-based diet. There are three main reasons why: adaptation, food addiction, and detoxification. During fasting, your body flips genetic survival switches that it has never flipped before and that's going to make you feel different. Most people are adapted to a diet that is high in animal protein and fat, sugar, salt, and caffeine. When you remove these things from your diet, you will experience physical withdrawal. If you have been in the habit of drinking diet sodas or chewing gum all day, you may also suffer withdrawal from food additives like aspartame.

The second reason you may feel bad when you fast or switch to a raw-food or a plant-based diet is the detoxification reaction. Your body stores toxins in fat. And during a fast, your body will break down toxic fat for energy. Some of these toxins are released into your bloodstream and circulate throughout your body before they are neutralized and eliminated. During this process, you're going to feel lousy. Some typical reactions caused by the adaptation process, food withdrawal, or detoxification are low energy, brain fog, headaches, dizziness, nausea, random aches and pains, pimples, rashes, and upset stomach. Every person has a different experience. In some cases, it could even trigger a fever, which could be beneficial. Your immune system ramps up into high gear when you have a fever, and a fever can wipe out a host of viruses, bacteria, and parasites in your body that you didn't even know you had. Note: If you develop a fever over 104°F, call your doctor and discontinue the fast.

If any of those reactions happen during a fast, it could be coincidental, but it's likely because there's some serious housecleaning happening in your body. Make sure you are super hydrated. Drink lots of water to help flush things out and power through it if you can. A water enema or a quick sweat in a sauna—20 minutes or less—can also help accelerate detoxification. Note: If you're taking prescription medication, fasting and/or saunas could be dangerous. Make sure that you are cautious with your approach and do it with supervision—medical, if necessary.

The typical scenario during a fast is low energy, and maybe a bit of a headache for a few days. If you start feeling bad, just remind yourself that it is part of the process. Most folks feel okay on day one, lousy and hungry on day two, and then turn a corner and lose their appetite and start to feel good on day three. When you get over that detoxification hump, usually after a few days, you should feel great. Every time I fast, there's always a point around day three of the fast where I am surprised at how much energy I have and how good I feel without being hungry.

A 24-hour water fast is an easy way to get your feet wet. However, a three-day water fast is considered to be the minimal length of time needed to get the benefits of autophagy and stem cell regeneration. If you are doing a three-day fast, I recommend doing it over a weekend. Start on a Friday morning—Thursday night would be your last meal—and don't eat again until Monday morning.

Most folks lose 1 to 2 pounds per day during a fast, but some of the weight returns once you resume eating. Fasting can jump-start weight loss, but the best way to lose weight and keep it off is by consistently eating a whole-food, plant-based diet. The more body fat you have, the longer you can fast. Obesity is the second leading cause of cancer, and getting rid of excess body fat is a very good thing. The powerful regenerative effects of fasting actually happen after the fast, when you resume eating after fasting for three to five days.

MASSIVE ACTION STEPS FOR DETOXIFICATION

➤ Stop putting artificial food loaded with man-made chemicals in your mouth

➤ Stop eating animal foods

➤ Buy organic produce

➤ Invest in a water purifier and a filter for your shower

➤ Replace your toxic makeup and body care with non-toxic brands

➤ Remove mercury fillings

➤ Keep your cell phone away from your head

➤ Turn off Wi-Fi at night and whenever possible

➤ Invest in an air purifier

➤ Replace your toxic cleaning supplies

➤ Consider a three- to five-day water fast or the ProLon five-day Fasting Mimicking Diet

LET'S GET PHYSICAL

*Those who think they have not time for bodily exercise
will sooner or later have to find time for illness.*
— EDWARD STANLEY, EARL OF DERBY

*If you can't fly, run. If you can't run, walk. If you can't walk, crawl.
But by all means, keep moving.*
— DR. MARTIN LUTHER KING, JR.

MANY PEOPLE ASSUME that health and fitness are synonymous, because typically when someone decides to get fit they start working out, eating better, and losing weight, and subsequently their health improves. But it is possible to be fit and unhealthy. It is also possible to be perfectly healthy but not very strong or fit. The goal is to achieve a balance of both. It's not unusual for athletes and fitness buffs to become so obsessed with performance and their physical appearance that they will put anything in their bodies to achieve their goals. Many eat large amounts of animal protein and take copious amounts of sports supplements and growth hormones to get big and ripped, or stronger and faster. Cancer survivor Mr. Livestrong himself, Lance Armstrong, admitted to using illegal drugs to win the Tour de France.

SITTING IS THE NEW SMOKING

Americans have become sedentary beings who spend on average 15.5 of our 16 to 17 waking hours per day sitting, and one-third of American children and two-thirds of American adults are either overweight or obese. According to recent estimates, half of Americans don't get enough physical activity, and over one-third of us are classified as "physically inactive." Lack of exercise is a major contributor to chronic diseases including cardiovascular diseases, diabetes, breast cancer, colon cancer, and endometrial cancer and increases your risk of 10 more cancers.[1,2] But you can reduce your risk by simply adding a little more movement to your life.

TOO MUCH OF A GOOD THING

Americans have the shortest life expectancies of any nation in the industrialized world, but professional athletes, who are at the opposite end of the exercise spectrum, have an even shorter life span. The average elite athlete dies by age 67, nine years before the average American coach potato, who has a life expectancy of about 78 (76 for men, 80 for women).

Exercise is definitely a good thing but, extreme exercise, including excessive weight training and endurance training for marathons and triathlons, may do more harm than good. This level of activity can also produce excessive levels of free radicals and high levels of the stress hormones adrenaline and cortisol, which can suppress immune function and raise your risk of infection or illnesses like colds and the flu.

Research done by David Nieman, Ph.D., and colleagues at Loma Linda University showed that marathon runners are six times more likely to become ill after a race due to impaired immune function. Extreme exercise creates excessive catabolic stress and increases the metabolism for prolonged periods of time, increasing free radicals and damaging cells. Marathons and intense aerobic exercise deplete existing antioxidants, suppress immunity, and break down muscle tissue.[3] Chronic physical stress from overtraining week after week, month after month, year after year without adequate recovery time keeps your body in an exhausted, depleted, and vulnerable state.

Exercise alone cannot produce optimal health. Jim Fixx, the "father of jogging" and author of the massive worldwide best-seller *The Complete Book of Running*, died of a heart attack after his morning run at the ripe old age of 52. His autopsy revealed complete blockage in one of his coronary arteries, 80 percent blockage in another, and signs of previous heart attacks.[4] Despite Jim's example and many others, the assumption that fitness equals health is still prevalent today.

Current research indicates that 90 minutes of intense exercise per day, or running 60 miles per week, is too much for most people. Consistent training at this level can keep you in a chronic state of exhaustion, inflammation, and adrenal depletion, all of which elevate your risk for developing disease. This is especially important for cancer patients. Some cancer patients with a strong will to live believe that if they punish their bodies with extreme exercise like long-distance running or triathlons, they are somehow beating back their cancer, but this kind of behavior can have the opposite effect. Extreme exercise creates excessive physical stress on the body that can suppress your immune system for up to 72 hours after each workout, increasing your risk of infections. A 2.5 hour run can drop your natural killer cell count by 50 percent.[5] Extreme exercise can also lead to injury and extended debilitation, during which you lose the benefits of daily exercise.

The internal repair required after extreme exercise can also monopolize valuable resources that the body needs to heal cancer. In addition to suppressing immune function, extreme exercise creates large amounts of lactic acid in the body, which can block key nutrients from reaching healthy cells, and even fuel cancer growth.

THE RIGHT AMOUNT OF EXERCISE

All movement, including light, moderate, and heavy exercise, can be beneficial as long as you get the balance right. For most folks, this means more exercise than you get sitting at a desk all day and less exercise than you would get training for the Olympics. While many people view exercise as a means to get stronger or to look better on the beach, the primary goal of exercise should be to increase your life span and your health span, which is your number of healthy years. Looking better on the beach is a bonus.

Daily moderate aerobic exercise like brisk walking, short running, bike riding, yoga, weight training, and dancing improves immune function by boosting T cell production, increases oxygenation of tissues, improves function of antioxidant enzymes, and triggers the release of endorphins that make you feel good. Exercise has been proven to be an effective antidepressant and to reduce anxiety.[6]

TIP:

If you work out at a public gym, don't touch your eyes, nose, or mouth, and make sure you wash your hands immediately afterward. Gyms are a breeding ground for pathogens and bacteria, which is why my wife and I jokingly refer to the gym as "the germ."

Exercise has also been shown to reverse the loss of muscle tissue and bone mass in cancer patients and the elderly. When you consistently lift heavy weights, you send signals to your body to strengthen your muscles and bones. Routinely lifting heavy weights is the best way to prevent and reverse osteoporosis, far better than taking calcium supplements.

Diet and exercise also affect how your genes express themselves, literally turning good genes on and bad genes off.[7] A Finnish study done on twins showed that exercise reduced mortality by 66 percent for people age 25 to 64, and numerous studies have shown the powerful effect that exercise can have on cancer care and recovery.[8] Breast cancer patients who exercised regularly (the equivalent of walking 30 minutes per day) and ate five or more servings of fruits and vegetables per day had half the recurrence rate after nine years compared to patients who didn't exercise or eat lots of fruits and veggies.[9] That's huge!

Another study found that after moderate- to high-intensity exercise, the blood of breast cancer patients dripped on cancer cells had more cancer stopping power than their pre-exercise blood.[10]

A study published in the *British Medical Journal* found that bicycling to work was associated with a 45 percent reduced risk of dying from cancer and a 46 percent reduced risk of heart disease.[11] There's nothing magic about cycling; it's just that those who rode their bike to work consistently hit the ideal target of health-promoting exercise, which is 30 minutes of moderate to vigorous aerobic exercise per day.

A 2014 study of over 4,600 Swedish men with early stage prostate cancer found that the men who engaged in walking or biking every day for 20 minutes or more had a 39 percent lower risk of dying from prostate cancer and a 30 percent lower risk of dying from any other cause compared to the men who were less active.[12]

A 2014 study published in the *Journal of Clinical Oncology* found that colon cancer patients who exercised seven hours per week or more were 31 percent less likely to die from any cause than those who did not exercise at all. The study also found that patients who averaged five hours of TV watching per day were 22 percent more likely to die than those who watched less than two hours per day.[13]

Exercise can reverse decades of damage caused by being sedentary. In a study of out-of-shape, middle-aged adults, two years of consistent aerobic exercise four to five days per week was found to reverse years of damage, significantly improving their heart health.[14]

Exercise keeps your immune system strong even in old age. Our immune systems decline as we age and as we become less active, which makes us more susceptible to health problems like infections and cancer, but surprising research published in 2018 found that long-distance cyclists in their 60s, 70s, and 80s were found to have the same level of T cells in their blood as people in their 20s![15]

HOW EXERCISE PROMOTES DETOXIFICATION

Every day you are bombarded with toxins in your environment and in your food, which is why detoxification is such a critical process in your body. If the detox process is hindered, toxins can build up, eventually causing acidity and toxemia. A critical component of your immune system hinges on your body's ability to efficiently detoxify via your lymphatic system, which includes your tonsils, thymus, bone marrow, spleen, lymphatic fluid, vessels, and lymph nodes. The thymus and bone marrow produce white blood cells called lymphocytes. Your blood vessels deliver oxygen and nutrients to your cells. Your lymph vessels are like blood vessels and they contain clear lymphatic fluid that carries white blood cells (B cell and T cell lymphocytes) throughout your body to attack invaders and infected cells. Your lymphatic fluid also carries dead cells, metabolic waste, and toxins away from healthy tissue to be eliminated through sweat, mucus, urine, and liver bile, which is carried out in your poop.

Lymph nodes are like holding stations that filter the lymph fluid and capture microbes for B and T cells to deal with. They are located in your armpits, groin, and neck and around the blood vessels of your chest and abdomen. You have about three times more lymphatic fluid than blood, but there's no pump in the lymphatic system. Instead, voluntary and involuntary muscle contractions in your body circulate the lymphatic fluid through a series of one-way valves.

One of the lesser known benefits of exercise is that it moves your lymphatic fluid, promoting detoxification in your body.

The more you move your body, the more you move your lymphatic fluid. When I first started researching, I read every natural cancer survival testimony I could find and I found many common threads, one of which was getting exercise by jumping on a mini-trampoline, aka "rebounding." I figured that since so many natural survivors and health practitioners were recommending it, there must be something to it, so I bought myself a rebounder.

Jumping on a trampoline creates increased G-force resistance (gravitational load) and is thought to positively stress every cell in your body and strengthen your entire musculoskeletal system: your bones, muscles, connective tissue, and even organs. Rebounding promotes lymphatic circulation by stimulating the millions of one-way valves in your lymphatic system. In addition, rebounding is low impact, is gentle on your joints, and improves strength and balance. Rebounding allows you to do jumping and aerobic exercises for much longer intervals than you could on solid ground.

The Three Basic Rebounding Exercises

To do the health bounce, you gently bounce up and down on a rebounder mini-trampoline without your feet leaving the mat. While this may not feel like exercise, it provides enough motion to effectively move your lymphatic system. Many folks can easily do this type of gentle bouncing for 30 minutes to an hour or more, even while watching TV.

The strength bounce involves jumping as high as you can. This movement strengthens primary and stabilizer muscles throughout your body, improves your balance, and moves your lymphatic system. Be careful with high jumping and work up to it gradually. If you jump too high, you could end up with your head stuck in the ceiling or come down wrong and injure yourself.

Aerobic bouncing is the most fun of the three. It consists of jumping jacks, twisting, jogging, or sprinting in place, bouncing on one leg at a time, dancing, and any other crazy maneuvers you can think of. Put on some music you enjoy, move your body, and have fun while you get your blood pumping and your sweat on.

My typical rebounder routine is warming up for a couple of minutes with gentle health bouncing, 5 to 10 minutes alternating between strength and aerobic bouncing, and then cooling down with a couple minutes of health bouncing. I often put on headphones and listen to workout/dance music, worship music, or healing scriptures while bouncing. It's pretty hard to overdo it with rebounding, but if you feel sensitivity or pain while doing it, take it easy. While healing cancer, I did this two to three times per day.

If you are too weak to jump, some rebounders include a stabilizer bar you can hold on to, or you can simply sit on the rebounder and bounce gently in a seated position. I bought my rebounder a few months after abdominal surgery and found it too painful to jump on at first, so I started with gentle health bouncing. As my body healed, the pain went away and I was eventually able to do the strength and aerobic bouncing.

Maximize Your Rebounding Workout

➤ Do it outside. Get fresh air and sunshine and connect with God and nature (if nature permits).

➤ Take at least 10 deep breaths while bouncing. Inhale through your nose, hold it for a few seconds, and then push it out through your mouth, fully emptying your lungs.

➤ Rebound with enough intensity to break a sweat at least once per day.

Sweating is super beneficial because it helps your body detoxify specific toxins including arsenic, cadmium, lead, and mercury.[16] Saunas are an effective way to sweat out toxins, but sweaty aerobic exercise is even better because exercise turns on cancer-protective genes in your body. Either way you'll need a shower after you get sweaty. The nice thing about rebounding is that you can still get a benefit from it even if you don't break a sweat, but try to get at least one sweaty workout per day. I like to rebound first thing in the morning before I shower for the day.

SUN LOVE

Epidemiological studies suggest that we could prevent roughly 30,000 U.S. cancer deaths per year just by getting more sunshine. Regular sunlight/vitamin D intake inhibits growth of breast and colon cancer cells and is also associated with substantial decreases in death rates from these two cancers, and metabolites of vitamin D have produced complete and partial clinical responses in lymphoma patients having high vitamin D metabolite receptor levels in tumor tissue.

Severe sunburn can cause melanoma, but long-term regular sun exposure inhibits melanoma. We've been conditioned to be afraid of the sun because sun exposure can increase the risk of skin cancers that have a 0.3 percent death rate, causing about 2,000 deaths per year. But regular sun exposure prevents cancers that have death rates from 20 to 65 percent, causing 138,000 U.S. deaths per year.[17] Fifteen minutes of daily sunshine is ideal but can be difficult in winter months. Vitamin D is one of the most important anti-cancer vitamins, and I take at least 1,000 IU of vitamin D3 in supplement form every day.

RETURN TO PLANET EARTH

The most underrated form of exercise that does not require any equipment or a gym membership is walking. Walking for 10 to 20 minutes two to three times a day will do wonders for you, and grounding yourself by walking barefoot on the grass, dirt, or sand will increase the benefits even more. Walking barefoot allows your body to absorb negative ions from the surface of the earth, which have amazing benefits in your body. These negative ions act as antioxidants and have been found to improve blood flow, calm your nervous system, normalize cortisol, reduce inflammation and pain, improve immune function, and speed healing.[18]

To take the benefits of walking a step further, studies have shown that forest bathing—a fancy term for spending a few hours in the woods—increases natural killer cell activity and reduces blood pressure and stress hormones.[19,20] Some of these benefits are thought to be from breathing in phytoncides, which are aromatic compounds released into the air by trees and plants, like the compounds that make cedar smell like cedar.[21]

GET A FITNESS TRACKING GIZMO

A health-promoting gadget that may be helpful is a fitness tracker, which will show you how much exercise you're getting (or not getting) each day. It can also give key insights into the quality of your sleep. Fitness trackers are a helpful tool that will give you feedback you can use to improve your routine and incorporate more movement into your day. Most importantly, they keep you accountable and give you a sense of accomplishment when you hit your daily goals. Some folks are wary of fitness trackers because they don't like the idea of wearing an electronic device on their body 24 hours per day. However, if a fitness tracker keeps you exercising every day, I think the benefits outweigh any risks. If you are concerned about avoiding EMFs produced by fitness trackers, many newer models can be put on "airplane mode" and only sync with your phone when you tell them to. Last year someone gave me a fitness tracker as a gift. I was curious to see what kind of feedback it would give me, so I wore it for three months. It was fun seeing how many steps I took each day, how much sleep I got each night—I average 8 hours and 25 minutes—and how much my exercise routine contributed to my daily activity score. The tracker showed me exactly how much movement and exercise I need in my daily life to stay in an optimal range.

MOVEMENT IS LIFE

Depending on your situation, if you are recovering from surgery or treatment or are extremely out of shape, you may not be able to exercise much right off the bat. That's okay. Don't be discouraged. Start with light exercise like walking and gentle rebounding. Then, when you are able, try to incorporate some moderate aerobic exercise into your life like bike riding, short runs, hiking, martial arts, or fitness classes like yoga, Zumba, Jazzercise, or Pilates. Any kind of exercise that moves your body, increases your heart rate, and makes you break a sweat is wonderful. Just find something you enjoy and do it.

The latest research has shown that movement throughout the day may even more beneficial than 30 to 60 minutes of deliberate exercise once per day. There are many easy ways to incorporate more natural movement into your life, like always parking at the far end of the parking lot and taking the stairs instead of the elevator. If you sit at a desk all day, set a reminder to notify you every hour to get up, stretch your legs, and take a quick lap around the office for a few minutes. I bought myself an adjustable standing desk with a treadmill underneath, and I've never been happier with my office arrangement. The purpose of a treadmill desk is not to get a workout while you work; it's mainly just to make sure you stay in motion. Walking is better for you than standing still. Even when I set my treadmill at the slowest pace, I still manage to walk several miles per day on it. Movement is life!

NO TIME TO REST

The flip side of exercise is rest. Too much of one and not enough of the other can create an unhealthy imbalance. You need an early bedtime and lots of sleep, because sleep is when your body heals. Six to eight hours of sleep per night is considered to be the ideal range for most people, but individual needs vary. According to the CDC, more than a third of American adults aren't getting enough sleep.[22] If you're getting less than seven hours of sleep per night, you may be sleep deprived. Not getting enough sleep night after night can create a "sleep debt" that keeps growing over time and can lead to a gradual degradation of your health.

Sleep deprivation can affect your mood and brain function, including your memory, learning, creativity, and emotions. And most importantly, it can affect your physical appearance. Lack of sleep directly affects your face, causing swollen and drooping eyelids, dark circles, wrinkles, and droopy corners of your mouth. The longer you are sleep deprived, the more permanent these changes become. Sleep deprivation can also lead to depression, weight gain, a weak immune system, diabetes, heart disease, cancer, and death.

During sleep, the body produces hormones called cytokines that help fight infections. Low levels of cytokines make sleep-deprived people more susceptible to everyday infections like colds and flu. Researchers at Carnegie Mellon University found that otherwise healthy men and women who slept less than seven hours a night were three times more likely to develop cold symptoms after exposure to a cold-causing virus than people who slept eight hours or more.[23]

Before the advent of electricity, our ancestors tended to go to sleep earlier, typically within a few hours after sunset. Their sleep habits were in harmony with nature and the cycle of the sun. They slept less in the summer and more in the winter. In the winter months, they often slept for as many as twelve hours in two shifts, with one to three hours of wakefulness in the middle of the night, during which they would busy themselves reading, writing, working, praying, socializing, and, of course, getting busy.

Historical documents refer to these two sleeping shifts as first sleep and second sleep.

Electrical lighting and our modern indoor living and working environments have reduced our exposure to sunlight during the day, increased our exposure to artificial light at night, and caused our circadian clocks to be out of sync with the light-dark cycle produced by the sun. We are living in disharmony with nature.

A 2013 study found that after just one week of no exposure to artificial light, campers with varying internal biological clocks all synchronized with the light-dark cycle of the sun. Before camping their bodies began producing melatonin around 10:30 P.M., with sleep starting at 12:30 A.M. and melatonin offset happening around 8 A.M. After a week of camping, all of the campers' internal clocks shifted two hours earlier. Their bodies began producing melatonin right around sundown, with peak melatonin in the middle of the solar night and melatonin offset beginning right after sunrise.[24] Their circadian rhythms became perfectly aligned with the cycle of the sun.

Melatonin, also known as "the hormone of darkness," is produced by your pineal gland when your body detects low light in the evening. It is an antioxidant that is five times more powerful than vitamin C, and it increases the effectiveness of your lymphocytes, killer cells that fight off foreign invaders and mutated cells. In addition, melatonin increases the activity of superoxide dismutase and glutathione, which are antioxidants and detoxifiers and help repair damaged cells. Melatonin has been shown to inhibit angiogenesis and metastasis, and to promote apoptosis (cell death) in many different types of cancer cells.[25,26] The physiological surge of melatonin in your body at night is considered a "natural restraint" on tumor initiation, promotion, and progression.[27]

Exposure to artificial light, especially blue light, between dusk and bedtime can interfere with your sleep and your body's production of melatonin. Researchers found that exposure to room light (<200 lux) in the late evening reduced pre-sleep melatonin levels by 71.4 percent, shortened nighttime melatonin duration by about 90 minutes compared to dim light (<3 lux), and reduced total daily levels of melatonin by about 12.5 percent in human subjects.[28] Another study found that just 15 seconds of bright light exposure at night caused circadian disruption in participants and delayed melatonin onset by an average of 34 minutes.[29]

In the 2011 Nurses' Health Study, researchers at Harvard reported a correlation between low melatonin levels in women who worked the night shift and an increased risk of breast cancer.[30] Shorter wavelength blue light emitted by LED and fluorescent lighting, as well as electronics like TVs, smartphones, computers, some alarm clocks, and LED street lights, suppresses melatonin more than any other type of light.[31] A 2018 study found that women in urban areas exposed to high levels of outdoor blue light at night had 1.5 higher risk of breast cancer and men had a twofold increase in prostate cancer risk compared to those who were less exposed.[32] A study by the University of Toronto found that night shift workers who wore glasses that blocked blue light wavelengths produced more melatonin than those who didn't.[33] Blind women have a 35 to 50 percent lower risk of breast cancer than women who can see.[34] They tend to sleep longer and have higher levels of melatonin and lower levels of estrogen, which is reduced by melatonin.

Substances that interfere with your body's melatonin production include caffeine, tobacco, alcohol, aspirin, Ibuprofen, beta blockers, benzodiazepines, corticosteroids, and drugs that regulate serotonin like Prozac. There are over 800 brand-name and generic drugs known to interact with melatonin.[35] If you are taking any prescription drugs, they could be inhibiting your body's production of melatonin, reducing the quality of your sleep, and affecting your health. Supplementation of 20 mg of melatonin per day (before bed) along with conventional treatments has been found to cause substantial improvements in tumor remission, one-year survival, and alleviation of side effects from radiotherapy and chemotherapy.[36]

LACK OF SLEEP CAN ELEVATE YOUR CANCER RISK

A Japanese study of nearly 24,000 women ages 40 to 79 found that women who slept less than six hours a night were more likely to develop breast cancer than those who slept longer.[37] A 2010 study at Case Western Reserve University found an increased risk for colon cancer in people who slept less than six hours per night.[38]

However, just like too much exercise, too much sleep could also be unhealthy. A 2017 study found that breast cancer patients who slept more than nine hours per night had a higher risk of death than those who slept between six and eight hours. Patients who reported difficulty falling asleep or staying asleep also had increased risk of death.[39,40]

Interrupted sleep can make cancer aggressive and speed its growth. In 2014 sleep apnea researchers at the University of Chicago found that cancerous tumors in mice whose sleep was gently interrupted every two minutes grew twice as large as the tumors in the mice who had slept normally without interruption.[41] And this was after only four weeks of interrupted sleep. Before you panic, four weeks of bad sleep for a mouse is roughly the equivalent of about 2.5 years of bad sleep for a human. Practitioners of Eastern medicine claim that every hour of sleep before midnight is twice as beneficial as every hour after midnight. Whether that's true or not, 11 P.M. to 1 A.M. has been identified as a critical recharge period for many internal systems, like your adrenals.

Sleeping pills are not the answer. Taking as few as 18 sleeping pills per year triples your risk of death and taking 2 to 3 pills per week increases your risk of death by a factor of five. The risk of death from taking sleep drugs including barbiturates, benzodiazepines like Xanax and Valium, and "Z" drugs like Ambien is nearly the same as the risk with smoking.[42]

The first step to getting more sleep is setting an earlier bedtime, within a few hours after the sun goes down. Depending on your living situation, this may involve rearranging your schedule. You'll definitely need the support of the people you share a roof with. On the plus side, going to bed early usually makes it easier to get up early, which means less stress trying to get out the door in the morning. This can create time for you to read a devotional, pray, meditate, juice, work out, or plan your to-do list and meals for the day.

Exposure to bright morning light helps reset your internal clock and normalize your circadian rhythm. A 2017 study found that breast cancer patients who were exposed to bright light from a light box for 30 minutes every morning for one month had significant improvements in sleep quality and sleep time and less chronic fatigue.[43] According to one of the study authors, cancer survivors and other individuals who spend most of their days indoors may not receive enough bright light to keep their biological rhythms synchronized. Researchers recommend spending time near windows with lots of natural light and keeping the indoor lighting as bright as possible during the morning.[44]

SLEEP DETOXIFIES YOUR BRAIN

While studying the brains of sleeping mice, scientists at the University of Rochester discovered a dramatic increase in the circulation of cerebrospinal fluid going in and out of the brain. Dr. Maiken Nedergaard, professor of neurosurgery and author of the study published in *Science*, likened the process to a dishwasher, forcefully washing out all of the toxic metabolic waste that accumulated in your brain that day. The longer you stay awake, the more toxins (like beta amyloid) accumulate in your brain.[45] These toxins influence your brain chemistry and affect your ability to think clearly and rationally.

Healthy Nighttime Rituals

Here's my list of nighttime rituals to help you get the best sleep possible and optimize your body's ability to repair, regenerate, and heal.

Eat an early dinner and go to bed on an empty stomach.

Eat all your meals within an 11-hour window or less, such as 8 A.M. to 7 P.M. Researchers found that breast cancer patients who fasted less than 13 hours per night had a 36 percent higher risk for recurrence compared to those who fasted 13 hours or more.[46] Don't eat a meal before bed, and definitely do not eat in the middle of the night. Eating late at night forces your body to use energy to digest food while you sleep instead of repairing itself.

Dim the lights around your house after sundown.

This prepares your body for sleep. Take a warm bath. Use essential oils like frankincense, myrrh, and lavender to calm yourself and relax. Reading before bed can help you relax as well and get your brain and body into sleep mode. Don't turn the lights back on to brush your teeth or to use the bathroom before bed.

Avoid anything stimulating.

Caffeine, sugar, social media, and work-related activities all turn on your brain, which can make it difficult to fall asleep quickly once you get into bed. Stop watching stressful television before bed. Especially the news. Also avoid intense dramas, mysteries, horror, action/adventure shows, and sports. All of these types of entertainment excite you and raise your stress hormones, which can keep you awake and contribute to chronic stress.

Don't worry about tomorrow.

Worry will keep you awake. Don't worry about the future or tomorrow. A proven method to reduce nighttime worry and anxiety is to write down tomorrow's to-do list every night before bed. This will make you feel more organized and in control of your life, and put your mind at ease as you doze off.

Make your bedroom a cave.

Your bedroom should be cool, quiet, and dark. The ideal temperature for sound sleep is between 60 and 70 degrees Fahrenheit. If your room is much warmer or cooler, or if your blankets are too heavy or too light, you may toss and turn during the night and not get enough deep, restful sleep. It may be helpful to black out your windows or wear a sleep mask. Light at night can interfere with your body's production of melatonin, one of the most powerful anti-cancer hormones in your body.

Devices That Can Improve Sleep

Blue blockers—The nerdiest of health-nerd accessories, these orange-tinted glasses block the blue light produced by fluorescent and LED lighting and the screens of TVs and electronic devices. I often wear them at night.

Sound machine—The white noise produced by a sound machine can help you stay asleep by masking random outside noises and things that go bump in the night that might disturb your sleep. There are also sound-machine smartphone apps.

Sleep music—An alternative to a sound machine is soothing instrumental music played at specific frequencies thought to resonate with the body and promote healing.

Air purifier—Since you're in your bedroom for 7 to 10 hours every night, it makes sense to ensure you are breathing the cleanest air possible by reducing or eliminating pollutants and allergens, including pollen, pet dander, dust mites, smoke, chemical gases, bacteria, and mold. Some air purifiers have an audible fan that can serve as a sound machine.

Grounding sheet—Like walking barefoot in the grass, using a grounding sheet connects your body to the free-flowing negative ions on the surface of the earth. I use a grounding pad under my keyboard while working at my desk, and I sleep on a grounding sheet as well.

Sunrise alarm clock—Unlike jarring buzzers or a blaring radio that shock you out of deep sleep, a sunrise alarm clock wakes you naturally by gradually filling the room with light over the course of several minutes.

Organic mattress—Most commercial mattresses are made with synthetic fibers and treated with toxic flame retardants, which can off-gas chemical fumes that you breathe in all night. An organic mattress is a big investment that may require saving up for, but it's worth it. We sleep on an organic latex foam mattress.

Sleep mask and ear plugs—If you can't get your room dark enough, or if you travel a lot, you might benefit from wearing ear plugs and/or a sleep mask over your eyes.

For an updated list of the products I use in my bedroom to optimize my sleep, go to www.chrisbeatcancer.com/sleep.

A DAY OF REST

The final component in rest is setting aside an entire day for it every week. A day of rest may seem strange in our culture obsessed with productivity and achievement, but this is a biblical principle dating back to Genesis, and it's even one of the Ten Commandments.

> Remember the sabbath day, to keep it holy. Six days you shall labor and do all your work, but the seventh day is a sabbath of the LORD your God; in it you shall not do any work, you or your son or your daughter, your male or your female servant or your cattle or your sojourner who stays with you. For in six days the LORD made the heavens and the earth, the sea and all that is in them, and rested on the seventh day; therefore the LORD blessed the sabbath day and made it holy. (Exodus 20:8–11) (NASB)

In Japan's competitive corporate culture, employees routinely work 60 to 100 hours per week, in some cases not taking days off for months. It's become such a problem that they even have a word for one of its tragic consequences: *karoshi*, which means death from overwork. The stress induced by working too much has been found to cause heart attacks and strokes as well as depression-related suicide.

So what does a day of rest look like? It is one day per week where you don't do physical or mental work and you don't require people to work for you. On our day of rest, we go to church, sometimes have lunch with friends or family, and then usually take naps and relax for the rest of the day. We might read, watch a movie, play a game with the kids, or have dinner with in-laws, but that's about it.

Doing nothing may be hard for you if you enjoy working or feel pressure to be productive, but your body and brain need a break. Don't think about work. Don't talk about work. Don't check your e-mail. Stay off the internet if it's work related. And just try to be at peace. The less physical energy you exert on your day of rest, the more benefit you will receive from it. Making yourself take a day of rest is important not only to maintain your health, but to restore it.

Massive Action Steps for Exercise and Rest

➤ Commit to 30 to 60 minutes of aerobic exercise per day six days per week (walking counts).

➤ Exercise outside in the fresh air and sunshine as much as possible.

➤ Get sweaty at least once per day six days per week.

➤ Get a few minutes of sunshine on your body every day.

➤ Walk barefoot in the grass for a few minutes every day.

➤ Spend a few hours in nature "forest bathing" at least once per week.

➤ Park farther away than you normally would and take the stairs instead of the elevator.

➤ Stand up every hour or so, take a walk around the office, and move your body.

➤ Consider investing in a treadmill desk.

➤ Eat your meals in an 11-hour window.

➤ Go to bed within a few hours of sundown.

➤ Make your bedroom cool, quiet, and dark.

➤ Consider investing in tools and devices to improve your exercise habits and sleep.

➤ Take one day of rest every week.

UNDER PRESSURE

Stress and Negative Emotions

Worry is a misuse of the imagination.

— DAN ZADRA

Worry never robs tomorrow of its sorrow. It only saps today of its joy.

— LEO BUSCAGLIA

WHEN I GRADUATED FROM COLLEGE, the countdown to marriage began. My wedding date was only six months away and I needed to get my act together. So, as I mentioned earlier, I took a job at a financial firm. It wasn't what I had planned on, but I had sales experience and a business degree, and the man who recruited me made it sound pretty lucrative. I started out in financial planning selling life insurance and annuities, with eventual plans to become a fully licensed investment broker. There was no salary. It was straight commission with a small weekly draw, and I was constantly stressed about finding new clients and whether I was going to make enough money to keep the job.

The following year I started buying rental properties and had to learn how to get houses renovated and rented, and how to manage tenants. I was having loads more fun investing in real estate than I ever did in the insurance business, but I was still stressed. I was working longer and harder than I had ever worked in my life. I was burning the candle at both ends, living on adrenaline, sugar, caffeine, and fast food, and I was not taking care of myself. The year after that, the abdominal pains started. Then in December came the cancer diagnosis.

Stress can make you sick. And kill you.

I've counseled a lot of people with cancer over the years, and the one thing they all have in common is stress. The human body is intelligently designed with a survival mechanism triggered by anything your mind perceives as threatening. This is known as a fight-or-flight response. Any time you find yourself in a thrilling, dangerous, or life-threatening situation, like riding a roller coaster, watching a scary movie, or looking down the barrel of a gun, your body automatically kicks into survival mode.

If you are confronted by a tiger, the first thing that happens is a sense: danger. Followed by a thought: *I'm about to be tiger food.* That thought triggers an emotion: fear. That emotion triggers the release of stress hormones (adrenaline and cortisol), which activate a physical response in your body. Simply put, these hormones divert all of your available energy to your muscles and the parts of your brain that can assist you in survival. Adrenaline gives you strength and power. Cortisol tells your body to dump glucose into your bloodstream, making you more alert and giving you a burst of energy to run faster and farther, or fight harder.

If a tiger came after you and you somehow managed to escape, your body would eventually shift out of fight-or-flight mode and back to normal operation. Once the stressful event is over, the stress hormones stop pumping, the fear subsides, your mind and body relax, and all of your other bodily functions that have been "paused," like digestion and immune function, come back online.

Have you ever been so upset that you can't think straight? Or sat down to take a test and your memory was blank? Or heard someone say they couldn't remember what happened after a traumatic event? Stress hormones did that. The reason stress hormones switch off your immune system, digestive system, reproductive system, and parts of your brain is simple: energy conservation. Your brain uses about 20 percent of your energy. Your digestive system uses about 15 percent of your energy—sometimes more, which is why eating a heavy meal can make you sleepy. Your body is brilliantly designed to direct energy to where it is needed most. In a true fight-or-flight situation, that would be your muscles.

The hormones produced by stress are a very good thing in the proper context and can help save your life. In a real fight-or-flight situation, they can help you escape from a swarm of bad guys, hightail it out of there, or even lift a car off someone trapped underneath, Superman style. That kind of stress is called acute stress—a short-term stressful situation with a beginning and an end. But acute stress events are few and far between, and very rare for most of us in first-world nations. Our problem is something very different. Our problem is chronic stress.

THE TIGER YOU CAN'T ESCAPE

Chronic stress is the grinding, day in, day out stress caused by the worries, fears, responsibilities, and conflicts we have in life. It is like the tiger that you can never get away from. It's always behind you—stalking you. You have to keep moving. And you can't rest for long. You are running from it every day, from the time you wake up until the time you go to sleep, and sometimes it even wakes you up in the middle of the night.

We are stressed to the max in our modern world, and stressors are coming at us from all sides: negative and dramatic media, financial difficulties, family demands and problems, toxic relationships, social pressures, work demands, bad lifestyle habits like self-abuse, lack of sleep, stimulants, and even too much exercise.

Stress starts in the mind and manifests in the body. Chronic stress produces elevated levels of adrenaline and cortisol, which keep you in a constant state of "flight-or-flight light" and can lead to all sorts of problems over time, like chronic fatigue from exhaustive depletion (adrenal failure); depression; nervousness; hypertension; a reduction in your body's ability to digest and absorb the nutrients in food; digestive problems like ulcers, Crohn's disease, and colitis; hormone problems; a decrease in male testosterone and sperm count; irregular menstrual cycles and fertility problems in women; and mostly importantly, immune suppression, which increases the likelihood of developing a chronic disease in the body, like cancer. Simply put, when stress hormones are up, your immune system is down.

Cortisol causes a release of sugar into your bloodstream for energy, but later causes intense sugar cravings to replenish glucose reserves. This leads to impulsive and irrational stress eating, which almost always involves extremely unhealthy, high-sugar "comfort foods" like pizza, pasta, ice cream, candy, snack foods, and sugary drinks. Prolonged elevated blood glucose promotes inflammation and fuels cancer growth if it is not used by muscle activity.

Stress also interferes with your brain function. When you are under stress, parts of your brain are switched off—affecting your ability to think rationally—and your lower brain stem (aka your reptilian brain) becomes dominant. The reptilian brain controls your instinctive survival responses like anger, aggressive dominant behavior, fear, revenge, tribalism, territorial behavior, and reproductive impulses. The reptilian brain is primitive, impulsive, and irrational, which is why people who are in a state of fear, worry, anxiety, anger, or sexual arousal often make impulsive, irrational, and really bad decisions. Extreme rage can make you temporarily insane.

In 2013 researchers reported that anti-cancer drugs didn't work as well in mice under stress because adrenaline turns off the mechanism that tells cancer cells to die. The mice were then given a beta blocker to block adrenaline production, which slowed down their heart rate, lowered their blood pressure, and restored their immune function. When adrenaline production was inhibited, the mice did not have accelerated tumor growth even when put under stress.[1] Another study found that mice put under stress had six times the spread of cancer.[2] According to study author and cancer biologist Dr. Erica Sloan, "Stress sends a signal into the cancer that allows tumor cells to escape from the cancer and spread through the body."[3]

Stress has the same effect on cancer in humans. Stress activates a gene in immune system cells called ATF3 that causes them to malfunction and help cancer cells spread throughout the body. Both breast cancer patients and mice with activated ATF3 in their immune cells were found to have lower survival rates than those without activated ATF3. This cancer-promoting stress gene can also be turned on by chemotherapy, radiation, and poor diet.[4]

Without exception, every single cancer patient I've met had major chronic stress in their life besides cancer. And in many cases, it wasn't just one thing. It was a combination of several significant stressors persisting in their life for many years. Many of us are teetering on the brink of disease. Then a major stressful event happens, which is the cancer trigger, the tipping point that pushes us over the edge. The death or disability of a loved one, betrayal, a divorce or bad breakup, the loss of a job, insults, injuries, and harassment. Even moving, marriage, and pregnancy fall into this category. Many patients I've talked to are able to pinpoint one or more traumatic cancer-trigger events that happened to them in the five years before their diagnosis. And of course, a cancer diagnosis only makes matters worse. A cancer diagnosis or recurrence is a stress bomb. The fear and worry that accompany a diagnosis can be profoundly immunosuppressant and a catalyst for accelerated cancer growth and metastasis in the body. This is why it is critical to identify and eliminate all the stresses in your life.

STRESS. OUT.

The first step in reducing stress is to stop worrying. Worrying is a bad habit that you can break. Stop worrying about your health, about other people, about the economy, about the government, about the future, and about events you cannot control. To worry is to live in fear.

As a Christian, I looked to the Bible for answers. The words of Jesus, Paul, and Peter gave me clarity and peace and showed me how to overcome fear, anxiety, and worry.

Jesus said, "Do not worry about your life, what you will eat or drink; or about your body, what you will wear . . . But seek first his kingdom and his righteousness, and all these things will be given to you as well. Therefore, do not worry about tomorrow, for tomorrow will worry about itself. Each day has enough trouble of its own." (Matthew 6:25–34) (NIV)

Paul said, "Don't worry about anything; instead, pray about everything. Tell God what you need, and thank him for all he has done. Then you will experience God's peace, which exceeds anything we can understand." (Philippians 4:6–7) (NIV)

Peter said, ". . . Humble yourselves under the mighty hand of God, that He may exalt you at the proper time, casting all your anxiety on Him, because He cares for you." (1 Peter 5:6–7) (NASB)

Worry and doubt are the opposite of faith. I realized that exercising my faith meant trusting God to lead me, to protect me, to provide for me and my family, and to heal me. Fully trusting Him meant letting go of my fear, choosing to believe and not to doubt.

As part of my daily routine, every time I felt worried and afraid, this is what I prayed:

> Lord, I am not going to be afraid. I am giving you my fear. Jesus, I am laying it at your feet. I trust you with my life, my health, my family, my finances, my future. I trust you. Thank you for leading me in the path of healing, for supplying all my needs, and for working everything out for my good. Amen.

THE LIFE-CHANGING MAGIC OF PROBLEM SOLVING

Marie Kondo wrote an international best-seller on how to get rid of clutter in your home called *The Life-Changing Magic of Tidying Up*. If you are one of the few people left on the planet who haven't read it, the premise is simple. One by one, go through every item you own and ask yourself whether or not it brings you joy. If it doesn't bring you joy, throw it out. The power of this method is that it requires you to systematically evaluate everything you own. In the same way, you need to focus your attention on identifying and dealing with the stress-producing problems in your life that you've been avoiding.

Many of the problems we have in life persist unnecessarily simply because we put off solving them. We avoid them, ignore them, procrastinate, and in some cases even deny they exist. Some problems and stressors in life resolve on their own, but others will not go away until you take action. Everyone has problems in their life that they need to solve. Now is the time to face your problems head-on, take Massive Action, and get busy solving them. And as you do, you will feel the weight of stress and anxiety lifted off you.

Make a two-column list with Problems on one side and Solutions on the other. In the left-hand column, list your problems and sources of stress. Ask yourself, *What am I worried about? What is causing me the most stress? Who is causing me the most stress?* Once that is done, review each stress-producer in your life and then ask yourself, *What do I need to do to remove this stress from my life?* Write your answer on the right-hand side of the list. This practice engages the creative problem-solving part of your brain. Most problems have a simple solution—not necessarily an easy solution, but a simple one. For example, if your problem is bitterness toward an ex, the solution is that you need to forgive. If your problem is that you are in an abusive relationship, the solution is that you need to leave and get help, and you need to forgive.

Identify the largest sources of stress on the list and tackle those first. Dealing with the big problems will give you the biggest bang for your buck in terms of stress reduction. Chronic stress will not only make you sick, but it will keep you sick. That's why it's imperative that you eliminate as many sources of stress and negativity from your life as quickly as possible. If friends or family members are stressing you out, tell them you need space or distance yourself from them for the time being. If you are trying to heal cancer or another chronic disease, this is a time to be a little selfish. It's okay. You have to take care of yourself first if you want to be around to take care of others. Finally, some of your problems are out of your control and cannot be solved by you. Those are the ones you give to God.

Massive Action Steps for Stress Reduction

➤ Identify the sources of stress in your life.

➤ Make a to-do list to eliminate every stress in your life.

➤ Get busy removing stresses and solving your problems.

➤ Stop worrying. Give your fears and worries to God daily and trust Him to take care of you.

➤ Read *How to Stop Worrying and Start Living* by Dale Carnegie.

➤ Laugh! One hour of stand-up comedy can boost your immune system for up to 12 hours.[5]

➤ Sing! Singing for an hour reduces stress hormones and boosts your immune system.[6]

SPIRITUAL
HEALING

Do not be wise in your own eyes.
Fear the LORD and turn away from evil.
It will be healing to your body and refreshment to your bones.

— PROVERBS 3:7-8 (NASB)

CANCER FORCED ME to step out in faith and trust God in a way that I never had before. I had never had a crisis like this in my life. I had never known this kind of desperation. I had never felt like my life was completely out of my control. Cancer threatened to cut my life short, and I knew I needed help from above. My faith and my relationship with God were a huge part of my healing journey.

I grew up in a Christian home. I came to know Jesus at a young age, but as I got older I saw some things in the church I didn't like, and I used that as an excuse to rebel. I gravitated toward other rebellious kids who were not good influences, and by the time I was 16, my relationship with God was practically nonexistent. When I was 21, in the midst of working, going to college, and seeing an emptiness in what the world had to offer, I decided to make my relationship with God a priority in my life. I got plugged into a local church and began attending Bible studies, going on church retreats, and growing in my faith. Five years later the colon cancer diagnosis happened. Micah and I had just celebrated our two-year anniversary and I was playing on the church worship team every Sunday. In the midst of the shock, fear, anxiety, confusion, frustration, and everything else that comes with a cancer diagnosis, I remembered Romans 8:28 (NIV):

> And we know that God works all things for the good of those who love Him, who have been called according to His purpose.

Cancer was not good news. I did not see it as a gift or a blessing. It was the worst thing that had ever happened to me. But I chose to believe that God was going to work this bad thing out for my good. In my fear I made the choice to believe and I said, "Okay, God, I don't understand why this is happening, but I'm going to believe that You are going to work this for my good."

As I read through the Bible looking for encouragement, I came across Psalm 34. The Sunday after I was diagnosed, my wife and I stood up in front of our church and I made the dreaded announcement. "Hi, everybody. I've been diagnosed with colon cancer . . . but I'm choosing to believe this promise in Psalm 34:19 (NIV):

> The righteous person may have many troubles, but the LORD delivers him from them all.

And I said, "This is my verse. God is going to deliver me from this."

After surgery I prayed and said, "God, if there's another way besides chemo, please show me . . ." Two days later I received the book *God's Way to Ultimate Health*, which helped me understand that it didn't make sense to pray and ask for healing while continuing to do the things that could be making me sick. I knew I needed to take Massive Action to change my life and rebuild my body as part of the process, and I believed that in doing so I would be delivered from my affliction.

There's a beautiful story in the Bible about a woman who came to Jesus for healing. She had what was described as "an issue of blood." She had a bleeding condition. And because of this, according to Jewish religious law, she was considered unclean and untouchable and had lived as an outcast from her own people for 12 years. And it said, "She had suffered a great deal under the care of many doctors and had spent all she had, yet instead of getting better she grew worse." (Mark 5:6) (NIV)

After hearing about Jesus, she came up in the crowd behind Him and touched His cloak, and immediately her bleeding stopped. Jesus, perceiving that power had gone out of Him, turned around in the crowd and said, "Who touched my garments?" And his disciples said, "The crowd is pressing in on you and you're asking who touched you?" Jesus looked around and saw the woman, and He knew that she was the one who had touched Him. She fell down trembling before Him and told him that she was sick and that she had come to touch His garment. And Jesus said to her, "Daughter, your faith has made you well. Go in peace and be healed of your affliction." (Matthew 9:18, Mark 5:24, Luke 8:41) (NASB)

I met a woman at a conference a few years ago who came up to me and said, "I was diagnosed with cancer. And in my prayer life, I became just like that woman who needed a touch from Jesus, and God healed me." She had experienced miraculous healing and her cancer was gone. I could barely keep it together as she told me her story—because I knew where she had been. I'd been there too—down on my knees, desperate for a touch from God. Yes, I radically changed my whole life. I took responsibility for my health, for my diet and lifestyle, and for my environment, but at the end of the day, I was depending on God to lead me and to heal me.

THE POWER OF I AM

Your thoughts and beliefs create your reality and shape your future. As you think, so you are. Even though this concept has been rebranded many times as the Power of Positive Thinking, the Law of Attraction, and the Secret, and may seem a bit cliché, it is timeless truth.

Your thoughts, beliefs, and expectations are much more powerful than you realize. Regardless of the type of treatment, patients who believe a therapy is going to work have a higher likelihood of getting well and are often the ones who defy the odds, while patients who don't believe a therapy is going to help them tend to do worse. Something incredible happens when you start thinking positively and seeing yourself in a way that you may not yet be. The process starts in your mind and translates into your body. Early in my healing journey I realized that I had nothing to lose, so I changed the way I thought and I started thinking of myself as I wanted to be: healed, healthy, and well.

The placebo effect is a pervasive medically documented phenomenon. Studies in both laboratory and clinical settings consistently show that when people ingest a pharmacologically inert substance (a placebo) but believe that it is an active substance, they experience both the subjective sensations and physiologic effects expected from that active substance.[1]

In nearly every drug trial, some patients who are given a sugar pill instead of the real medication get the same benefit because they believed they would. There are also numerous documented cases of patients who got better after a fake surgery that they thought was real. A systematic review of 53 placebo-controlled surgeries found that in 51 percent of the trials, the measurable benefit in the fake surgery group was the exact same as the surgery group! The other 49 percent of placebo surgery trials reported that real surgery was more beneficial than fake surgery, but only generally by a small margin.[2]

The flip side of the placebo effect is called the nocebo effect. Some patients who expect a medication or treatment to cause them harm or have negative side effects, even if they are taking a placebo, end up experiencing those negative side effects. As a result of these phenomena, some patients who believe that chemotherapy will cure them are cured by the placebo effect. And others who believe chemo will not cure them and will cause them more harm may be amplifying its harmful effects. Your attitude, expectations, and beliefs can be more powerful than drugs or surgery. That's why it's so important to choose to think positively.

Positive thinking and affirmations may remind you of Al Franken's *Saturday Night Live* skits from the '90s, where Stuart Smalley looks at himself in the mirror and says, "I'm good enough. I'm smart enough. And doggone it, people like me." As silly as this may seem, don't discount affirmations. They can be a transformative, life-changing practice. You will be amazed at how good you feel when you make it a daily practice to encourage yourself, think positively, and see yourself as well.

No one talks to you more than *you*. Instead of depending on encouragement from others, which you may or may not get, start encouraging yourself. You can apply this to every area of your life. "I am smart. I am strong. I am courageous. I am loved. I am worthy of love. I am blessed. I am attractive. I am successful. I belong here. I am valuable. I am healed. I am healthy. I am well. And doggone it, people like me!" Stop criticizing yourself and encourage yourself instead. And talk to your body. Talk to your organs. Tell them to be healed and to be well. Choose to love yourself.

One of the most famous healing scriptures in the Bible is Isaiah 53:5 (NKJV), where the prophet Isaiah, predicting Jesus the Messiah, says "He was wounded for our transgressions. He was bruised for our iniquities. The chastisement for our peace was upon Him. And by His stripes we are healed."

Every day throughout the day, I would meditate on this verse and pray it out loud over my body, over and over again. I would say, "By Your stripes I am healed, I am healthy, and I am well, in the name of Jesus." I was exercising my faith and trusting in the redeeming work that Jesus did on the cross, and I was speaking life and health into my body.

DEALING WITH DOUBT

In John 14 (NASB) Jesus says, "Whatever you ask in My name, I will do, that the Father may be glorified in the Son. If you ask Me anything in My name, I will do it." And that's why when I prayed and asked for healing, I did it in the name of Jesus.

"Father, I'm asking for healing in the name of Jesus. And I'm believing You're going to do it, because You said that whatever I ask in Your Name You will do. I'm holding You to Your word. And I'm choosing to believe that, and that only. And I'm not going to doubt it."

Doubt can creep in, but doubt is just a thought, and you can change your thoughts. Faith is a choice. It is a practice and a discipline. Every person needs to work on this, and I still work on it daily. When doubts creep in, I just say to myself, *No, I'm not going to doubt. I'm going to believe.*

When I was struggling with fear and doubt, I often put worship music on in my headphones or in my car, sang along, got choked up, and let the emotions flow. What I found in my spiritual journey was that the very act of worship, of focusing my attention on God and not on my problems, encouraged me, strengthened my faith, and became an antidote for fear and doubt.

FAITH VERSUS FEAR

As a culture we have been conditioned to put our faith, hope, and trust in doctors first. But I want to encourage you to put your faith, hope, and trust in God first.

You need to make faith-based decisions, not fear-based decisions.

Don't let anyone use fear to motivate you, because fear-based decisions are often irrational, emotional, and unwise decisions. And fear-based decisions are often the wrong ones.

A powerful thing to ask God in prayer besides "Show me what I need to do" is "Show me what I need to change." If you ask God to show you what you need to change in your life, He will. Things will come to mind that you know are wrong and that you need to address. Ask and listen. Then take action and make those changes.

WHY ME?

A question a lot of cancer patients ask, especially if they are people of faith, is "Why did God allow this to happen?"

At the time of my diagnosis, I couldn't help but think, *This is so unfair. There are thieves and rapists and murderers . . . evil people doing evil things every day. They deserve cancer! I don't deserve cancer. I'm one of the good guys! I'm playing music in church every Sunday morning, for Pete's sake! I'm not lying, cheating, and stealing from people. I've tried to put God first in my life for the last five years and now I've got cancer? Come on!*

I know "life isn't fair," but cancer at 26 felt especially unfair. Throughout my life I had heard people say, "Whatever happens is God's will." If they were right, then that meant God wanted me to have cancer, a proposition that I didn't like and that didn't line up with the God I knew. So rather than accept that belief, I decided to study the scriptures to find out for myself whether it was God's will for me to be sick, or whether it was His will for me to be well. And what I found ignited my faith and restored my hope that I would be healed.

Psalm 103 (NIV) says, "Praise the LORD, my soul and forget not all His benefits, who forgives all your sins and heals all your diseases, who redeems your life from the pit, and crowns you with love and compassion, who satisfies your desires with good things, so that your youth is renewed like the eagle's."

I found promises of health and healing throughout the Bible. When I looked at the life and ministry of Jesus with fresh eyes, I realized that Jesus wasn't just a teacher. Jesus was a healer.

Jesus spent most of his time with the poor and the outcasts of society, the people no one cared about. He taught them about the Kingdom of God and about right and wrong, and showed them love by His actions. He performed miracles and He healed the sick over, and over, and over again. Jesus demonstrated God's great love for us in the way He served the needy and by taking the punishment for our sins on the cross. Here are just a few of the many accounts of Jesus healing the sick, documented in the book of Matthew, that ignited my faith.

"When evening came, they brought to Him many who were demon-possessed, and He cast out the spirits with a word, and healed all who were ill." (Matthew 8:16) (NASB)

In Matthew, Chapter 12, Jesus says to a man with a crippled hand, "Stretch out your hand." The man stretched it out and it was restored to normal, like his other hand. After that, the religious leaders conspired against Jesus on how to destroy Him. Jesus was aware of this, so he left. And many people followed Him, and He healed them all, and warned them not to tell who He was. (Matthew 12:9–16) (NASB)

"When Jesus went ashore, He saw a large crowd and felt compassion for them and healed their sick." (Matthew 14:14) (NASB)

"Large crowds came to Jesus, bringing with them those who were lame, crippled, blind, mute, and many others, and they laid them down at his feet; and He healed them." (Matthew 15:30) (NASB)

HEALING YOUR HEART

Bitterness, resentment, and unforgiveness are three of the most destructive emotional states, and they will rot you from the inside out and destroy your health. Now is the time to exercise your forgiveness muscle and forgive everyone who has ever hurt you.

Get into a quiet, prayerful state and close your eyes. Next search your memory for all the people who have hurt you. Think through your life chronologically. Go back as far you can—all the way back to your childhood. Family members, friends, schoolmates, strangers, co-workers . . .

Even seemingly insignificant events from your childhood may have caused deep emotional wounds that need to be healed. If you can still remember the offense, there's a chance it may still be affecting you today. If the memory triggers an emotion, that's a signal that there may be some forgiveness that needs to happen.

Take time to remember every single person who has hurt you and forgive each and every one of them, by name.

Revisiting all the times you've been hurt is something most people don't do and don't want to do. I know it's hard. But this is a critical step. Do not skip this part of the healing process. The thing you want to do least is usually the thing you need to do most. Bitterness can be a barrier to healing. You can radically change your diet and lifestyle and do all the therapies in the world, but if you don't forgive the people who have hurt you and let go of your anger and bitterness toward them, you may not get well.

When you let go of the past and choose to forgive, God will heal your heart and change you. When you pray to forgive, don't just think it. Say it out loud. Speak it out of your mouth. It's powerful. As you are thinking of each person who hurt you, pray this way:

> God. You know what they did. And you know how I feel about it. They hurt me . . . but today, right now, I'm choosing to forgive them. I am letting them go. And I am giving them to you. I am not going to carry this anger and bitterness anymore. I am laying it at your feet. It's all yours. Thank you for forgiving me, and for healing my heart and healing my body. And I'm asking you to have mercy on them and to bless them, in Jesus' name. Amen.

Love them? Bless them? Pray for them? Believe me, that's the last thing I want to do for someone who has hurt me. When someone wrongs me, I want justice, vengeance—that's human nature. But remember: we reap what we sow. When you plant a seed in the ground, you don't grow another seed; you harvest a plant with hundreds or thousands of seeds. People who sow bad seeds in life will reap an exponential harvest of bad things on themselves, much more than they sowed.

I find tremendous comfort in knowing that people will eventually get what they deserve. That makes it easier to let the offenses go. And in the meantime, I just follow Jesus' instructions and ask God to have mercy on the people who have hurt me and to bless them. Jesus emphasized the importance of forgiveness throughout his ministry. When He taught his disciples how to pray, he instructed them to pray, "Forgive us our sins as we forgive those who sin against us." It doesn't matter if you don't feel like it or if you don't feel sincere when you pray to forgive someone. Just keep on forgiving.

FORGIVENESS IS NOT A FEELING

Forgiveness is a decision. You choose to forgive despite your feelings. *I'll forgive them when they're sorry and when they apologize.* Nope. That's not going to work. Because some people will never be sorry and never apologize. The act of forgiveness is not for them; it is for you.

Forgiveness is not a one-shot deal. It is a choice for life. It is choosing to no longer hold what someone did against them. Forgiveness is choosing to show them love by letting it go, forever. If you decided to eat healthy for one week and then went back to junk food, how much would it benefit you? Forgiveness works the same way. It only works if you stick with it.

Some memories may still cause you grief and pain after you've made the decision to forgive. If that happens, you must remind yourself that you made a decision to forgive and that you're sticking with your decision. Don't let those old hurts and emotions get a foothold in your mind. Continue giving them back to God, and I assure you there will come a point in time when the forgiveness will be complete in your heart. You will see them in a new way and the pain will be gone. Going forward, make a decision to forgive new offenses quickly.

ASKING OTHERS FOR FORGIVENESS

The next part of the process is asking for forgiveness from the people that you have hurt. This is an okay place to play your cancer card if you have one. A conversation could go something like this:

"Hey, John. It's Chris . . . I don't know if you've heard, but I was diagnosed with cancer recently . . . It's made me realize that I need make some things right . . . I'm calling to ask you to forgive me for [insert offense here]. What I did was wrong and I am truly sorry. I also wanted to ask if there was anything I can do to make it up to you . . ."

Some people may graciously forgive you and others may not. They may even unleash a verbal assault on you that they think you deserve. And maybe you do deserve it. If the latter happens, don't defend yourself, don't argue, and definitely don't try to justify your actions or tell them that they were wrong too. Just let them say what they need to say. The most important thing is that you humble yourself, admit you were wrong, ask for forgiveness, and exit the conversation gracefully. This can be a powerful first step to mending a broken relationship.

GOD IS WILLING TO FORGIVE YOU

Guilt and shame about mistakes you've made in the past can lead to depression and self-hatred, which will make you miserable and sick. If you've cheated people, stolen from them, betrayed their trust, used them, and hurt them, you can push those memories aside and forget about them for a while, but ultimately you can never get away from them. Unresolved spiritual and emotional issues stay in your subconscious, raising your overall anxiety and unhappiness, and often lead to self-medication and destructive behaviors.

When you are born, your heart is pure and innocent, like a glass of purified water. One sin, the first lie you ever told, is like a tiny drop of sewage in the glass. One drop renders the water impure—polluted and undrinkable. Now imagine every bad thing you've thought or done in your life as another drop of sewage in that glass, or, to put it another way, as a black spot on your heart. We've all done shameful things that have polluted and corrupted our hearts, and we all need forgiveness.

Sin separates us from God, but Jesus Christ took the punishment for our sins on the cross, making a bridge between us and God. When God forgives you, He wipes the slate clean. Your hardened, black heart is transplanted with a new heart. And the most beautiful thing of all is that you simply have to turn to Him and ask. He loves you so much and is willing to forgive you and will not hold your past mistakes against you. Knowing that God loves you and is quick to forgive makes it possible to forgive yourself and let go of the guilt and shame you've been carrying.

One of the last things Jesus said when he was dying on the cross, innocent of any wrongdoing, was "Father forgive them, for they know not what they do."

If Jesus was able to forgive those who conspired against Him and those who beat Him, whipped Him, spit on Him, nailed Him to a cross, and mocked Him while He was dying, you can forgive the people in your life who have hurt you.

In my search for answers, all the roads I ventured down brought me to the same place. Whether God struck me with cancer or it was the result of my choices or the choices of others became irrelevant, and I realized that I had only one appropriate response—to surrender. Once I made that act of surrender, it opened the door to some of the sweetest and most powerful times in my life. He gave me peace in the middle of the storm, and He carried me through to the other side. I don't view cancer as a gift or a blessing, but God worked it for my good and used it to bless my life.

JUST ASK

If you don't know God, if you don't know if there is a God, all you have to do is reach out and ask. Just get alone, get quiet, and say, "Okay, God, here I am. I'm ready. I'm open. I'm willing to believe. Just reveal Yourself to me. I want to know You." I'm certain that if you continue to pray that way, God will reveal Himself to you and He will speak to you. Amazing, incredible, supernatural things will happen in your life. You just have to humble yourself and ask.

*"Ask and it will be given to you; seek and you will find;
knock and the door will be opened to you."*
— MATTHEW 7:7 (NIV)

Finally, find a Bible and read about the life and the words of
Jesus. Read the books of Matthew, Mark, Luke, and John. If you
want to know God's heart, you'll see it in Jesus.

Massive Action Steps to Spiritual Healing

➤ Choose faith over fear and doubt.

➤ Give your fears, worries, and anxiety to God and trust Him
to lead you.

➤ Catch yourself when you are thinking negatively and choose
to think positively.

➤ Always look for the silver lining in every situation.

➤ Encourage yourself every day.

➤ Visualize yourself being well.

➤ Speak life and health into your body.

➤ Forgive everyone who has ever hurt you.

➤ Ask for forgiveness from those you have hurt.

➤ Be quick to forgive going forward.

➤ Get right with God. Surrender. Reach out and ask for
forgiveness, help, and healing.

➤ Ask God to show you what you need to do and what you
need to change.

➤ Find a Bible and read Matthew, Mark, Luke, and John.

EPILOGUE

LIFE IS A JOURNEY full of obstacles, roadblocks, detours, and miracles. Sometimes you find yourself traveling with companions, and sometimes your journey separates you from the people you care about and you have to travel alone. Sometimes your paths intersect again down the road. Sometimes they don't. Sometimes you realize you're going the wrong way and you have to turn around and retrace your steps. Sometimes you have to completely abandon your path and start a new one.

In his poem "The Road Not Taken," Robert Frost reflects on his choice to take the road less traveled and how it "made all the difference." In my Robert Frost moment, the popular path—the conventional road—was enticing. It was easy.

Conventional cancer treatment required nothing from me except to show up. It was a permission slip to not change, to keep living the life that was killing me. Chemo put God in a box. He was either going to cure me with chemo or He wasn't—it was not up to me. I was tempted to get on the conventional train, relinquish control of my life, and be a passenger. It appealed to my reluctance to examine my life, to face my faults and my flaws, and to admit my mistakes. It appealed to my narcissism that I was just unlucky, a victim, and that nothing that happened to me was ever my fault. That's not to say conventional treatment or chemotherapy is wrong for everyone, but those are the reasons it was wrong for me.

The alternate path—the road less traveled—was hard. And it was lonely. I had no idea where it would take me, and I knew it would be challenging, but I sensed it would make me stronger and wiser. Deep in my core, it made the most sense. Despite the opinions of many people around me, I knew this was the path I had to take. I didn't like who I was, and I didn't want to change. But I knew I had to change to survive. I embraced the fear of failure, the fear of the unknown, the fear of death, and the adventure of it all. I savored the thrill of being alive and the freedom to live or die on my own terms. And I felt powerful. Once I made the decision to step out in faith, into the unknown, I had peace. And I knew that if I made it through the jungle, I could show others the way.

Maybe you are at the same crossroad. Fighting doubt and fear. Trying to decide what to do next and frustrated because there are no good options, no guarantees. Maybe your instincts are telling you to do the opposite of everyone else, but maybe you are afraid of criticism and rejection. Maybe you are afraid of failure. Maybe you've been telling yourself you aren't worthy of health or success or happiness. You are. Now is the time to start telling yourself that you are. Now is the time to stop criticizing yourself and start encouraging yourself. Your thoughts and actions create your reality and your future. Changing your thoughts and actions can change the course of your life.

This is your journey. You are the navigator. You are the author of your story. Don't let anyone rush you into things you don't understand. Don't do anything that doesn't make sense to you. Don't let anyone take the wheel from you. Don't let anyone manipulate you with fear. Make decisions that are based on facts and faith, not fear. Listen to your instincts and intuition. Listen to your gut. Listen to the Holy Spirit. Pray. Reach out. Ask God for help. Ask for signs. Ask for direction. Ask God to show you what you need to do, and what you need to change. Both faith and doubt are a choice. Choose faith. Be strong and courageous.

Epilogue

You may be afraid, but courage cannot exist without fear. Courage is the decision to move forward in spite of fear. Fear is the darkness that courage shines through. Now is the time to start your healing adventure. It just takes one step . . .

May you prosper in good health even as your soul prospers.

RESOURCES

THE END OF THIS BOOK is just the beginning. I have so much more to share with you! For bonus content and resources, including my free patient guide *20 Questions for Your Oncologist*, interviews with holistic survivors, access to our community of thrivers, helpful links, and more, please visit

www.chrisbeatcancer.com/bookresources

ENDNOTES

CHAPTER 1: Into the Jungle

1. University of Chicago Medicine, "Evidence Mounts for Link Between Opioids and Cancer Growth," *UChicago Medicine* (Mar 2012). http://www .uchospitals.edu/news/2012/20120321-opioid.html (accessed Apr 2018).

2. Jay Soong-Jin Lee et al, "New Persistent Opioid Use Among Patients with Cancer After Curative-Intent Surgery," *Journal of Clinical Oncology* 35.36 (Oct 2017): 4042–49. http://ascopubs.org/doi/abs/10.1200/JCO.2017.74.1363 (accessed Apr 2018).

3. The American Cancer Society Medical and Editorial Content Team, "Survival Rates for Colorectal Cancer, by Stage," *The American Cancer Society* (Feb 2018). https://www.cancer.org/cancer/colon-rectal-cancer/detection -diagnosis-staging/survival-rates.html (accessed Apr 2018).

4. Christopher H. Lieu et al, "Association of Age with Survival in Patients with Metastatic Colorectal Cancer: Analysis from the ARCAD Clinical Trials Program," *Journal of Clinical Oncology* 32.27 (Sep 2014): 2975–82. https:// www.ncbi.nlm.nih.gov/pmc/articles/PMC4809210/ (accessed Apr 2018).

5. Robert Preidt, "Colon Cancer Hits Younger Adults Especially Hard, Study Finds," *HealthDay* (Oct 2013). https://consumer.healthday.com/senior -citizen-information-31/misc-aging-news-10/colon-cancer-hits-younger -adults-especially-hard-study-finds-680634.html (accessed Apr 2018).

6. National Cancer Institute, "Colon Cancer Treatment (PDQ®)–Health Professional Version," *NIH* (Apr 2018). https://www.cancer.gov/types/ colorectal/hp/colon-treatment-pdq#section/all (accessed Apr 2018).

7. Chang Hyun Kim et al, "Prognostic Comparison Between Number and Distribution of Lymph Node Metastases in Patients with Right-Sided Colon

Cancer," *Annals of Surgical Oncology* 21.4 (Apr 2014): 1361–68. https://link .springer.com/article/10.1245/s10434-013-3426-3 (accessed Apr 2018).

8. Robert Preidt, "Colon Cancer's Location May Be Factor in Survival," *WebMD* (2015). https://www.webmd.com/colorectal-cancer/news/20150224/colon -cancers-location-may-be-factor-in-survival (accessed Apr 2018).

9. Fausto Petrelli et al, "Prognostic Survival Associated with Left-Sided vs Right-Sided Colon Cancer: A Systematic Review and Meta-Analysis," *JAMA Oncology* 3.2 (Oct 2017): 211–19. https://www.ncbi.nlm.nih.gov/ pubmed/27787550 (accessed Apr 2018).

CHAPTER 2: Survival of the Sickest

1. Rosalie A. David and Michael R. Zimmerman, "Cancer: An Old Disease, a New Disease or Something in Between?" *Nature Reviews Cancer* 10.10 (Oct 2010): 728–33. https://www.ncbi.nlm.nih.gov/pubmed/20814420 (accessed Apr 2018).

2. William H. Goodson et al, "Assessing the Carcinogenic Potential of Low-Dose Exposures to Chemical Mixtures in the Environment: The Challenge Ahead," *Carcinogenesis* 36.1 (Jun 2015): S254–96. https://www.ncbi.nlm.nih .gov/pmc/articles/PMC4480130/ (accessed Apr 2018).

3. International Agency for Research on Cancer, "IARC: Diesel Engine Exhaust Carcinogenic," *World Health Organization* (Jun 2012). http://www.iarc.fr/en/ media-centre/pr/2012/pdfs/pr213_E.pdf (accessed Apr 2018).

4. Jeffrey Switchenko et al, "Resolving Uncertainty in the Spatial Relationships Between Passive Benzene Exposure and Risk of Non-Hodgkin Lymphoma," *Cancer Epidemiology* 41 (Jul 2016): 139–51. https://www.ncbi.nlm.nih.gov/ pmc/articles/PMC4946246/ (accessed Apr 2018).

5. Goodson et al, "Assessing the Carcinogenic Potential."

6. Michael J. McGinnis and William H. Foege, "The Immediate vs. the Important," *JAMA* 291.10 (Mar 2004): 1263–64. https://jamanetwork.com/ journals/jama/article-abstract/198333 (accessed Apr 2018).

7. Michael J. McGinnis and William H. Foege, "Actual Causes of Death in the United States," *JAMA* 270.18 (Nov 1993): 2207–12. https://jamanetwork .com/journals/jama/article-abstract/409171?redirect=true (accessed Apr 2018).

8. Song Wu et al, "Substantial Contribution of Extrinsic Risk Factors to Cancer Development," *Nature* 529.7584 (Jan 2016): 43–47. https://www.nature.com/ articles/nature16166 (accessed Apr 2018).

9. Doug Irving, "Chronic Conditions in America: Price and Prevalence," *RAND Review* (Jul 2017). https://www.rand.org/blog/rand-review/2017/07/chronic -conditions-in-america-price-and-prevalence.html (accessed Apr 2018).

Endnotes

10. Paul D. Loprinzi et al, "Healthy Lifestyle Characteristics and Their Joint Association with Cardiovascular Disease Biomarkers in US Adults," *Mayo Clinic Proceedings* 91.4 (Apr 2016): 432–42. http://www .mayoclinicproceedings.org/article/S0025-6196%252816%252900043-4/ abstract (accessed Apr 2018).

11. Julie Beck, "Less Than 3 Percent of Americans Live a 'Healthy Lifestyle,'" *The Atlantic* (Mar 2016). https://www.theatlantic.com/health/archive/2016/03/ less-than-3-percent-of-americans-live-a-healthy-lifestyle/475065/ (accessed Apr 2018).

12. Seung Hee Lee-Kwan et al, "Disparities in State-Specific Adult Fruit and Vegetable Consumption—United States, 2015," MMWR 66.45 (Nov 2017): 1241–47. https://www.cdc.gov/mmwr/volumes/66/wr/mm6645a1.htm (accessed Apr 2018).

13. Michael Greger, "Calculate Your Healthy Eating Score," *Nutrition Facts* (Aug 2011). https://nutritionfacts.org/video/calculate-your-healthy-eating-score/ (accessed Apr 2018).

14. M. F. McCarty, "Proposal for a Dietary Phytochemical Index," *Medical Hypotheses* 63.5 (2004): 813–17. https://www.ncbi.nlm.nih.gov/ pubmed/15488652 (accessed 2018).

15. National Cancer Institute, Epidemiology and Genomics Research Program, "Sources of Energy among the U.S. Population, 2005–06," *Epidemiology and Genomics Research Program*. National Cancer Institute (Updated April 2016). http://epi.grants.cancer.gov/diet/foodsources/energy/ (accessed April 2018).

16. Anette Christ et al, "Western Diet Triggers NLRP3-Dependent Innate Immune Reprogramming," *Cell* 172.1–2 (Jan 2018): 162–75.e14. http://www.cell.com/ cell/abstract/S0092-8674(17)31493-9 (accessed Apr 2018).

17. Thibault Fiolet et al, "Consumption of Ultra-Processed Foods and Cancer Risk: Results from NutriNet-Santé Prospective Cohort," *BMJ* 360 (Feb 2018): k322. https://www.bmj.com/content/360/bmj.k322 (accessed Apr 2018).

18. Allison M. Hodge et al, "Consumption of Sugar-Sweetened and Artificially Sweetened Soft Drinks and Risk of Obesity-Related Cancers," *Public Health Nutrition* (Feb 2018): 1–9. https://www.cambridge.org/core/journals/public -health-nutrition/article/consumption-of-sugarsweetened-and-artificially -sweetened-soft-drinks-and-risk-of-obesityrelated-cancers/14DB5E863485356 0209984B07CED68B1 (accessed Apr 2018).

19. Noelle K. LoConte et al, "Alcohol and Cancer: A Statement of the American Society of Clinical Oncology," *Journal of Clinical Oncology* 36.1 (Jan 2018): 83–93. https://www.ncbi.nlm.nih.gov/pubmed/29112463 (accessed Apr 2018).

20. "Millennials 'set to be fattest generation,'" *BBC News* (Feb 2018). http://www .bbc.com/news/health-43195977 (accessed Apr 2018).

21. Centers for Disease Control and Prevention, "Behavioral Risk Factor Surveillance System," *CDC* (reviewed Mar 2018). https://www.cdc.gov/brfss/ (accessed Apr 2018).

22. Brooke C. Steele et al, "Vital Signs: Trends in Incidence of Cancers Associated with Overweight and Obesity—United States, 2005–2014," *Morbidity and Mortality Weekly Report* 66.39 (Oct 2017): 1052–58. https://www.cdc.gov/ mmwr/volumes/66/wr/mm6639e1.htm (accessed Apr 2018).

23. Béatrice Lauby-Secretan et al, "Body Fatness and Cancer—Viewpoint of the IARC Working Group," *The New England Journal of Medicine* 375.8 (Aug 2016): 794–98. http://www.nejm.org/doi/full/10.1056/NEJMsr1606602 (accessed Apr 2018).

24. American Association for Cancer Research, "High Body Fat Levels Associated with Increased Breast Cancer Risk in Women with Normal BMI," *ScienceDaily* (Jan 2018) www.sciencedaily.com/releases/2018/01/180126085442.htm (accessed Apr 2018).

25. D. Chakraborty et al, "Fibroblast Growth Factor Receptor Is a Mechanistic Link Between Visceral Adiposity and Cancer," *Oncogene* 36.48 (Nov 2017): 6668–79. https://www.ncbi.nlm.nih.gov/pubmed/28783178 (accessed Apr 2018).

26. C. Stephen et al, "Association of Leisure-Time Physical Activity with Risk of 26 Types of Cancer in 1.44 Million Adults," *JAMA Internal Medicine* 176.6 (Jun 2016): 816–25. https://www.ncbi.nlm.nih.gov/pubmed/27183032 (accessed Apr 2018).

27. Rachel Rettner, "Exercise May Reduce the Risk of These 13 Cancers," *LiveScience* (May 2016). https://www.livescience.com/54749-exercise-reduces -cancer-risk.html (accessed Apr 2018).

28. Center for Nutrition Policy and Promotion, "Nutrient Content of the U.S. Food Supply, 1909–2010," *United States Department of Agriculture* (Mar 2014). https://www.cnpp.usda.gov/USFoodSupply-1909-2010 (accessed Apr 2018).

29. Michael F. Jacobson, "Carcinogenicity and Regulation of Caramel Colorings," *International Journal of Occupational and Environmental Health* 18.3 (Jul–Sep 2012): 254–59. https://www.ncbi.nlm.nih.gov/pubmed/23026009 (accessed Apr 2018).

30. Rudolf Kaaks, "Nutrition, Insulin, IGF-1 Metabolism and Cancer Risk: A Summary of Epidemiological Evidence," *Novartis Foundation Symposium* 262 (2004): 247–60. https://www.ncbi.nlm.nih.gov/pubmed/15562834 (accessed Apr 2018).

31. Samuel S. Epstein, "Re: Role of the Insulin-Like Growth Factors in Cancer Development and Progression," *Journal of the National Cancer Institute* 93.3 (Feb 2001): 238. https://academic.oup.com/jnci/article/93/3/238/2909702 (accessed Apr 2018).

32. American Institute for Cancer Research, "AICR's Foods That Fight Cancer: Whole Grains," *AICR.* http://www.aicr.org/foods-that-fight-cancer/whole -grains.html (accessed Apr 2018).

33. Celine Gasnier et al, "Glyphosate-Based Herbicides Are Toxic and Endocrine Disruptors in Human Cell Line," *Toxicology* 262 (Aug 2009): 184–91. https:// www.ncbi.nlm.nih.gov/pubmed/19539684 (accessed Apr 2018).

34. Anthony Samsel and Stephanie Seneff, "Glyphosate, Pathways to Modern Diseases II: Celiac Sprue and Gluten Intolerance," *Interdisciplinary Toxicology* 6.4 (Dec 2013): 159–84. https://www.ncbi.nlm.nih.gov/pmc/articles/ PMC3945755/ (accessed Apr 2018).

35. Paolo Bofetta, Enzo Merler, and Harri Vainio, "Carcinogenicity of Mercury and Mercury Compounds," *Scandinavian Journal of Work, Environment & Health* 19.1 (Feb 1993): 1–7. https://www.jstor.org/stable/i40043315 (accessed Apr 2018).

36. Environmental Working Group, "First Ever U.S. Tests of Farmed Salmon Show High Levels of Cancer-Causing PCBs," *EWG* (Jul 2003). https://www .ewg.org/news/news-releases/2003/07/30/first-ever-us-tests-farmed-salmon -show-high-levels-cancer-causing-pcbs#.WnDIWiPMw_M (accessed Apr 2018).

37. Mary E. Cogswell et al, "Sodium and Potassium Intakes Among US Adults: NHANES 2003–2008," *American Journal of Clinical Nutrition* 96.3 (Jul 2012): 647–57. https://www.ncbi.nlm.nih.gov/pmc/articles/PMC3417219/ (accessed Apr 2018).

38. Center for Nutrition Policy and Promotion, "Nutrient Content of the U.S. Food Supply, 1909–2010."

39. International Agency for Research on Cancer, "Section of Infections— Infections and Cancer Biology Group," *World Health Organization* (2018). https://www.iarc.fr/en/research-groups/ICB/index.php (accessed Apr 2018).

40. Jeffrey I. Cohen, "Epstein-Barr Virus Vaccines," *Clinical & Translational Immunology* 4.32 (Jan 2015): 1–6. http://www.nature.com/cti/journal/v4/n1/ full/cti201427a.html (accessed Apr 2018).

41. Stephen Starko Francis et al, "In Utero Cytomegalovirus Infection and Development of Childhood Acute Lymphoblastic Leukemia," *Blood* 129.12 (Mar 2017): 1680–84. https://www.ncbi.nlm.nih.gov/pmc/articles/ PMC5364339/ (accessed Apr 2018).

42. "91% of Women Do Not Know about CMV," *National CMV Foundation.* (2018). https://www.nationalcmv.org/home.aspx (accessed Apr 2018).

43. U.S. Department of Agriculture, "Bovine Leukosis Virus (BLV) on U.S. Dairy Operations, 2007," *USDA* (2008). https://www.aphis.usda.gov/animal_ health/nahms/dairy/downloads/dairy07/Dairy07_is_BLV.pdf (accessed Apr 2018).

44. Gertrude Case Buehring et al, "Humans Have Antibodies Reactive with Bovine Leukemia Virus," *AIDS Research and Human Retroviruses* 19.12 (Dec

2003): 1105–13. https://www.ncbi.nlm.nih.gov/pubmed/14709247 (accessed Apr 2018).

45. Gertrude Case Buehring et al, "Exposure to Bovine Leukemia Virus Is Associated with Breast Cancer: A Case-Control Study," *PLoS ONE* 10.9 (Sep 2015): e0134304. http://journals.plos.org/plosone/article?id=10.1371/journal.pone.0134304%20 (accessed Apr 2018).

46. Gertrude Case Buehring et al, "Bovine Leukemia Virus DNA in Human Breast Tissue," *Emerging Infectious Diseases* 20.5 (May 2014): 772–82. https://www.ncbi.nlm.nih.gov/pmc/articles/PMC4012802/ (accessed Apr 2018).

47. Buehring et al, "Exposure to Bovine Leukemia Virus Is Associated with Breast Cancer: A Case-Control Study."

48. D. C. Wilcox et al, "The Okinawan Diet: Health Implications of a Low-Calorie, Nutrient-Dense, Antioxidant-Rich Dietary Pattern Low in Glycemic Load," *The Journal of the American College of Nutrition* 28 (Aug 2009): 500–16. https://www.ncbi.nlm.nih.gov/pubmed/20234038 (accessed Apr 2018).

49. International Agency for Research on Cancer, "GLOBOCAN 2012: Estimated Cancer Incidence, Mortality and Prevalence Worldwide in 2012," *World Health Organization* (2012). http://globocan.iarc.fr (accessed Apr 2018).

50. S. J. O'Keefe et al. "Why Do African Americans Get More Colon Cancer Than Native Africans?" *Journal of Nutrition* 131.1 (Jan 2007): 175–82. https://www.ncbi.nlm.nih.gov/pubmed/17182822 (accessed Apr 2018).

CHAPTER 3: Doctor's Orders

1. Gabrielle Glaser, "Unfortunately, Doctors Are Pretty Good at Suicide," *NCP Journal of Medicine* (Aug 2015). https://www.ncnp.org/journal-of-medicine/1601-unfortunately-doctors-are-pretty-good-at-suicide.html (accessed Apr 2018).

2. Nicholas A. Yaghmour et al, "Causes of Death of Residents in ACGME-Accredited Programs 2000–2014: Implications for the Learning Environment," *Academic Medicine* 92.7 (May 2017): 976–83. https://www.ncbi.nlm.nih.gov/pmc/articles/PMC5483979/ (accessed Apr 2018).

3. Keith H. Berge, Marvin D. Seppala, and Agnes M. Schipper, "Chemical Dependency and the Physician," *Mayo Clinic Proceedings* 84.7 (Jul 2009): 625–31. http://www.mayoclinicproceedings.org/article/S0025-6196(11)60751-9/fulltext (accessed Apr 2018).

4. Barbara Starfield, "Is US Health Really the Best in the World?" *JAMA* 284.4 (Jul 2000): 483–85. https://jamanetwork.com/journals/jama/article-abstract/192908?redirect=true (accessed Apr 2018).

5. Vanessa McMains, "Johns Hopkins Study Suggests Medical Errors Are Third-Leading Cause of Death in U.S.," *HUB* (May 2016). https://hub.jhu.edu/2016/05/03/medical-errors-third-leading-cause-of-death/ (accessed Apr 2018).

6. Donald W. Light, Joel Lexchin, and Jonathan J. Darrow, "Institutional Corruption of Pharmaceuticals and the Myth of Safe and Effective Drugs," *The Journal of Law, Medicine & Ethics* 41.3 (Oct 2013): 590–600. http://journals.sagepub.com/doi/abs/10.1111/jlme.12068 (accessed Apr 2018).

7. Michael O. Schroeder, "Death by Prescription," *U.S. News & World Report* (Sep 2016). https://health.usnews.com/health-news/patient-advice/articles/2016-09-27/the-danger-in-taking-prescribed-medications (accessed Apr 2018).

8. John T. James, "A New, Evidence-Based Estimate of Patient Harms Associated with Hospital Care," *Journal of Patient Safety* 9.3 (Sep 2013): 122–28. https://www.ncbi.nlm.nih.gov/pubmed/23860193 (accessed Apr 2018).

9. Gary Null et al, "Death by Medicine," *WebDC* (2004). http://www.webdc.com/pdfs/deathbymedicine.pdf (accessed Apr 2018).

10. Gary Null et al, "Death by Medicine," *Life Extension Magazine* (2004). http://www.lifeextension.com/Magazine/2004/3/awsi_death/Page-02 (accessed Apr 2018).

11. Matthew Semler et al, "Balanced Crystalloids versus Saline in Critically Ill Adults," *The New England Journal of Medicine* 378.9 (Mar 2018): 829–839. https://www.nejm.org/doi/full/10.1056/NEJMoa1711584; https://www.ncbi.nlm.nih.gov/pubmed/29485925 (accessed May 2018).

12. Michelle Castillo, "Study Shows Annual Mammograms Don't Save Lives," *CBS News* (Feb 2014). https://www.cbsnews.com/news/canadian-study-shows-annual-mammograms-dont-reduce-breast-cancer-death-rate/ (accessed Apr 2018).

13. Archie Bleyer and H. Gilbert Welch, "Effect of Three Decades of Screening Mammography on Breast-Cancer Incidence," *The New England Journal of Medicine* 367 (Nov 2012): 1998–2005. http://www.nejm.org/doi/full/10.1056/NEJMoa1206809 (accessed Apr 2018).

14. Louise Davies and H. Gilbert Welch, "Current Thyroid Cancer Trends in the United States," *JAMA Otolaryngology-Head & Neck Surgery* 140.4 (Apr 2014): 317–22. https://jamanetwork.com/journals/jamaotolaryngology/article-abstract/1833060 (accessed Apr 2018).

15. Laura J. Esserman, Ian M. Thompson Jr., and Brian Reid, "Overdiagnosis and Overtreatment in Cancer: An Opportunity for Improvement," *JAMA* 310.8 (Jul 2013): 797–98. https://pdfs.semanticscholar.org/d900/94298f78dd262302506473254858060126fb.pdf (accessed Apr 2018).

16. Edward F. Patz et al, "Overdiagnosis in Low-Dose Computed Tomography Screening for Lung Cancer," *JAMA* 174.2 (Jul 2014): 269–74. https://www.ncbi.nlm.nih.gov/pmc/articles/PMC4040004/.

17. Jane C. Weeks et al, "Patients' Expectations about Effects of Chemotherapy for Advanced Cancer," *The New England Journal of Medicine* 367 (Oct 2012):

1616–25. http://www.nejm.org/doi/full/10.1056/NEJMoa1204410 (accessed Apr 2018).

18. Candice M. Wenzell et al, "Outcomes in Obese and Overweight Acute Myeloid Leukemia Patients Receiving Chemotherapy Dosed According to Actual Body Weight," *American Journal of Hematology* 88.10 (Oct 2013): 906–9. https://www.ncbi.nlm.nih.gov/pubmed/23828018 (accessed Apr 2018).

19. Ulrich Abel, "Chemotherapy of Advanced Epithelial Cancer–a Critical Review," *Journal of Biomedicine & Pharmacotherapy* 46.10 (Feb 1992): 439–52. https://www.ncbi.nlm.nih.gov/pubmed/1339108 (accessed Apr 2018).

20. "Lung Cancer Fact Sheet," *American Lung Association* (2016), http://www .lung.org/lung-health-and-diseases/lung-disease-lookup/lung-cancer/ resource-library/lung-cancer-fact-sheet.html (accessed Apr 2018).

21. National Cancer Institute, "SEER Cancer Statistics Review, 1975–2013," *NIH* (Sep 2016). https://seer.cancer.gov/archive/csr/1975_2013/ (accessed Apr 2018).

22. Hesborn Wao et al, "Survival of Patients with Non–Small Cell Lung Cancer Without Treatment: A Systematic Review and Meta-Analysis," *Systematic Reviews* 2 (Feb 2013): 10. https://www.ncbi.nlm.nih.gov/pmc/articles/ PMC3579762/ (accessed Apr 2018).

23. N. Bernards et al, "No Improvement in Median Survival for Patients with Metastatic Gastric Cancer Despite Increased Use of Chemotherapy," *Annals of Oncology* 24.12 (Dec 2013): 3056–60. https://academic.oup.com/annonc/ article/24/12/3056/172397 (accessed Apr 2018).

24. Holly G. Prigerson et al, "Chemotherapy Use, Performance Status, and Quality of Life at the End of Life," *JAMA Oncology* 1.6 (Jul 2015): 778–84. https://www.ncbi.nlm.nih.gov/pubmed/26203912 (accessed Apr 2018).

CHAPTER 4: Making a Killing

1. R. Jeffrey Smith and Jeffrey H. Birnbaum, "Drug Bill Demonstrates Lobby's Pull," *Washington Post* (Jan 2007). http://www.washingtonpost.com/wp-dyn/ content/article/2007/01/11/AR2007011102081.html (accessed Apr 2018).

2. Gardiner Harris, "Waste in Cancer Drugs Costs $3 Billion a Year, a Study Says," *The New York Times* (Mar 2016). https://www.nytimes .com/2016/03/01/health/waste-in-cancer-drugs-costs-3-billion-a-year-a -study-says.html (accessed Apr 2018).

3. Jackie Judd, "Taxpayers End Up Funding Drug Companies," *ABC News* (Jun 2012). http://abcnews.go.com/WNT/YourMoney/story?id=129651 (accessed Apr 2018).

4. M. D. Kesselheim et al, "The High Cost of Prescription Drugs in the United States Origins and Prospects for Reform," *JAMA* 316.8 (Aug 2016): 858–71. https://www.ncbi.nlm.nih.gov/pubmed/27552619 (accessed Apr 2018).

5. Marcia Angell, "Drug Companies and Doctors: A Story of Corruption," *The New York Review of Books* (Jan 2009). http://www.nybooks.com/articles/ archives/2009/jan/15/drug-companies-doctorsa-story-of-corruption/ (accessed Apr 2018).

6. Centers for Disease Control and Prevention, "Prescription Painkiller Overdoses in the US," *CDC* (Nov 2011). http://www.cdc.gov/vitalsigns/ PainkillerOverdoses/index.html (accessed Apr 2018).

7. Irving Kirsch, "Antidepressants and the Placebo Effect," *Zeitschrift Für Psychologie* 222.3 (2014): 128–34. https://www.ncbi.nlm.nih.gov/pmc/ articles/PMC4172306/ (accessed Apr 2018).

8. C. Glenn Begley and Lee M. Ellis, "Drug Development: Raise Standards for Preclinical Cancer Research," *Nature* 483 (Mar 2012): 531–33. https://www .ncbi.nlm.nih.gov/pubmed/22460880 (accessed Apr 2018).

9. Sharon Begley, "In Cancer Science, Many 'Discoveries' Don't Hold Up," *Reuters* (Mar 2012). https://www.reuters.com/article/us-science-cancer/ in-cancer-science-many-discoveries-dont-hold-up-idUSBRE82R12P20120328 (accessed Apr 2018).

10. Florian Prinz, Thomas Schlange, and Khusru Asadullah, "Believe It or Not: How Much Can We Rely on Published Data on Potential Drug Targets?" *Nature Reviews Drug Discovery* 10.9 (Aug 2011): 712. http://www.nature.com/ articles/nrd3439-c1 (accessed Apr 2018).

11. Daniele Mandrioli, Cristin E Kearns, and Lisa A. Bero, "Relationship Between Research Outcomes and Risk of Bias, Study Sponsorship, and Author Financial Conflicts of Interest in Reviews of the Effects of Artificially Sweetened Beverages on Weight Outcomes: A Systematic Review of Reviews," *PLoS ONE* 11.9 (Sep 2016): e0162198. http://journals.plos.org/plosone/ article?id=10.1371/journal.pone.0162198 (accessed Apr 2018).

12. C. Ferric et al, "Misconduct Accounts for the Majority of Retracted Scientific Publications," *Proceedings of the National Academy of Sciences* 109.42 (Sep 2012): 17028–33. http://www.pnas.org/content/109/42/17028 (accessed Apr 2018).

13. Richard Horton, "Offline: What Is Medicine's 5 Sigma?" *The Lancet* 385.9976 (Apr 2015): 1380. http://www.thelancet.com/journals/lancet/article/ PIIS0140-6736(15)60696-1/fulltext (accessed Apr 2018).

14. Angell, "Drug Companies and Doctors: A Story of Corruption."

15. Hope S. Rugo et al, "Randomized Phase III Trial of Paclitaxel Once Per Week Compared With Nanoparticle Albumin-Bound Nab-Paclitaxel Once Per Week or Ixabepilone With Bevacizumab As First-Line Chemotherapy for Locally Recurrent or Metastatic Breast Cancer: CALGB 40502/NCCTG N063H (Alliance)," *Journal of Clinical Oncology* 33.21 (2014): 2361–69. https://www .ncbi.nlm.nih.gov/pubmed/26056183 (accessed Apr 2018).

16. "Study Confirms Taxol Better Than Ixempra or Abraxane for Locally Advanced or Metastatic Disease," *BreastCancer.org* (Jun 2015). http://www .breastcancer.org/research-news/taxol-better-than-ixempra-or-abraxane (accessed Apr 2018).

17. Courtney Davis et al, "Availability of Evidence of Benefits on Overall Survival and Quality of Life of Cancer Drugs Approved by European Medicines Agency: Retrospective Cohort Study of Drug Approvals 2009–13," *BMJ* 359 (Oct 2017). https://www.bmj.com/content/359/bmj.j4530 (accessed Apr 2018).

18. "No Clear Evidence That Most New Cancer Drugs Extend or Improve Life." *BMJ Newsroom* (Oct 2017). http://www.bmj.com/company/newsroom/ no-clear-evidence-that-most-new-cancer-drugs-extend-or-improve-life/ (accessed Apr 2018).

19. Margaret Hamburg, "FDA Pulls Approval for Avastin in Breast Cancer," *Cancer Discovery* (Nov 2011). http://cancerdiscovery.aacrjournals.org/ content/candisc/early/2011/11/21/2159-8290.CD-ND112311OL-08.full.pdf (accessed Apr 2018).

20. Vishal Ranpura, Sanjaykumar Hapani, and Shenhong Wu, "Treatment-Related Mortality with Bevacizumab in Cancer Patients: A Meta-Analysis," *JAMA* 305.5 (2011): 487–94. https://jamanetwork.com/journals/jama/ fullarticle/645368 (accessed Apr 2018).

21. National Cancer Institute, "When Combined with Chemotherapy, Bevacizumab Is Associated with Increased Risk of Death," *NCI* (Mar 2011). https://www.cancer.gov/types/colorectal/research/bevacizumab-severe-side -effects (accessed Apr 2018).

22. Ed Silverman, "Drug Makers Pay $67 Million for Misleading Docs About Cancer Drug Survival Data," *STAT News* (Jun 2016). https://www.statnews .com/pharmalot/2016/06/06/drug-makers-pay-67m-misleading-docs-cancer -drug-survival-data/ (accessed Apr 2018).

23. Office of Public Affairs, "Pharmaceutical Companies to Pay $67 Million To Resolve False Claims Act Allegations Relating to Tarceva," *United States Department of Justice* (Jun 2016). https://www.justice.gov/opa/pr/ pharmaceutical-companies-pay-67-million-resolve-false-claims-act -allegations-relating-tarceva (accessed Apr 2018).

24. Graeme Morgan, Robyn Ward and Michael Barton, "The Contribution of Cytotoxic Chemotherapy to 5-Year Survival in Adult Malignancies," *Journal of Clinical Oncology* 16.8 (2004): 549–60. http://www.clinicaloncologyonline .net/article/S0936-6555(04)00222-5/abstract (accessed Apr 2018).

25. Chris Kahlenborn et al, "Oral Contraceptive Use as a Risk Factor for Premenopausal Breast Cancer: A Meta-Analysis," *Mayo Clinic Proceedings* 81.10 (Oct 2006): 1290–302. https://www.ncbi.nlm.nih.gov/ pubmed/17036554 (accessed Apr 2018).

26. Yu Sun et al, "Treatment-Induced Damage to the Tumor Microenvironment Promotes Prostate Cancer Therapy Resistance Through WNT16B," *Nature Medicine* 18.9 (Sep 2012): 1359–68. https://www.ncbi.nlm.nih.gov/pmc/articles/PMC3677971/ (accessed Apr 2018).

27. Beth Israel Deaconess Medical Center, "Double-Edged Sword: Killing Cancer Cells Can Also Drive Tumor Growth," *EurekAlert!* (Nov 2017). https://www.eurekalert.org/pub_releases/2017-11/bidm-dsk113017.php (accessed Apr 2018).

28. Gali Weinreb, "Research: Chemotherapy Can Cause Metastasis," *Globes* (Dec 2016). http://www.globes.co.il/en/article-technion-research-finds-chemotherapy-can-cause-metastasis-1001164952 (accessed Apr 2018).

29. Fred Hutchinson Cancer Research Center, "Long-Term Tamoxifen Use Increases Risk of an Aggressive, Hard to Treat Type of Second Breast Cancer," *ScienceDaily* (Aug 2009). https://www.sciencedaily.com/releases/2009/08/090825150954.htm (accessed Apr 2018).

30. Christina Izzo, "Weighing the Risks and Benefits of Tamoxifen as Chemoprevention in High-Risk Women," *Cancer Updates, Research & Education* (Jan 2015). https://www.curetoday.com/articles/weighing-the-risks-and-benefits-of-tamoxifen-as-chemoprevention-in-high-risk-women (accessed Apr 2018).

31. Shezad Malik, "Taxotere Permanent Hair Loss Lawsuit," *The Legal Examiner* (Mar 2016). http://fortworth.legalexaminer.com/fda-prescription-drugs/taxotere-permanent-hair-loss-lawsuit/ (accessed Apr 2018).

32. Nathan Gay and Vinay Prasad, "Few People Actually Benefit from 'Breakthrough' Cancer Immunotherapy," *STAT News* (Mar 2017). https://www.statnews.com/2017/03/08/immunotherapy-cancer-breakthrough/ (accessed Apr 2018).

33. James Larkin, "Combined Nivolumab and Ipilimumab or Monotherapy in Untreated Melanoma," *The New England Journal of Medicine* 373.1 (Jul 2015): 23–34. http://www.nejm.org/doi/full/10.1056/NEJMoa1504030 (accessed Apr 2018).

34. Zosia Chustecka, "New Immunotherapy Costing $1 Million a Year," *Medscape* (Jun 2015). https://www.medscape.com/viewarticle/845707 (accessed Apr 2018).

35. Megan Molteni, "The Most Promising Cancer Treatments in a Century Have Arrived—but Not for Everyone," *Wired* (Nov 2017). https://www.wired.com/story/cancer-immunotherapy-has-arrived-but-not-for-everyone/ (accessed Apr 2018).

36. Janet M. Busey et al, "Patient Knowledge and Understanding of Radiation from Diagnostic Imaging," *JAMA Internal Medicine* 173.3 (Feb 2013): 239–41. https://jamanetwork.com/journals/jamainternalmedicine/fullarticle/1487286 (accessed Apr 2018).

37. "Radiation Dose in X-Ray and CT Exams," *Radiology Info* (Feb 2017). https://www.radiologyinfo.org/en/info.cfm?pg=safety-xray (accessed Apr 2018).

38. Andrew J. Einstein, "Beyond the Bombs: Cancer Risks from Low-Dose Medical Radiation," *Lancet* 380.9840 (Jun 2012): 455–57. https://www.ncbi.nlm.nih.gov/pmc/articles/PMC3674023/ (accessed Apr 2018).

39. Amy Berrington de Gonzalez et al, "Projected Cancer Risks from Computed Tomographic Scans Performed in the United States in 2007," *JAMA Internal Medicine* 169.22 (Dec 2009): 2071–77. https://www.ncbi.nlm.nih.gov/pubmed/20008689 (accessed Apr 2018).

40. David B. Larson et al, "Rising Use of CT in Child Visits to the Emergency Department in the United States, 1995–2008," *Radiology* 259.3 (Jun 2011): 793–801. https://www.ncbi.nlm.nih.gov/pubmed/21467249 (accessed Apr 2018).

41. Mark S. Pearce, "Radiation Exposure from CT Scans in Childhood and Subsequent Risk of Leukaemia and Brain Tumours: A Retrospective Cohort Study," *Lancet* 380.9840 (Aug 2012): 499–505. http://www.thelancet.com/journals/lancet/article/PIIS0140-6736(12)60815-0/abstract (accessed Apr 2018).

42. Geoffrey R. Oxnard et al, "Variability of Lung Tumor Measurements on Repeat Computed Tomography Scans Taken Within 15 Minutes," *Journal of Clinical Oncology* 29.23 (Jul 2011): 3114–19. https://www.ncbi.nlm.nih.gov/pmc/articles/PMC3157977/ (accessed Apr 2018).

43. Carrie Printz, "Radiation Treatment Generates Therapy-Resistant Cancer Stem Cells from Less Aggressive Breast Cancer Cells," *Cancer* 118.13 (Jun 2012): 3225. https://onlinelibrary.wiley.com/doi/full/10.1002/cncr.27701 (accessed Apr 2018).

44. Chann Lagadec et al, "Radiation-Induced Reprogramming of Breast Cancer Cells," *Stem Cells* 30.5 (May 2012): 833–44. https://www.ncbi.nlm.nih.gov/pmc/articles/PMC3413333/ (accessed Apr 2018).

45. Syed Wamique Yusuf, Shehzad Sami, and Iyad N. Daher, "Radiation-Induced Heart Disease: A Clinical Update," *Cardiology Research and Practice* 2011 (Dec 2010): 317659. https://www.hindawi.com/journals/crp/2011/317659/ (accessed Apr 2018).

46. Manisha Palta et al, "The Use of Adjuvant Radiotherapy in Elderly Patients with Early-Stage Breast Cancer: Changes in Practice Patterns After Publication of Cancer and Leukemia Group B 9343," *Cancer* 121.2 (Jan 2015): 188–93. https://www.ncbi.nlm.nih.gov/pubmed/25488523 (accessed Apr 2018).

47. Elizabeth B. Claus et al, "Dental X-Rays and Risk of Meningioma," *Cancer* 118.18 (Apr 2012): 4530–37. https://www.ncbi.nlm.nih.gov/pmc/articles/PMC3396782/ (accessed Apr 2018).

48. American Dental Association Council on Scientific Affairs, "The Use of Dental Radiographs: Update and Recommendations." *Journal of the American Dental Association* 137.9 (Sep 2006): 1304–12. http://jada.ada.org/article/S0002-8177(14)64322-1/fulltext (accessed Apr 2018).

CHAPTER 5: It's Not Like I Need Your Business

1. Louis S. Goodman et al, "Nitrogen Mustard Therapy: Use of Methyl-Bis(Beta-Chloroethyl)amine Hydrochloride and Tris(Beta-Chloroethyl)amine Hydrochloride for Hodgkin's Disease, Lymphosarcoma, Leukemia and Certain Allied and Miscellaneous Disorders," *JAMA* 132.3 (Sep 1946): 126–32. https://jamanetwork.com/journals/jama/article-abstract/288442?redirect=true (accessed Apr 2018).

2. Tom Reynolds, "Salary a Major Factor for Academic Oncologists, Study Shows," *Journal of the National Cancer Institute* 93.7 (Apr 2001): 491. https://academic.oup.com/jnci/article/93/7/491/2906507 (accessed Apr 2108).

3. Mireille Jacobsone et al, "How Medicare's Payment Cuts for Cancer Chemotherapy Drugs Changed Patterns of Treatment," *Health Affairs* 29.7 (Jul 2010): 1394–402. https://www.healthaffairs.org/doi/abs/10.1377/hlthaff.2009.0563 (accessed Apr 2018).

4. Jean M. Mitchell, "Urologists' Use of Intensity-Modulated Radiation Therapy for Prostate Cancer," *New England Journal of Medicine* 369.17 (Oct 2013): 1629–637. http://www.nejm.org/doi/full/10.1056/NEJMsa1201141 (accessed Apr 2018).

5. Lee N. Newcomer, "Changing Physician Incentives for Affordable, Quality Cancer Care: Results of an Episode Payment Model." *Journal of Oncology Practice* 10 (Jul 2014): 322–26. http://ascopubs.org/doi/abs/10.1200/jop.2014.001488 (accessed Apr 2018).

6. Matthew Herper, "The Truly Staggering Cost of Inventing New Drugs," *Forbes* (Feb 2012). https://www.forbes.com/sites/matthewherper/2012/02/10/the-truly-staggering-cost-of-inventing-new-drugs/#41ee3fa44a94 (accessed Apr 2018).

7. Rosie Taylor and Jim Giles, "Cash Interests Taint Drug Advice," *Nature* 437 (Oct 2005): 1070–71. http://www.nature.com/articles/4371070a (accessed Apr 2018).

8. Caroline Riveros et al, "Timing and Completeness of Trial Results Posted at ClinicalTrials.gov and Published in Journals," *PLoS Medicine* 10.12 (Dec 2013): e1001566. http://journals.plos.org/plosmedicine/article?id=10.1371/journal.pmed.1001566 (accessed Apr 2018).

9. Bob Grant, "Merck Published Fake Journal," *The Scientist Magazine* (Apr 2009). https://www.the-scientist.com/?articles.view/articleNo/27376/title/Merck-published-fake-journal/ (accessed Apr 2018).

10. Jim Edwards, "Merck Created Hit List to 'Destroy,' 'Neutralize' or 'Discredit' Dissenting Doctors," *CBS News* (May 2009). https://www.cbsnews.com/news/merck-created-hit-list-to-destroy-neutralize-or-discredit-dissenting-doctors/ (accessed Apr 2018).

11. Laura B. Vater et al, "Trends in Cancer-Center Spending on Advertising in the United States, 2005 to 2014," *JAMA Internal Medicine* 176.8 (Aug 2016): 1214–16. https://jamanetwork.com/journals/jamainternalmedicine/fullarticle/2532786 (accessed Apr 2018).

12. Laura B. Vater et al, "What Are Cancer Centers Advertising to the Public?: A Content Analysis," *Annals of Internal Medicine* 160.12 (Jun 2014): 813–20. https://www.ncbi.nlm.nih.gov/pmc/articles/PMC4356527/ (accessed Apr 2018).

13. Scott D. Ramsey et al, "Washington State Cancer Patients Found to Be at Greater Risk for Bankruptcy Than People without a Cancer Diagnosis," *Health Affairs* 32.6 (May 2013): 1143–52. https://www.ncbi.nlm.nih.gov/pmc/articles/PMC4240626/ (accessed Apr 2018).

CHAPTER 6: The Elephant in the Waiting Room

1. Michael J. Thun and Ahmedin Jemal, "How Much of the Decrease in Cancer Death Rates in the United States Is Attributable to Reductions in Tobacco Smoking?" *Tobacco Control* 15.5 (Oct 2006): 345–47. https://www.ncbi.nlm.nih.gov/pmc/articles/PMC2563648/ (accessed Apr 2018).

2. Peter M. Ravdin et al, "The Decrease in Breast-Cancer Incidence in 2003 in the United States," *The New England Journal of Medicine* 356.16 (Apr 2007): 1670–74. http://www.nejm.org/doi/full/10.1056/NEJMsr070105 (accessed Apr 2018).

3. Collaborative Group on Epidemiological Studies of Ovarian Cancer, "Menopausal Hormone Use and Ovarian Cancer Risk: Individual Participant Meta-Analysis of 52 Epidemiological Studies," *The Lancet* 385.9980 (May 2015): 1835–42. https://www.ncbi.nlm.nih.gov/pubmed/25684585 (accessed Apr 2018).

4. Odette Wegwarth, Wolfgang Gaissmaier, and Gerd Gigerenzer, "Deceiving Numbers: Survival Rates and Their Impact on Doctors' Risk Communication," *Medical Decision Making* 31.3 (Dec 2010): 386–94. http://journals.sagepub.com/doi/abs/10.1177/0272989X10391469 (accessed Apr 2018).

5. Steven A. Narod et al, "Breast Cancer Mortality After a Diagnosis of Ductal Carcinoma in Situ," *JAMA Oncology* 1.7 (Oct 2015): 888–96. https://www.ncbi.nlm.nih.gov/pubmed/26291673 (accessed Apr 2018).

6. Allison W. Kurian, "Recent Trends in Chemotherapy Use and Oncologists' Treatment Recommendations for Early-Stage Breast Cancer," *Journal of the National Cancer Institute* (Dec 2017): djx239. http://ascopubs.org/doi/abs/10.1200/JCO.2017.35.15_suppl.541 (accessed Apr 2018).

7.   Fatima Cardoso et al. "70-Gene Signature as an Aid to Treatment Decisions
      in Early-Stage Breast Cancer," *The New England Journal of Medicine* 375 (Aug
      2016): 717–29. http://www.nejm.org/doi/full/10.1056/NEJMoa1602253
      (accessed Apr 2018).

CHAPTER 8: Plants versus Zombies

1.   William W. Li et al, "Tumor Angiogenesis as a Target for Dietary Cancer
      Prevention," *Journal of Oncology* 2012 (Jul 2011): 1–23. https://www.hindawi
      .com/journals/jo/2012/879623/ (accessed Apr 2018).

2.   Jie Sun et al, "Antioxidant and Antiproliferative Activities of Common
      Fruits," *Journal of Agricultural and Food Chemistry* 50.25 (Dec 2002): 7449–54.
      https://www.ncbi.nlm.nih.gov/pubmed/12452674 (accessed Apr 2018).

3.   Katherine M. Weh, Jennifer Clarke, and Laura A. Kresty, "Cranberries and
      Cancer: An Update of Preclinical Studies Evaluating the Cancer Inhibitory
      Potential of Cranberry and Cranberry Derived Constituents," *Antioxidants* 5.3
      (Aug 2016): 27. https://www.ncbi.nlm.nih.gov/pmc/articles/PMC5039576/
      (accessed Apr 2018).

4.   Navindra P. Seeram et al, "Total Cranberry Extract versus Its Phytochemical
      Constituents: Antiproliferative and Synergistic Effects against Human Tumor
      Cell Lines," *Journal of Agricultural and Food Chemistry* 52.9 (Apr 2004): 2512–
      17. https://pubs.acs.org/doi/abs/10.1021/jf0352778 (accessed Apr 2018).

5.   Lisa S. McAnulty et al, "Effect of Blueberry Ingestion on Natural Killer Cell
      Counts, Oxidative Stress, and Inflammation Prior To and After 2.5 H of
      Running," *Applied Physiology, Nutrition, and Metabolism* 36.6 (Nov 2011):
      976–84. http://www.nrcresearchpress.com/doi/abs/10.1139/h11-120#
      .WsOH47CG-hc (accessed Apr 2018).

6.   Gordon J. McDougall, "Extracts Exert Different Antiproliferative Effects
      against Cervical and Colon Cancer Cells Grown In Vitro," *Journal of
      Agricultural and Food Chemistry* 56.9 (Apr 2008): 3016–23. https://www.ncbi
      .nlm.nih.gov/pubmed/18412361 (accessed Apr 2018).

7.   Marie E. Olsson et al, "Antioxidant Levels and Inhibition of Cancer Cell
      Proliferation In Vitro by Extracts from Organically and Conventionally
      Cultivated Strawberries," *Journal of Agricultural and Food Chemistry* 54.4 (Feb
      2006): 1248–55. https://www.ncbi.nlm.nih.gov/pubmed/16478244 (accessed
      Apr 2018).

8.   Chen, Tong et al, "Randomized Phase II Trial of Lyophilized Strawberries
      in Patients with Dysplastic Precancerous Lesions of the Esophagus," *Cancer
      Prevention Research* 5.1 (Jan 2012): 41–50. https://www.ncbi.nlm.nih.gov/
      pubmed/22135048 (accessed Apr 2018).

9.   Brian S. Shumway et al, "Effects of a Topically Applied Bioadhesive Berry
      Gel on Loss of Heterozygosity Indices in Premalignant Oral Lesions," *Cancer
      Prevention Research* 14.8 (Nov 2008): 2421–30. https://www.ncbi.nlm.nih
      .gov/pmc/articles/PMC3498466/ (accessed Apr 2018).

10. C. Ngamkitidechakul et al, "Antitumour Effects of Phyllanthus emblica L.: Induction of Cancer Cell Apoptosis and Inhibition of In Vivo Tumour Promotion and In Vitro Invasion of Human Cancer Cells," *Phytotherapy Research* 24.9 (Sep 2010): 1405–13. https://www.ncbi.nlm.nih.gov/pubmed/20812284 (accessed Apr 2018).

11. Muhammad S. Akhtar, "Effect of Amla Fruit (Emblica officinalis Gaertn.) on Blood Glucose and Lipid Profile of Normal Subjects and Type 2 Diabetic Patients," *International Journal of Food Sciences and Nutrition* 62.6 (Apr 2011): 609-616. https://www.ncbi.nlm.nih.gov/pubmed/21495900 (accessed Apr 2018).

12. Dominique Boivin et al, "Antiproliferative and Antioxidant Activities of Common Vegetables: A Comparative Study," *Food Chemistry* 112.2 (Jan 2009): 374–80. https://www.sciencedirect.com/science/article/pii/S0308814608006419 (accessed Apr 2018).

13. Yi-Fang Chu et al, "Antioxidant and Antiproliferative Activities of Common Vegetables," *Journal of Agricultural and Food Chemistry* 50.23 (Dec 2002): 6910–16. https://www.researchgate.net/publication/8665499_Antioxidant_and_Antiproliferative_Activities_of_Common_Vegetables (accessed Apr 2018).

14. Cai-Xia Zhang et al, "Greater Vegetable and Fruit Intake Is Associated with a Lower Risk of Breast Cancer Among Chinese Women," *International Journal of Cancer* 125.1 (Jul 2009): 181 –88. (Zhang) https://www.ncbi.nlm.nih.gov/pubmed/19358284 (accessed Apr 2018).

15. Victoria A. Kirsh et al, "Prospective Study of Fruit and Vegetable Intake and Risk of Prostate Cancer," *Journal of the National Cancer Institute* 99.15 (Aug 2007): 1200–1209. https://www.ncbi.nlm.nih.gov/pubmed/17652276 (accessed Apr 2018).

16. Shiuan Chen et al, "Anti-Aromatase Activity of Phytochemicals in White Button Mushrooms (Agaricus bisporus)," *Cancer Research* 66.24 (Dec 2006): 12026–34. https://www.ncbi.nlm.nih.gov/pubmed/17178902 (accessed Apr 2018).

17. Sang Chul Jeong, Sundar Rao Koyyalamudi, and Gerald Pang, "Dietary Intake of *Agaricus bisporus* White Button Mushroom Accelerates Salivary Immunoglobulin A Secretion in Healthy Volunteers," *Nutrition* 28.5 (May 2012): 527–31. http://www.nutritionjrnl.com/article/S0899-9007(11)00302-9/abstract (accessed Apr 2018).

18. N. N. Miura et al, "Blood Clearance of (1-->3)-beta-D-glucan in MRL lpr/lpr Mice," *FEMS Immunology and Medical Microbiology* 13.1 (Feb 1996): 51–57. https://www.researchgate.net/publication/14384731_Blood_clearance_of_1--3-beta-D-glucan_in_MRL_lprlpr_mice (accessed Apr 2018).

19. David C. Nieman, "Exercise Effects on Systemic Immunity," *Immunology and Cell Biology* 78.5 (Oct 2000): 496–501. https://www.researchgate.net/publication/274166266_Exercise_effects_on_systemic_immunity (accessed Apr 2018).

20. Min Zhang et al, "Dietary Intakes of Mushrooms and Green Tea Combine to Reduce the Risk of Breast Cancer in Chinese Women," *International Journal of Cancer* 124.6 (Mar 2008): 1404–8. https://www.ncbi.nlm.nih.gov/pubmed/19048616 (accessed Apr 2018).

21. Amanda Hutchins-Wolfbrandt and Anahita M. Mistry, "Dietary Turmeric Potentially Reduces the Risk of Cancer," *Asian Pacific Journal of Cancer Prevention* 12.12 (Jan 2011): 3169–73. https://www.researchgate.net/publication/223984006_Dietary_Turmeric_Potentially_Reduces_the_Risk_of_Cancer (accessed Apr 2018).

22. S. Bengmark, M. D. Mesa, and A. Gil, "Plant-Derived Health: The Effects of Turmeric and Curcuminoids," *Nutrición Hospitalaria* 24.3 (May–Jun 2009): 273–81. https://www.ncbi.nlm.nih.gov/pubmed/19721899 (accessed Apr 2018).

23. Noor Hasima and Bharat B. Aggarwal, "Cancer-Linked Targets Modulated by Curcumin," *International Journal of Biochemistry and Molecular Biology* 3.4 (Dec 2012): 328–51. https://www.ncbi.nlm.nih.gov/pmc/articles/PMC3533886/ (accessed Apr 2018).

24. Bharat B. Aggarwal, A. Kumar, and A. C. Bharti, "Anticancer Potential of Curcumin: Preclinical and Clinical Studies," *Anticancer Research* 23.1a (Jan–Feb 2003): 363–98. https://www.ncbi.nlm.nih.gov/pubmed/12680238 (accessed Apr 2018).

25. Christopher D. Lao et al, "Dose Escalation of a Curcuminoid Formulation," *BMC Complementary and Alternative Medicine* 6:10 (Feb 2006). https://www.researchgate.net/publication/7234027_Dose_escalation_of_a_curcuminoid_formulation_BMC_Complement_Altern_Med_610 (accessed Apr 2018).

26. Subash C. Gupta, Sridevi Patchva, and Bharat B. Aggarwal, "Therapeutic Roles of Curcumin: Lessons Learned from Clinical Trials," *The AAPS Journal* 15.1 (Jan 2013): 195–218. https://www.ncbi.nlm.nih.gov/pmc/articles/PMC3535097/ (accessed Apr 2018).

27. Abbas Zaidi, Maggie Lai, and Jamie Cavenagh, "Long-Term Stabilisation of Myeloma with Curcumin," *BMJ Case Reports* 2017 (Apr 2017). http://casereports.bmj.com/content/2017/bcr-2016-218148.abstract (accessed Apr 2018).

28. Guido Shoba et al, "Influence of Piperine on the Pharmacokinetics of Curcumin in Animals and Human Volunteers," *Planta Medica* 64.4 (May 1998): 353–56. https://www.ncbi.nlm.nih.gov/pubmed/96191201 (accessed Apr 2018).

29. I. Savini et al, "Origanum vulgare Induces Apoptosis in Human Colon Cancer Caco2 Cells," *Nutrition and Cancer* 61.3 (Feb 2009): 381–89. https://www.researchgate.net/publication/24284438_Origanum_Vulgare_Induces_Apoptosis_in_Human_Colon_Cancer_Caco_2_Cells (accessed Apr 2018).

30. Ladislav Vaško et al, "Comparison of Some Antioxidant Properties of Plant Extracts from Origanum vulgare, Salvia officinalis, Eleutherococcus senticosus

and Stevia rebaudiana," *In Vitro Cellular & Developmental Biology—Animal* 50.7 (Aug 2014): 614–22. https://www.ncbi.nlm.nih.gov/pubmed/24737278 (accessed Apr 2018).

31. Federation of American Societies for Experimental Biology (FASEB), "Component of Pizza Seasoning Herb Oregano Kills Prostate Cancer Cells," *ScienceDaily* (Apr 2012). www.sciencedaily.com/releases/2012/04/120424162224.htm (accessed Apr 2018).

32. National Cancer Institute, "Garlic and Cancer Prevention," (Jan 2008). https://www.cancer.gov/about-cancer/causes-prevention/risk/diet/garlic-fact-sheet (accessed Apr 2018).

33. Shunsuke Kimura, "Black Garlic: A Critical Review of Its Production, Bioactivity, and Application," *Journal of Food and Drug Analysis* 25.1 (Jan 2017): 62–70. https://www.sciencedirect.com/science/article/pii/S1021949816301727 (accessed Apr 2018).

34. Ruth Clark and Seong-Ho Lee, "Anticancer Properties of Capsaicin Against Human Cancer," *Anticancer Research* 36.3 (Feb 2016): 837–43. http://ar.iiarjournals.org/content/36/3/837.abstract (accessed Apr 2018).

35. Kristin L. Kamerud, Kevin A. Hobbie, and Kim A. Anderson. "Stainless Steel Leaches Nickel and Chromium into Foods During Cooking," *Journal of Agriculture and Food Chemistry* 61.39 (Aug 2013): 9495–501. https://pubs.acs.org/doi/abs/10.1021/jf402400v (accessed Apr 2018).

36. Dugald Seely et al, "In Vitro Analysis of the Herbal Compound Essiac," *Anticancer Research* 27.6b (Nov–Dec 2007): 3875–82. https://www.ncbi.nlm.nih.gov/pubmed/18225545 (accessed Apr 2018).

37. Yan Sun et al, "Immune Restoration and/or Augmentation of Local Graft versus Host Reaction by Traditional Chinese Medicinal Herbs," *Cancer* 52.1 (Jul 1983): 70–73. https://www.ncbi.nlm.nih.gov/pubmed/6336578 (accessed Apr 2018).

38. Yan San et al, "Herbaline—(Special Spice)," *Jason Winters International.* https://sirjasonwinters.com/scientific-documentation-herbalene/ (accessed Apr 2018).

39. Jian-Ming Lü et al, "Molecular Mechanisms and Clinical Applications of Nordihydroguaiaretic Acid (NDGA) and Its Derivatives: An Update," *Medical Science Monitor* 16.5 (Aug 2010): RA93–100. https://www.ncbi.nlm.nih.gov/pmc/articles/PMC2927326/ (accessed Apr 2018).

40. Xiaoxia Li et al, "A Review of Recent Research Progress on the Astragalus Genus," *Molecules* 19.11 (Nov 2014): 18850–80. https://www.ncbi.nlm.nih.gov/pubmed/25407722 (accessed Apr 2018).

41. Arash Khorasani Esmaeili et al, "Antioxidant Activity and Total Phenolic and Flavonoid Content of Various Solvent Extracts from In Vivo and In Vitro Grown Trifolium pratense L. (Red Clover)," *BioMed Research*

International 2015 (Apr 2015): 643285. https://www.hindawi.com/journals/
bmri/2015/643285/ (accessed Apr 2018).

42. Yun Wang et al, "The Red Clover (Trifolium pratense) Isoflavone Biochanin A
    Inhibits Aromatase Activity and Expression," *British Journal of Nutrition* 99.2
    (May 2008): 303–10. https://www.researchgate.net/publication/6079305_
    The_red_clover_Trifolium_pratense_isoflavone_biochanin_A_inhibits_
    aromatase_activity_and_expression (accessed Apr 2018).

43. Pamela Ovadje et al, "Dandelion Root Extract Affects Colorectal Cancer
    Proliferation and Survival Through the Activation of Multiple Death
    Signalling Pathways," *Oncotarget* 7.45 (Nov 2016): 73080–100. https://www
    .ncbi.nlm.nih.gov/pmc/articles/PMC5341965/ (accessed Apr 2018).

44. Sophia C. Sigstedt et al, "Evaluation of Aqueous Extracts of Taraxacum
    officinale on Growth and Invasion of Breast and Prostate Cancer Cells,"
    International Journal of Oncology 32.5 (May 2008): 1085–90. https://www.ncbi
    .nlm.nih.gov/pubmed/18425335 (accessed Apr 2018).

45. Pamela Ovadje et al, "Selective Induction of Apoptosis Through Activation
    of Caspase-8 in Human Leukemia Cells (Jurkat) by Dandelion Root Extract,"
    Journal of Ethnopharmacology 133.1 (Jan 2011): 86–91. https://www.ncbi.nlm
    .nih.gov/pubmed/20849941 (accessed Apr 2018).

46. S. J. Chatterjee et al, "The Efficacy of Dandelion Root Extract in Inducing
    Apoptosis in Drug-Resistant Human Melanoma Cells," *Evidence-Based
    Complementary and Alternative Medicine* 2011 (Dec 2010): 129045. https://
    www.hindawi.com/journals/ecam/2011/129045/ (accessed Apr 2018).

47. Pamela Ovadje et al, "Selective Induction of Apoptosis and Autophagy
    Through Treatment with Dandelion Root Extract in Human Pancreatic
    Cancer Cells," *Pancreas* 41.7 (Oct 2012): 1039–47. https://www.ncbi.nlm.nih
    .gov/pubmed/22647733 (accessed Apr 2018).

48. Long-Gang Zhao et al, "Green Tea Consumption and Cause-Specific
    Mortality: Results from Two Prospective Cohort Studies in China," *Journal of
    Epidemiology* 27.1 (2017): 36–41. https://www.ncbi.nlm.nih.gov/pmc/articles/
    PMC5328738/ (accessed Apr 2018).

49. Gong Yang et al, "Green Tea Consumption and Colorectal Cancer Risk: A
    Report from the Shanghai Men's Health Study," *Carcinogenesis* 32.11 (Nov
    2011): 1684–88. https://www.ncbi.nlm.nih.gov/pubmed/21856996 (accessed
    Apr 2018).

50. Hui-Hsuan Lin, Jing-Hsien Chen, and Chau-Jong Wang, "Chemopreventive
    Properties and Molecular Mechanisms of the Bioactive Compounds
    in Hibiscus Sabdariffa Linne," *Current Medicinal Chemistry* 18.8 (Feb
    2011): 1245–54. https://www.researchgate.net/publication/49807880_
    Chemopreventive_Properties_and_Molecular_Mechanisms_of_the_Bioactive_
    Compounds_in_Hibiscus_Sabdariffa_Linne (accessed Apr 2018).

CHAPTER 9: Heroic Doses

1. Richard J. Bloomer et al, "A 21 Day Daniel Fast Improves Selected Biomarkers of Antioxidant Status and Oxidative Stress in Men and Women," *Nutrition and Metabolism* 8.17 (Mar 2011). https://www.ncbi.nlm.nih.gov/pubmed/21414232 (accessed Apr 2018).

2. Dean Ornish et al, "Intensive Lifestyle Changes May Affect the Progression of Prostate Cancer," *The Journal of Urology* 174 (Sep 2005): 1065–70. https://www.ncbi.nlm.nih.gov/pubmed/16094059 (accessed Apr 2018).

3. G. A. Saxe, "Can Diet in Conjunction with Stress Reduction Affect the Rate of Increase in Prostate Specific Antigen after Biochemical Recurrence of Prostate Cancer?" *The Journal of Urology* 166.1 (Dec 2001): 2202–7. https://www.ncbi.nlm.nih.gov/pubmed/11696736 (accessed Apr 2018).

4. R. J. Barnard et al, "Effects of a Low-Fat, High-Fiber Diet and Exercise Program on Breast Cancer Risk Factors In Vivo and Tumor Cell Growth and Apoptosis In Vitro," *Nutrition and Cancer* 55.1 (Feb 2006): 28–34. https://www.ncbi.nlm.nih.gov/pubmed/16965238 (accessed Apr 2018).

5. Véronique Bouvard et al, "Carcinogenicity of Consumption of Red and Processed Meat," *The Lancet Oncology* 16.16 (Oct 2015): 1599–1600. http://www.thelancet.com/journals/lanonc/article/PIIS1470-2045(15)00444-1/abstract (accessed Apr 2018).

6. Giuseppe Lippi, Camilla Mattiuzzi, and Gianfranco Cervellin, "Meat Consumption and Cancer Risk: A Critical Review of Published Meta-Analyses," *ScienceDirect* 97 (Jan 2016): 1–14. https://www.ncbi.nlm.nih.gov/pubmed/26633248 (accessed Apr 2018); Jeanine M. Genkinger and Anita Koushik,"Meat Consumption and Cancer Risk" *PLoS Medicine* 4.12 (Dec 2007): e345. https://www.ncbi.nlm.nih.gov/pmc/articles/PMC2121650 (accessed May 2018).

7. R. J. Barnard et al, "Effects of a Low-Fat, High-Fiber Diet and Exercise Program on Breast Cancer Risk Factors In Vivo and Tumor Cell Growth and Apoptosis In Vitro," *Nutrition and Cancer* 55.1 (Feb 2006): 28–34. https://www.ncbi.nlm.nih.gov/pubmed/16965238 (accessed Apr 2018).

8. Barbara C. Halpern et al, "The Effect of Replacement of Methionine by Homocystine on Survival of Malignant and Normal Adult Mammalian Cells in Culture," *Proceedings of the National Academy of Sciences of the United States of America* 71.4 (Apr 1974): 1133–36. https://www.ncbi.nlm.nih.gov/pmc/articles/PMC388177/ (accessed Apr 2018).

9. Paul Cavuoto and Michael F. Fenech, "A Review of Methionine Dependency and the Role of Methionine Restriction in Cancer Growth Control and Life-Span Extension," *Cancer Treatment Reviews* 38.6 (Oct 2012): 726–36. https://www.ncbi.nlm.nih.gov/pubmed/22342103 (accessed Apr 2018).

Endnotes

10. I. Vucenik and A. M. Shamsuddin, "Protection Against Cancer by Dietary IP6 and Inositol," *Nutrition and Cancer* 55.2 (Feb 2006): 109–25. https://www.ncbi.nlm.nih.gov/pubmed/17044765 (accessed Apr 2018).

11. Morgan E. Levine, "Low Protein Intake Is Associated with a Major Reduction in IGF-1, Cancer, and Overall Mortality in the 65 and Younger but Not Older Population," *Cell Metabolism* 19.3 (Mar 2014): 407–17. https://www.ncbi.nlm.nih.gov/pubmed/24606898 (accessed Apr 2018).

12. Jae Jeng Yang et al, "Dietary Fat Intake and Lung Cancer Risk: A Pooled Analysis," *Journal of Clinical Oncology* 35.26 (Jul 2017): 3055–64. https://www.ncbi.nlm.nih.gov/pubmed/28742456 (accessed Apr 2018).

13. Semir Beyaz et al, "High Fat Diet Enhances Stemness and Tumorigenicity of Intestinal Progenitors," *Nature* 531.7592 (Mar 2016): 53–58. https://www.ncbi.nlm.nih.gov/pmc/articles/PMC4846772/ (accessed Apr 2018).

14. F. K. Tabung, S. E. Steck, and J. Zhang, "Dietary Inflammatory Index and Risk of Mortality: Findings from the Aerobics Center Longitudinal Study." Poster presented at American Institute for Cancer Research (AICR) Annual Research Conference, November 7, 2013, Bethesda, MD. https://www.ncbi.nlm.nih.gov/pubmed/24718872 (accessed Apr 2018).

15. Abina Sieri et al, "Dietary Fat Intake and Development of Specific Breast Cancer Subtypes," *Journal of the National Cancer Institute* 106.5 (Apr 2014): dju068. https://www.ncbi.nlm.nih.gov/pubmed/24718872 (accessed Apr 2018).

16. E. H. Allot et al, "Saturated Fat Intake and Prostate Cancer Aggressiveness: Results from the Population-Based North Carolina-Louisiana Prostate Cancer Project," *Prostate Cancer and Prostatic Diseases* 20 (Mar 2017): 48–54. https://www.ncbi.nlm.nih.gov/pubmed/27595916 (accessed Apr 2018).

17. Mary H. Ward, "Heme Iron from Meat and Risk of Adenocarcinoma of the Esophagus and Stomach," *European Journal of Cancer Prevention* 21.2 (Mar 2012): 134–38. https://www.ncbi.nlm.nih.gov/pmc/articles/PMC3261306/ (accessed Apr 2018).

18. Nadia M. Bastide, Fabrice H. F. Pierre, and Denis E. Corpet, "Heme Iron from Meat and Risk of Colorectal Cancer: A Meta-Analysis and a Review of the Mechanisms Involved," *Cancer Prevention Research* 4.2 (Feb 2011): 177–84. https://www.ncbi.nlm.nih.gov/pubmed/21209396 (accessed Apr 2018).

19. Nathalie M. Scheers et al, "Ferric Citrate and Ferric EDTA but Not Ferrous Sufate Drive Amphiregulin-Mediated Activation of the MAP Kinase ERK in Gut Epithelial Cancer Cells," *Oncotarget* 9 (Jul 2008): 996–1002. http://www.oncotarget.com/index.php?journal=oncotarget&page=article&op=view&path%5b%5d=24899 (accessed May 2018).

20. Leo R. Zacharski, "Decreased Cancer Risk after Iron Reduction in Patients with Peripheral Arterial Disease: Results from a Randomized Trial," *Journal of the National Cancer Institute* 100.14 (2018): 17066–17077. https://www.ncbi.nlm.nih.gov/pubmed/18612130 (accessed Apr 2018).

21. Dagfinn Aune et al, "Fruit and Vegetable Intake and the Risk of Cardiovascular Disease, Total Cancer and All-Cause Mortality—A Systematic Review and Dose-Response Meta-Analysis of Prospective Studies," *International Journal of Epidemiology* 46.3 (Jun 2017): 1029–56. https://www .ncbi.nlm.nih.gov/pubmed/28338764 (accessed Apr 2018).

22. Sarah Boseley, "Forget Five a Day, Eat 10 Portions of Fruit and Veg to Cut Risk of Early Death," *The Guardian* (Feb 2017). https://www.theguardian .com/society/2017/feb/23/five-day-10-portions-fruit-veg-cut-early-death (accessed Apr 2018).

23. S. De Flora, M. Bagnasco, and H. Vainio, "Modulation of Genotoxic and Related Effects by Carotenoids and Vitamin A in Experimental Models: Mechanistic Issues," *Mutagenesis* 14.2 (Mar 1999): 153–72. https://www.ncbi .nlm.nih.gov/pubmed/10229917 (accessed Apr 2018).

24. L. P. Christensen, "Aliphatic C(17)-Polyacetylenes of the Falcarinol Type as Potential Health Promoting Compounds in Food Plants of the Apiaceae Family," *Recent Patents on Food, Nutrition & Agriculture* 3.1 (Jan 2011): 64–77 . https://www.ncbi.nlm.nih.gov/pubmed/21114468 (accessed Apr 2018).

25. Ohio State University, "The Compound in the Mediterranean Diet That Makes Cancer Cells 'Mortal,'" *EurekAlert!* (May 2013). https://www.eurekalert .org/pub_releases/2013-05/osu-tci052013.php (accessed Apr 2018).

26. Rachel S. Rosenberg et al. "Modulation of Androgen and Progesterone Receptors by Phytochemicals in Breast Cancer Cell Lines," *Biochemical and Biophysical Research Communications* 248.3 (Aug 1998): 935–39. https://www .researchgate.net/publication/13581330_Modulation_of_Androgen_and_ Progesterone_Receptors_by_Phytochemicals_in_Breast_Cancer_Cell_Lines (accessed Apr 2018).

27. Xin Cai and Xuan Liu, "Inhibition of Thr-55 Phosphorylation Restores p53 Nuclear Localization and Sensitizes Cancer Cells to DNA Damage," *Proceedings of the National Academy of Sciences of the United States of America* 105.44 (Nov 2008): 16958–63. http://www.pnas.org/content/105/44/16958 (accessed Apr 2018).

28. M. Noroozi, W. J. Angerson, and M. E. Lean, "Effects of Flavonoids and Vitamin C on Oxidative DNA Damage to Human Lymphocytes," *The American Journal of Clinical Nutrition* 67.6 (Jun 1998): 1210–18. https://www .ncbi.nlm.nih.gov/pubmed/9625095 (accessed Apr 2018).

29. Theodore Fotsis et al, "Flavonoids, Dietary-Derived Inhibitors of Cell Proliferation and In Vitro Angiogenesis," *Cancer Research* 57.14 (Jul 1997): 2916–21. https://www.ncbi.nlm.nih.gov/pubmed/9230201 (accessed Apr 2018).

30. Hiroe Kikuzaki and Nobuji Nakatani, "Antioxidant Effects of Some Ginger Constituents," *Journal of Food Science* 58.6 (Nov 1993): 1407–10. https://www .researchgate.net/publication/227851087_Antioxidant_Effects_of_Some_ Ginger_Constituents (accessed Apr 2018).

Endnotes

31. H. Y. Zhou et al, "Experimental Study on Apoptosis Induced by Elemene in Glioma Cells," *Ai Zheng* 22.9 (Sep 2003): 959–63. http://europepmc.org/abstract/med/12969529 (accessed Apr 2018).

32. Manjeshwar S. Baliga et al, "Update on the Chemopreventive Effects of Ginger and Its Phytochemicals," *Critical Reviews in Food Science and Nutrition* 51.6 (Jul 2011): 499–23 https://www.ncbi.nlm.nih.gov/pubmed/21929329 (accessed Apr 2018).

33. Magdalena Szejk, Joanna Kolodziejczyk-Czepas, and Halina Małgorzata Żbikowska, "Radioprotectors in Radiotherapy—Advances in the Potential Application of Phytochemicals," *Postepy Higieny* 70 (Jun 2016): 722–34. http://europepmc.org/abstract/med/27356603 (accessed Apr 2018).

34. Yue Zhou et al, "Dietary Natural Products for Prevention and Treatment of Liver Cancer," *Nutrients* 8.3 (Mar 2016): 156. https://www.ncbi.nlm.nih.gov/pmc/articles/PMC4808884/ (accessed Apr 2018).

35. Aesun Shin, Jeongseon Kim, and Sohee Park. "Gastric Cancer Epidemiology in Korea," *Journal of Gastric Cancer* 11.3 (Sep 2011): 135–40. https://www.ncbi.nlm.nih.gov/pmc/articles/PMC3204471/ (accessed Apr 2018).

36. Onica LeGendre, Paul A. S. Breslin, and David A. Foster, "(-)-Oleocanthal Rapidly and Selectively Induces Cancer Cell Death via Lysosomal Membrane Permeabilization," *Molecular & Cellular Oncology* 2.4 (Oct–Dec 015): e1006077. https://www.ncbi.nlm.nih.gov/pmc/articles/PMC4568762/ (accessed Apr 2018).

37. J. Gopal, "Authenticating Apple Cider Vinegar's Home Remedy Claims: Antibacterial, Antifungal, Antiviral Properties and Cytotoxicity Aspect," *National Product Research* 2017 (Dec 2017): 1–5. https://www.ncbi.nlm.nih.gov/pmc/articles/PMC4568762/ (accessed Apr 2018).

38. Anne Berit, C. Samuelsen, Jürgen Schrezenmeir, and Svein H. Knutsen, "Effects of Orally Administered Yeast-Derived Beta-glucans: A Review," *Molecular Nutrition and Food Research* 58.1 (Sep 2013): 183–93. https://onlinelibrary.wiley.com/doi/full/10.1002/mnfr.201300338 (accessed Apr 2018).

39. V. Vetvicka, B. P. Thornton, and G. D. Ross, "Targeting of Natural Killer Cells to Mammary Carcinoma via Naturally Occurring Tumor Cell-Bound iC3b and Beta-glucan-primed CR3 (CD11b/CD18)," *The Journal of Immunology* 159.2 (Jul 1997): 599–605. https://www.ncbi.nlm.nih.gov/pubmed/9218574 (accessed Apr 2018).

40. Gokhan Demir et al, "Beta glucan Induces Proliferation and Activation of Monocytes in Peripheral Blood of Patients with Advanced Breast Cancer," *International Immunopharmacology* 7.1 (Jan 2007): 113–16. https://www.ncbi.nlm.nih.gov/pubmed/17161824 (accessed Apr 2018).

41. Erdinc Yenidogan et al, "Effect of β-Glucan on Drain Fluid and Amount of Drainage Following Modified Radical Mastectomy," *Advances in Therapy*

31.1 (Jan 2014): 130–39. https://www.ncbi.nlm.nih.gov/pubmed/24421054 (accessed Apr 2018).

42. Soo Young Kim et al, "Biomedical Issues of Dietary Fiber β-Glucan," *Journal of Korean Medical Science* 21.5 (Oct 2006): 781–89. https://www.ncbi.nlm.nih .gov/pmc/articles/PMC2721983/ (accessed Apr 2018).

43. Temidayo Fadelu et al, "Nut Consumption and Survival in Patients with Stage III Colon Cancer: Results from CALGB 89803 (Alliance)," *Journal of Clinical Oncology* 36.11 (Apr 2018): 1112–1120. https://www.ncbi.nlm.nih .gov/pubmed/29489429 (accessed May 2018).

44. I. Garrido et al, "Polyphenols and Antioxidant Properties of Almond Skins: Influence of Industrial Processing," *Journal of Food Science* 3.2 (Mar 2008): C106–115. https://www.ncbi.nlm.nih.gov/pubmed/18298714 (accessed May 2018).

45. P. A. Brandt and L. J. Schouten, "Relationship of Tree Nut, Peanut and Peanut Butter Intake with Total and Cause-Specific Mortality: A Cohort Study and Meta-Analysis," *International Journal of Epidemiology* 44.3 (Jun 2015): 1038–1049. doi:10.1093/ije/dyv039 (accessed May 2018).

CHAPTER 10: Building a New Body

1. S. J. O'Keefe et al, "Rarity of Colon Cancer In Africans Is Associated with Low Animal Product Consumption, Not Fiber," *American Journal of Gastroenterology* 94.5 (May 1999): 1373–80. https://www.ncbi.nlm.nih.gov/ pubmed/10235221 (accessed Apr 2018).

2. Fernando P. Carvalho, João M. Oliveira, and Margarida Malta, "Radionuclides in Deep-Sea Fish and Other Organisms from the North Atlantic Ocean," *ICES Journal of Marine Science* 68.2 (Dec 2010): 333–40. https://www.researchgate .net/publication/273028830_Radionuclides_in_deep-sea_fish_and_other_ organisms_from_the_North_Atlantic_Ocean (accessed Apr 2018).

3. Alphonse Kelecom and Rita de Cássia dos Santos Gouvea, "Increase of Po-210 Levels in Human Semen Fluid After Mussel Ingestion," *Journal of Environmental Radioactivity* 102.5 (Feb 2011): 443–47. https://www .researchgate.net/publication/49812789_Increase_of_Po-210_levels_in_ human_semen_fluid_after_mussel_ingestion (accessed Apr 2018).

4. Daniel J. Madigan, Zofia Baumann, and Nicholas S. Fisher, "Pacific Bluefin Tuna Transport Fukushima-Derived Radionuclides from Japan to California," *Proceedings of the National Academy of Sciences of the United States of America* 109.24 (Jun 2012): 9483–86. https://www.ncbi.nlm.nih.gov/ pubmed/22645346 (accessed Apr 2018).

5. *Consumer Reports*, "Talking Turkey: Our New Tests Show Reasons for Concern," *Consumer Reports* (Jun 2013). https://www.consumerreports.org/ cro/magazine/2013/06/consumer-reports-investigation-talking-turkey/index .htm (accessed Apr 2018).

6. Food and Drug Administration, "2011 Retail Meat Report," *FDA* (2013). https://www.fda.gov/downloads/AnimalVeterinary/SafetyHealth/ AntimicrobialResistance/NationalAntimicrobialResistanceMonitoringSystem/ UCM334834.pdf (accessed Apr 2018).

7. Campaign on Human Health and Industrial Farming, "Record-High Antibiotic Sales for Meat and Poultry Production," *The PEW Charitable Trusts* (Feb 2013). http://www.pewtrusts.org/en/research-and-analysis/ analysis/2013/02/06/recordhigh-antibiotic-sales-for-meat-and-poultry -production (accessed Apr 2018).

8. Clett Erridge, "The Capacity of Foodstuffs to Induce Innate Immune Activation of Human Monocytes *In Vitro* Is Dependent on Food Content of Stimulants of Toll-Like Receptors 2 and 4," *British Journal of Nutrition* 105.1 (Jan 2011): 15–23. https://www.ncbi.nlm.nih.gov/pubmed/20849668 (accessed Apr 2018).

9. Rupali Deopurkar et al, "Differential Effects of Cream, Glucose, and Orange Juice on Inflammation, Endotoxin, and the Expression of Toll-Like Receptor-4 and Suppressor of Cytokine Signaling-3," *Diabetes Care* 33.5 (May 010): 991–97. https://www.ncbi.nlm.nih.gov/pmc/articles/PMC2858203/ (accessed Apr 2018).

10. C. R. Daniel et al, "Large Prospective Investigation of Meat Intake, Related Mutagens, and Risk of Renal Cell Carcinoma," *The American Journal of Clinical Nutrition* 95.1 (Jan 2012): 155–162. https://www.ncbi.nlm.nih.gov/ pubmed/22170360 (accessed May 2018).

11. J. Wang et al, "Carcinogen Metabolism Genes, Red Meat and Poultry Intake, and Colorectal Cancer Risk," *International Journal of Cancer* 130.8 (Apr 2012): 1898–1907. https://www.ncbi.nlm.nih.gov/pubmed/21618522 (accessed May 2018).

12. E. de Stefani et al, "Meat Consumption, Meat Cooking and Risk of Lung Cancer Among Uruguayan Men," *Asian Pacific Journal of Cancer Prevention* 11.6 (2010): 1713–1717. https://www.ncbi.nlm.nih.gov/pubmed/21338220 (accessed May 2018).

13. Esther M. John et al, "Meat Consumption, Cooking Practices, Meat Mutagens and Risk of Prostate Cancer," *Nutrition and Cancer* 63.4 (2011): 525–537. https://www.ncbi.nlm.nih.gov/pmc/articles/PMC3516139 (accessed May 2018).

14. K. E. Anderson et al, "Pancreatic Cancer Risk: Associations with Meat-Derived Carcinogen Intake in the Prostate, Lung, Colorectal, and Ovarian Cancer Screening Trial (PLCO) Cohort," *Molecular Carcinogenesis* 51.1 (Jan 2012): 128–137. https://www.ncbi.nlm.nih.gov/pubmed/22162237 (accessed May 2018).

15. Donghui Li et al, "Dietary Mutagen Exposure and Risk of Pancreatic Cancer," *Cancer Epidemiology, Biomarkers & Prevention* 16.4 (Apr 2007): 655–661. https://www.ncbi.nlm.nih.gov/pubmed/17416754 (accessed May 2018).

16. K. Puangsombat et al, "Occurrence of Heterocyclic Amines in Cooked Meat Products," *Meat Science* 90.3 (Mar 2012): 739–746. https://www.ncbi.nlm.nih .gov/pubmed/22129588 (accessed May 2018).

17. Ola Viegas et al, "Inhibitory Effect of Antioxidant-Rich Marinades on the Formation of Heterocyclic Aromatic Amines in Pan-Fried Beef," *Journal of Agricultural and Food Chemistry* 60.24 (Jun 2012): 6235–40. https://www.ncbi .nlm.nih.gov/pubmed/22642699 (accessed Apr 2018).

18. J. S. Smith, F. Ameri, and P. Gadgil, "Effect of Marinades on the Formation of Heterocyclic Amines in Grilled Beef Steaks," *Journal of Food Science* 73.6 (2008): 100–105. https://www.ncbi.nlm.nih.gov/pubmed/19241593 (accessed Apr 2018).

19. Afsaneh Farhadian et al, "Effects of Marinating on the Formation of Polycyclic Aromatic Hydrocarbons (Benzo[a]pyrene, Benzo[b]uoranthene and Fluoranthene) in Grilled Beef Meat," *Food Control* 28.2 (Dec 2012): 420–25. https://www.researchgate.net/publication/257398846_Effects_ of_marinating_on_the_formation_of_polycyclic_aromatic_hydrocarbons_ benzoapyrene_benzobfluoranthene_and_fluoranthene_in_grilled_beef_meat (accessed Apr 2018).

20. Timothy J. Key et al, "Cancer Incidence in Vegetarians: Results from the European Prospective Investigation into Cancer and Nutrition," *The American Journal of Clinical Nutrition* 89.5 (May 2009): 1620–26. https://www .ncbi.nlm.nih.gov/pubmed/19279082 (accessed Apr 2018).

CHAPTER 11: Take Out the Trash

1. Hyun-Wook Lee et al, "E-cigarette Smoke Damages DNA and Reduces Repair Activity in Mouse Lung, Heart, and Bladder as well as in Human Lung and Bladder Cells," *Proceedings of the National Academy of Sciences of the United States of America* (Jan 2018). http://www.pnas.org/content/ early/2018/01/25/1718185115 (accessed Apr 2018).

2. Anthony Samsel and Stephanie Seneff, "Glyphosate's Suppression of Cytochrome P450 Enzymes and Amino Acid Biosynthesis by the Gut Microbiome: Pathways to Modern Diseases," *Entropy* 15.4 (Apr 2013): 1416– 63. http://www.mdpi.com/1099-4300/15/4/1416 (accessed Apr 2018).

3. Siriporn Thongprakaisang et al, "Glyphosate Induces Human Breast Cancer Cells Growth via Estrogen Receptors," *Food and Chemical Toxicology* 59 (Jun 2013): 129–36. https://www.researchgate.net/publication/237146763_ Glyphosate_induces_human_breast_cancer_cells_growth_via_estrogen_ receptors (accessed Apr 2018).

4. Carey Gillam, "Weedkiller Found in Granola and Crackers, Internal FDA Emails Show," *The Guardian* (Apr 2018). https://www.theguardian.com/ us-news/2018/apr/30/fda-weedkiller-glyphosate-in-food-internal-emails (accessed May 2018).

5. Liza Oates et al, "Reduction in Urinary Organophosphate Pesticide Metabolites in Adults After a Week-Long Organic Diet," *Journal of Environmental Research* 132 (Jun 2014): 105–11. https://www.ncbi.nlm.nih.gov/pubmed/24769399 (accessed Apr 2018).

6. Asa Bradman et al, "Effect of Organic Diet Intervention on Pesticide Exposures in Young Children Living in Low-Income Urban and Agricultural Communities," *Environmental Health Perspectives* 123.10 (Oct 2015): 1086–93. https://www.ncbi.nlm.nih.gov/pubmed/25861095 (accessed Apr 2018).

7. Zhi-Yong Yang et al, "Effects of Home Preparation on Pesticide Residues in Cabbage," *Food Control* 18.12 (Dec 2007): 1484–1487. https://www.sciencedirect.com/science/article/pii/S0956713506002696 (accessed May 2018).

8. "Citizen Petition in re: Use of Hydrofluorosilic Acid in Drinking Water Systems of the United States," *EPA* (Apr 2013). https://www.epa.gov/sites/production/files/documents/tsca_21_petition_hfsa_2013-04-22.pdf (accessed May 2018).

9. Sherri A. Mason, Victoria Welch, and Joseph Neratko, "Synthetic Polymer Contamination in Bottled Water," *Fredonia* (2018). https://orbmedia.org/sites/default/files/FinalBottledWaterReport.pdf (accessed Apr 2018).

10. R. Vogt et al, "Cancer and Non-Cancer Health Effects from Food Contaminant Exposures for Children and Adults in California: A Risk Assessment," *Environmental Health* 11 (Nov 2012): 83. https://www.ncbi.nlm.nih.gov/pubmed/23140444 (accessed May 2018).

11. Chris Exley, "Strong Evidence Linking Aluminum and Alzheimer's," *Hippocratic Post* (Dec 2016). https://www.hippocraticpost.com/mental-health/strong-evidence-linking-aluminium-alzheimers/ (accessed Apr 2018).

12. Mike Adams, "Natural Consumer Products Found Contaminated with Cancer-Causing 1,4-Dioxane in Groundbreaking Analysis Released by OCA," *Organic Consumers Association* (Mar 2008). https://www.organicconsumers.org/news/natural-consumer-products-found-contaminated-cancer-causing-14-dioxane-groundbreaking-analysis (accessed Apr 2018).

13. P. D. Darbre, "Aluminium, Antiperspirants and Breast Cancer," *Journal of Inorganic Biochemistry* 99.9 (Sep 2005): 1912–19. https://www.ncbi.nlm.nih.gov/pubmed/16045991 (accessed Apr 2018).

14. G. M. Richardson et al, "Mercury Exposure and Risks from Dental Amalgam in the US Population, Post-2000," *Science of the Total Environment* 409.20 (Sep 2011): 4257–68. https://www.ncbi.nlm.nih.gov/pubmed/21782213 (accessed Apr 2018).

15. José G. Dórea et al, "Speciation of Methyl- and Ethyl-Mercury in Hair of Breastfed Infants Acutely Exposed to Thimerosal-Containing Vaccines," *Clinica Chimica Acta* 412.17–18 (Aug 2011): 1563–66. https://www.ncbi.nlm.nih.gov/pubmed/21782213 (accessed Apr 2018).

16. Brian C. McDonald et al, "Volatile Chemical Products Emerging as Largest Petrochemical Source of Urban Organic Emissions," *Science* 359.6377 (Feb 2018): 760–64. http://science.sciencemag.org/content/359/6377/760 (accessed Apr 2018).

17. The American Cancer Society medical and editorial content team, "Radon and Cancer," *The American Cancer Society* (Sep 2015). https://www.cancer.org/cancer/cancer-causes/radiation-exposure/radon.html (accessed Apr 2018).

18. Wikipedia contributors, "NASA Clean Air Study," *Wikipedia, The Free Encyclopedia* (Jan 2018). https://en.wikipedia.org/w/index.php?title=NASA_Clean_Air_Study&oldid=821719488 (accessed Jan 2018).

19. B. C. Wolverton, Rebecca C. McDonald, and E. A. Watkins Jr., "Foliage Plants for Removing Indoor Air Pollutants from Energy-Efficient Homes," *JSTOR*, 38.2 (Apr–Jun 1984): 224–28. https://www.jstor.org/stable/4254614 (accessed Apr 2018).

20. Orianne Dumas et al, "Occupational Exposure to Disinfectants and Asthma Control in US Nurses," *European Respiratory Journal* 50.4 (Oct 2017): 700237. https://www.ncbi.nlm.nih.gov/pubmed/28982772 (accessed Apr 2018). "Occupational exposure to disinfectants and COPD incidence in US nurses: a prospective cohort study," The air indoor pollution session, 08.30–0.30 hours CEST, Monday 11 September, Brown 1+2 (south).

21. Øistein Svanes et al, "Cleaning at Home and at Work in Relation to Lung Function Decline and Airway Obstruction," *American Journal of Respiratory and Critical Care Medicine* (2018). http://www.thoracic.org/about/newsroom/press-releases/resources/women-cleaners-lung-function.pdf (accessed Apr 2018).

22. University of Washington, "Scented Laundry Products Emit Hazardous Chemicals Through Dryer Vents," *EurekAlert!* (Aug 2011). https://www.eurekalert.org/pub_releases/2011-08/uow-slp082311.php (accessed Apr 2018).

23. Euro Pukkala et al, "Occupation and Cancer—Follow-up of 15 Million People in Five Nordic Countries," *Acta Oncologica* 48.5 (2009): 646–90. https://www.ncbi.nlm.nih.gov/pubmed/19925375 (accessed Apr 2018).

24. Andrea't Mannetje, Amanda Eng, and Neil Pearce, "Farming, Growing Up on a Farm, and Haematological Cancer Mortality," *Occupational & Environmental Medicine* 69.2 (Feb 2012): 126–32. https://www.ncbi.nlm.nih.gov/pubmed/2179574 (accessed Apr 2018).

25. Gregory J. Tranah, Paige M. Bracci, and Elizabeth A. Holly, "Domestic and Farm-Animal Exposures and Risk of Non-Hodgkin Lymphoma in a Population-Based Study in the San Francisco Bay Area," *Cancer Epidemiological, Biomarkers & Preventions* 17.9 (Sep 2008): 2382–87. https://www.ncbi.nlm.nih.gov/pmc/articles/PMC2946322/ (accessed Apr 2018).

26. Samuel Milham, "Historical Evidence That Electrification Caused the 20th Century Epidemic of 'Diseases of Civilization,'" *Medical Hypotheses* 74.2 (Feb

2010): 337–45. http://www.sammilham.com/historical%20evidence.pdf (accessed Apr 2018).

27. N. Wertheimer and E. Leeper, "Electrical Wiring Configurations and Childhood Cancer," *American Journal of Epidemiology* 109.3 (Mar 1979): 273–84. https://www.ncbi.nlm.nih.gov/pubmed/453167 (accessed Apr 2018).

28. Martin L. Pall, "Wi-Fi Is an Important Threat to Human Health," *Environmental Research* 164 (Jul 2018): 405–416. https://www.sciencedirect.com/science/article/pii/S0013935118300355?via=ihub (accessed May 2018).

29. Ali H. Mokdad et al, "Trends and Patterns of Disparities in Cancer Mortality Among US Counties, 1980–2014," *JAMA* 317.4 (Jan 2017): 388–406. https://www.ncbi.nlm.nih.gov/pmc/articles/PMC5617139/ (accessed Apr 2018).

30. "Cancer Stat Facts: Brain and Other Nervous System," *National Cancer Institute: Surveillance, Epidemiology, and End Results Program*. https://seer.cancer.gov/statfacts/html/brain.html (accessed May 2018).

31. Alasdair Philips et al, "Brain Tumours: Rise in Glioblastoma Multiforme Incidence in England 1995–2015 Suggests an Adverse Environmental or Lifestyle Factor," *Journal of Environmental and Public Health* (May 2018). https://www.hindawi.com/journals/jeph/aip/7910754/ (accessed May 2018).

32. Suzanne Wu, "Fasting Triggers Stem Cell Regeneration of Damaged, Old Immune System," *USC News* (Jun 2014). https://news.usc.edu/63669/fasting-triggers-stem-cell-regeneration-of-damaged-old-immune-system/ (accessed Apr 2018).

33. C. Lee et al, "Fasting Cycles Retard Growth of Tumors and Sensitize a Range of Cancer Cell Types to Chemotherapy," *Science Translational Medicine* 4.124 (Mar 2012): 124ra27. https://www.ncbi.nlm.nih.gov/pmc/articles/PMC3608686/ (accessed Apr 2018).

34. Tanya B. Dorff et al, "Safety and Feasibility of Fasting in Combination with Platinum-Based Chemotherapy," *BMC Cancer* 16.360 (Jun 2016): 1–9. https://bmccancer.biomedcentral.com/articles/10.1186/s12885-016-2370-6 (accessed Apr 2018).

35. Min Wei et al, "Fasting-Mimicking Diet and Markers/Risk Factors for Aging, Diabetes, Cancer, and Cardiovascular Disease," *Science Translational Medicine* 9.377 (Feb 2017): eaai8700. https://www.ncbi.nlm.nih.gov/pubmed/28202779 (accessed Apr 2018).

CHAPTER 12: Let's Get Physical

1. Frank W. Booth, Christian K. Roberts, and Matthew J. Laye, "Lack of Exercise Is a Major Cause of Chronic Diseases," *Comprehensive Physiology* 2.2 (Jan 2012): 1143–211. https://www.ncbi.nlm.nih.gov/pmc/articles/PMC4241367/ (accessed Apr 2018).

2. National Cancer Institute, "Physical Activity and Cancer," *NIH* (Jan 2017). https://www.cancer.gov/about-cancer/causes-prevention/risk/obesity/physical-activity-fact-sheet (accessed Apr 2018).

3. L. Packer, "Oxidants, Antioxidant Nutrients and the Athlete," *Journal of Sports Science* 15.3 (Jun 1997): 353–63. https://www.ncbi.nlm.nih.gov/pubmed/9232561 (accessed Apr 2018).

4. Jake Emmett, "The Physiology of Marathon Running," *Marathon and Beyond* (2007). http://www.marathonandbeyond.com/choices/emmett.htm (accessed Apr 2018).

5. Roy J. Shephard and Pang N. Shek, "Potential Impact of Physical Activity and Sport on the Immune System—a Brief Review," *British Journal of Sports Medicine* 28.4 (Dec 1994): 247–55. https://www.ncbi.nlm.nih.gov/pubmed/7894956 (accessed Apr 2018).

6. Brett R. Gordon et al, "The Effects of Resistance Exercise Training on Anxiety: A Meta-Analysis and Meta-Regression Analysis of Randomized Controlled Trials," *Sports Medicine* 47.12 (Aug 2017): 2521–32. https://www.researchgate.net/publication/318102093_The_Effect_of_Resistance_Exercise_Training_on_Anxiety_Symptoms_A_Systematic_Review_and_Meta-Analysis (accessed Apr 2018).

7. R. Barrès et al, "Acute Exercise Remodels Promoter Methylation in Human Skeletal Muscle," *Cell Metabolism* 15.3 (Mar 2012): 405–11. https://www.ncbi.nlm.nih.gov/pubmed/22405075 (accessed Apr 2018).

8. Urho M. Kujala, "Relationship of Leisure-Time Physical Activity and Mortality: The Finnish Twin Cohort," *JAMA* 279.6 (Feb 1998): 440–44. https://www.ncbi.nlm.nih.gov/pubmed/9466636 (accessed Apr 2018).

9. John P. Pierce, "Greater Survival After Breast Cancer in Physically Active Women with High Vegetable-Fruit Intake Regardless of Obesity," *Journal of Clinical Oncology* 25.17 (Jun 2007): 2345–51. https://www.ncbi.nlm.nih.gov/pmc/articles/PMC2274898/ (accessed Apr 2018).

10. Christine Dethlefsen, "Exercise-Induced Catecholamines Activate the Hippo Tumor Suppressor Pathway to Reduce Risks of Breast Cancer Development," *Cancer Research* 77.18 (Sep 2017): 4894–904. http://cancerres.aacrjournals.org/content/early/2017/09/07/0008-5472.CAN-16-3125 (accessed Apr 2018).

11. Carlos A. Celis-Morales et al, "Association Between Active Commuting and Incident Cardiovascular Disease, Cancer, and Mortality: Prospective Cohort Study," *BMJ* 357 (Apr 2017): j1456. https://www.bmj.com/content/357/bmj.j1456 (accessed Apr 2018).

12. Stephanie E. Bonn et al, "Physical Activity and Survival Among Men Diagnosed with Prostate Cancer," *Cancer Epidemiology, Biomarkers & Prevention* 24.1 (Dec 2014): 57–64. http://cebp.aacrjournals.org/content/early/2014/11/26/1055-9965.EPI-14-0707 (accessed Apr 2018).

13. Hannah Arem et al, "Pre- and Postdiagnosis Physical Activity, Television Viewing, and Mortality Among Patients with Colorectal Cancer in the National Institutes of Health–AARP Diet and Health Study," *Journal of Clinical Oncology* 33.2 (Jan 2015): 180–88. https://www.ncbi.nlm.nih.gov/pmc/articles/PMC4279238/ (accessed Apr 2018).

14. Erin J. Howden et al, "Reversing the Cardiac Effects of Sedentary Aging in Middle Age—a Randomized Controlled Trial: Implications for Heart Failure Prevention," *Circulation* 137.14 (Jan 2018): 1–18. http://circ.ahajournals.org/content/early/2018/01/03/CIRCULATIONAHA.117.030617 (accessed Apr 2018).

15. Niharika Arora Duggal, "Major Features of Immunesenescence, Including Reduced Thymic Output, Are Ameliorated by High Levels of Physical Activity in Adulthood," *Aging Cell* 17.2 (Mar 2018): e12750. https://onlinelibrary.wiley.com/doi/full/10.1111/acel.12750 (accessed Apr 2018).

16. Margaret E. Sears, Kathleen J. Kerr, and Riina I. Bray, "Arsenic, Cadmium, Lead, and Mercury in Sweat: A Systematic Review," *Journal of Environmental and Public Health* 2012 (2012): 1–10. https://www.hindawi.com/journals/jeph/2012/184745/ (accessed Apr 2018).

17. H. G. Ainsleigh, "Beneficial Effects of Sun Exposure on Cancer Mortality," *Preventative Medicine* 22.1 (Jan 1993): 132–40. https://www.ncbi.nlm.nih.gov/pubmed/8475009 (accessed Apr 2018).

18. James L. Oschman, Gaétan Chevalier, and Richard Brown, "The Effects of Grounding (Earthing) on Inflammation, the Immune Response, Wound Healing, and Prevention and Treatment of Chronic Inflammatory and Autoimmune Diseases," *Journal of Inflammation Research* 8 (Mar 2015): 83–96. https://www.ncbi.nlm.nih.gov/pmc/articles/PMC4378297/ (accessed Apr 2018).

19. Q. Li et al, "Forest Bathing Enhances Human Natural Killer Activity and Expression of Anti-Cancer Proteins," *International Journal of Immunopathology and Pharmacology* 20.2 (Apr–Jun 2007): 3–8. https://www.ncbi.nlm.nih.gov/pubmed/17903349 (accessed Apr 2018).

20. Q. Li et al, "Acute Effects of Walking in Forest Environments on Cardiovascular and Metabolic Parameters," *European Journal of Applied Physiology* 111.11 (Nov 2011): 2845–53. https://www.ncbi.nlm.nih.gov/pubmed/21431424 (accessed Apr 2018).

21. Q. Li et al, "Effect of Phytoncide from Trees on Human Natural Killer Cell Function," *International Journal of Immunopathology and Pharmacology* 22.4 (Oct –Dec 2009): 951–59. https://www.ncbi.nlm.nih.gov/pubmed/20074458 (accessed Apr 2018).

22. Centers for Disease Control and Prevention, "1 in 3 Adults Don't Get Enough Sleep," *CDC* (reviewed Feb 2016). https://www.cdc.gov/media/releases/2016/p0215-enough-sleep.html (accessed Apr 2018).

23. Sheldon Cohen et al, "Sleep Habits and Susceptibility to the Common Cold," *Archives of Internal Medicine* 169.1 (Jan 2009): 62–67. https://www.ncbi.nlm .nih.gov/pmc/articles/PMC2629403/ (accessed Apr 2018).

24. Kenneth P. Wright, Jr. et al, "Entrainment of the Human Circadian Clock to the Natural Light-Dark Cycle," *Current Biology* 23.16 (Aug 2013): 1554–58. https://www.ncbi.nlm.nih.gov/pubmed/23910656 (accessed Apr 2018)

25. Ya Li et al, "Melatonin for the Prevention and Treatment of Cancer," *Oncotarget* 8.24 (Jun 2017): 39896–921. https://www.ncbi.nlm.nih.gov/pmc/ articles/PMC5503661/ (accessed Apr 2018).

26. M. Sánchez-Hidalgo et al, "Melatonin, a Natural Programmed Cell Death Inducer in Cancer," *Current Medicinal Chemistry* 19.22 (2012): 3805–21. https://www.ncbi.nlm.nih.gov/pubmed/22612707 (accessed Apr 2018).

27. Mariangela Rondanelli et al, "Update on the Role of Melatonin in the Prevention of Cancer Tumorigenesis and in the Management of Cancer Correlates, Such as Sleep-Wake and Mood Disturbances: Review and Remarks," *Aging Clinical and Experimental Research* 25.5 (Oct 2013): 499–510. https://www.ncbi.nlm.nih.gov/pubmed/24046037 (accessed Apr 2018).

28. Joshua J. Gooley et al, "Exposure to Room Light before Bedtime Suppresses Melatonin Onset and Shortens Melatonin Duration in Humans," *The Journal of Clinical Endocrinology & Metabolism* 96.3 (Mar 2011): E463–72. https:// academic.oup.com/jcem/article/96/3/E463/2597236 (accessed Apr 2018).

29. Shadab A. Rahman et al, "Circadian Phase Resetting by a Single Short-Duration Light Exposure," *JCI Insight* 2.7 (Apr 2017): e89494. https://www .ncbi.nlm.nih.gov/pmc/articles/PMC5374060 (accessed May 2018).

30. Eva S. Schernhammer and Susan E. Hankinson, "Urinary Melatonin Levels and Postmenopausal Breast Cancer Risk in the Nurses' Health Study Cohort," *Cancer Epidemiology, Biomarkers and Prevention* 18.1 (Jan 2009): 74–79. https:// www.ncbi.nlm.nih.gov/pmc/articles/PMC3036562/ (accessed Apr 2018).

31. Harvard Medical School, "Blue Light Has a Dark Side," *Harvard Health Publishing* (May 2012). https://www.health.harvard.edu/staying-healthy/ blue-light-has-a-dark-side (accessed Apr 2018).

32. Ariadna Garcia-Saenz et al, "Evaluating the Association between Artificial Light-at-Night Exposure and Breast and Prostate Cancer Risk in Spain (MCC-Spain Study)," *Environmental Health Perspectives* 126.4 (Apr 2018). https:// ehp.niehs.nih.gov/ehp1837 (accessed May 2018).

33. Alina Bradford, "How Blue LEDs Affect Sleep," *Live Science* (Feb 2016). https://www.livescience.com/53874-blue-light-sleep.html (accessed Apr 2018).

34. J. Kliukiene, T. Tynes, and A. Andersen, "Risk of Breast Cancer Among Norwegian Women with Visual Impairment," *British Journal of Cancer* 84.3 (Feb 2001): 397–99. https://www.ncbi.nlm.nih.gov/pmc/articles/ PMC2363754/ (accessed Apr 2018).

35. "Melatonin Drug Interactions," *Drugs.com* (updated Mar 2018). https://www
    .drugs.com/drug-interactions/melatonin.html (accessed Apr 2018).

36. Ye-min Wang et al,"The Efficacy and Safety of Melatonin in Concurrent
    Chemotherapy or Radiotherapy for Solid Tumors: A Meta-Analysis of
    Randomized Controlled Trials," *Cancer Chemotherapy and Pharmacology* 69.5
    (May 2012): 1213–20. https://www.ncbi.nlm.nih.gov/pubmed/22271210
    (accessed Apr 2018).

37. Jane Brody, "Cheating Ourselves of Sleep," *New York Times* (Jun 2013).
    https://well.blogs.nytimes.com/2013/06/17/cheating-ourselves-of-sleep/
    (accessed Apr 2018).

38. Cheryl L. Thompson et al, "Short Duration of Sleep Increases Risk of
    Colorectal Adenoma,"" *Cancer* 117.4 (Feb 2011): 841–47. https://www.ncbi
    .nlm.nih.gov/pmc/articles/PMC3021092/ (accessed Apr 2018).

39. Claudia Trudel-Fitzgerald et al, "Sleep and Survival Among Women with
    Breast Cancer: 30 Years of Follow-up within the Nurses' Health Study," *British
    Journal of Cancer* 116 (Apr 2017): 1239–46. https://www.ncbi.nlm.nih.gov/
    pubmed/28359077 (accessed Apr 2018).

40. Dave Levitan, "Longer Sleep Linked to Increased Mortality Risk in Breast
    Cancer," *Cancer Network* (Apr 2017). http://www.cancernetwork.com/breast
    -cancer/longer-sleep-linked-increased-mortality-risk-breast-cancer (accessed
    Apr 2018).

41. Fahed Hakim et al, "Fragmented Sleep Accelerates Tumor Growth and
    Progression Through Recruitment of Tumor-Associated Macrophages and
    TLR4 Signaling," *Cancer Research* 74.5 (Mar 2014): 1329–37. https://www
    .ncbi.nlm.nih.gov/pmc/articles/PMC4247537/ (accessed Apr 2018).

42. Daniel F. Kripke, "Hypnotic Drug Risks of Mortality, Infection, Depression,
    and Cancer: But Lack of Benefit," *F1000Research* 5 (May 2016): 918. https://
    www.ncbi.nlm.nih.gov/pmc/articles/PMC4890308/ (accessed Apr 2018).

43. Lisa M. Wu et al, "The Effect of Systematic Light Exposure on Sleep in a
    Mixed Group of Fatigued Cancer Survivors," *Journal of Clinical Sleep Medicine*
    14.1 (Jan 2017): 31–39. https://www.ncbi.nlm.nih.gov/pmc/articles/
    PMC5734890/ (accessed Apr 2018).

44. Lisa Rapaport, "Bright Light Therapy May Help Fatigued Cancer Survivors
    Sleep Better," *Reuters* (2017). https://www.reuters.com/article/us-health
    -cancer-sleep/bright-light-therapy-may-help-fatigued-cancer-survivors-sleep
    -better-idUSKBN1FF2QY (accessed Apr 2018).

45. U.S. Department of Health and Human Services, "How Sleep Clears the
    Brain," *NIH* (Oct 2013). https://www.nih.gov/news-events/nih-research
    -matters/how-sleep-clears-brain (accessed Apr 2018).

46. Catherine R. Marinac et al, "Prolonged Nightly Fasting and Breast Cancer
    Prognosis," *JAMA Oncology* 2.8 (Aug 2016): 1049–55. https://www.ncbi.nlm
    .nih.gov/pmc/articles/PMC4982776/ (accessed Apr 2018).

CHAPTER 13: Under Pressure

1. Sazzad Hassan et al, "Behavioral Stress Accelerates Prostate Cancer Development in Mice," *The Journal of Clinical Investigation* 123.2 (Feb 2013): 874–86. https://www.ncbi.nlm.nih.gov/pmc/articles/PMC3561807/ (accessed Apr 2018).

2. Caroline P. Le et al, "Chronic Stress in Mice Remodels Lymph Vasculature to Promote Tumour Cell Dissemination," *Nature Communications* 7 (Mar 2016): 10634. https://www.ncbi.nlm.nih.gov/pmc/articles/PMC4773495/ (accessed Apr 2018).

3. Alice Donaldson, "Stress Can Allow Cancer to Spread Faster Through the Body, New Research on Mice Shows," *ABC News* (Jun 2016). http://www.abc.net.au/news/2016-06-28/stress-can-speed-up-spread-of-cancer-in-body-scientists-say/7548024 (accessed Apr 2018).

4. Ohio State University, "The Stress and Cancer Link: 'Master-Switch' Stress Gene Enables Cancer's Spread," *ScienceDaily* (Aug 2013). www.sciencedaily.com/releases/2013/08/130822194143.htm (accessed Apr 2018).

5. L. S. Berk et al, "Modulation of Neuroimmune Parameters During the Eustress of Humor-Associated Mirthful Laughter," *Alternative Therapies in Health and Medicine* 7.2 (Mar 2001): 62–72, 74–76. https://www.ncbi.nlm.nih.gov/pubmed/11253418 (accessed May 2018).

6. Daisy Fancourt et al, "Singing Modulates Mood, Stress, Cortisol, Cytokine and Neuropeptide Activity in Cancer Patients and Carers," *Ecancermedicalscience* 10 (Apr 2016): 631. https://www.ncbi.nlm.nih.gov/pmc/articles/PMC4854222/ (accessed Apr 2018).

CHAPTER 14: Spiritual Healing

1. W. A. Brown, "Expectation, the Placebo Effect and the Response to Treatment," *Rhode Island Medical Journal* 98.5 (May 2015): 19–21. https://www.ncbi.nlm.nih.gov/pubmed/25938400 (accessed May 2018).

2. K. Wartolowska et al, "Use of Placebo Controls in the Evaluation of Surgery: Systematic Review," *BMJ* 348 (May 2014): g3253. https://www.ncbi.nlm.nih.gov/pubmed/24850821 (accessed May 2018).

INDEX

Index

ACKNOWLEDGMENTS

THIS BOOK TOOK ME MANY YEARS, much longer than it should have, because I am an excellent procrastinator and prefer sprints over marathons. A finished book might be my biggest miracle of all.

Thank you to all of the amazing death-defying cancer survivors, integrative medical doctors, and holistic healers I have ever interviewed. You have taught me so much about health and healing and you inspire me every day.

While writing this book, before I had an agent (still don't) or a publisher, I had a dream, a vision, a premonition, a prophecy—I don't know what to call it—that I would not have to play the traditional publishing game, i.e., convincing an agent to represent me and convincing a publisher to publish my book. I sensed that the perfect publisher would come to me at the perfect time. And that is exactly what happened. Thank you Liana Werner-Gray. You were instrumental in that perfect timing.

Thank you to Perry Wilson for introducing me to Howie Klausner. Thank you to Howie for introducing me to Matt West. Thank you to Matt West, for taking my sprawling mess of a manuscript, dissecting it piece by piece, and helping me develop it into something that actually resembled a book. You saw the forest for the trees. You have an amazing gift, my brother.

To my Hay House Family. Thank you to Reid Tracy and Patty Gift at Hay House for believing in me and my message and for publishing this book! Thank you to my editor, Lisa Cheng, for your enthusiastic support and gracious encouragement in the refinement process. And to everyone else at Hay House—thank you for all the work you did behind the scenes to bring this baby to life.

Thank you to Rev. George Malkmus, Dr. Richard Schulze, Dr. Lorraine Day, Anne and David Frahm, Dr. Hulda Clark, and Dr. Max Gerson. Your books and tapes were all I had in the beginning, and they gave me the courage to step out into the unknown and start my healing adventure. I stand on your shoulders. Thank you to John Smothers and the late Roy Page, M.D., your support meant the world to me in my darkest hour.

Thank you to Dr. Michael Greger at nutritionfacts.org. Your commitment to bring evidence-based nutritional science to the masses has had a profound impact on my life and my work, including the content of this book, and is changing the world.

To my dear friends in the health and wellness world who have helped me reach more people, Ty and Charlene Bollinger, Kevin Gianni, Robyn Openshaw, Dr. Eric Zielinski, John Robbins, Ocean Robbins, Dr. Kelly Turner, James Colquhoun, and so many others—thank you.

To Mark Rogers, I am grateful for your friendship and partnership in helping me share the SQUARE ONE Program with hundreds of thousands of people around the world. If we ever meet in person, it's going to be weird for me.

To my family, Mom and Dad, David and Catharine Wark, for loving me unconditionally, always supporting me, and believing in me when I didn't believe in myself. To my sister, Lindsay Bean, and my drummer/brother-in-law/best man Brad Bean, and to my wonderful in-laws, Ernie and Lynn, Kathy, Donna, Ashley and Josh, Beth and Jeremy, David and Liza, Meredith and Alan, Rob, Melody, Lucas, Meryl, and all of your significant others, thank you for graciously adopting me into your big fun family. Thank you for your prayers. I love you all so much. Aunt Connie, you are dearly missed.

Acknowledgments

To my beautiful and brilliant daughters, Marin and Mackenzie, you bring me so much joy. I am so proud of you both. I am blessed beyond words to be your dad and to be alive to watch you grow up. You make me a rich man.

And to the love of my life, my dream girl and wonderful wife, Micah. Twenty-two years and counting! Thank you for loving me, accepting me for who I am, sticking with me when I was sick and broke, and for putting up with me and all my crazy health obsessions over the years. See, it was worth it! We've weathered the storm and created an amazing life and family together. I love you with all my heart, and I can't imagine life without you. Let's grow old together and die at the same time.

And finally, a massive thank-you to you, my friends, fans, followers, and readers. Without your support, I would have not been able to sustain this mission. I measure my success not by the number of dollars I make, or the number of books I sell, but by the number of people I'm able to encourage, inspire, inform, empower, and ultimately save. You all have been instrumental in my success. Thank you for helping me spread the message of hope—that cancer can be healed.

ABOUT
THE AUTHOR

CHRIS WARK is an author, speaker, patient advocate, and wellness crusader. He was diagnosed with stage III colon cancer in 2003 at 26 years old. He had surgery, but instead of chemotherapy, he used nutrition and natural therapies to heal himself. Chris has made many appearances on radio and television and was featured in the award-winning documentary film *The C Word*. Chris inspires countless people to take control of their health and reverse disease with a radical transformation of diet and lifestyle. You can visit him online at www.chrisbeatcancer.com.

We hope you enjoyed this Hay House book. If you'd like to receive
our online catalog featuring additional information on Hay House
books and products, or if you'd like to find out more about the
Hay Foundation, please contact:

Hay House, Inc., P.O. Box 5100, Carlsbad, CA 92018-5100
(760) 431-7695 or (800) 654-5126
(760) 431-6948 (fax) or (800) 650-5115 (fax)
www.hayhouse.com® • www.hayfoundation.org

———

Published in Australia by:
Hay House Australia Pty. Ltd., 18/36 Ralph St., Alexandria NSW 2015
Phone: 612-9669-4299 • *Fax:* 612-9669-4144 • www.hayhouse.com.au

Published in the United Kingdom by:
Hay House UK, Ltd., Astley House, 33 Notting Hill Gate, London W11 3JQ
Phone: 44-20-3675-2450 • *Fax:* 44-20-3675-2451 • www.hayhouse.co.uk

Published in India by: Hay House Publishers India,
Muskaan Complex, Plot No. 3, B-2, Vasant Kunj, New Delhi 110 070
Phone: 91-11-4176-1620 • *Fax:* 91-11-4176-1630 • www.hayhouse.co.in

———

Access New Knowledge.
Anytime. Anywhere.

Learn and evolve at your own pace
with the world's leading experts.

www.hayhouseU.com

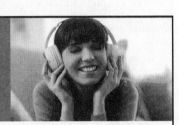

Hay House Podcasts
Bring Fresh, Free Inspiration Each Week!

Hay House Meditations Podcast

Features your favorite Hay House authors guiding you through meditations designed to help you relax and rejuvenate. Take their words into your soul and cruise through the week!

Dr. Wayne W. Dyer Podcast

Discover the timeless wisdom of Dr. Wayne W. Dyer, world-renowned spiritual teacher and affectionately known as "the father of motivation." Each week brings some of the best selections from the 10-year span of Dr. Dyer's talk show on HayHouseRadio.com.

Hay House World Summit Podcast

Over 1 million people from 217 countries and territories participate in the massive online event known as the Hay House World Summit. This podcast offers weekly mini-lessons from World Summits past as a taste of what you can hear during the annual event, which occurs each May.

Hay House Radio Podcast

Listen to some of the best moments from HayHouseRadio.com, featuring expert authors such as Dr. Christiane Northrup, Anthony William, Caroline Myss, James Van Praagh, and Doreen Virtue discussing topics such as health, self-healing, motivation, spirituality, positive psychology, and personal development.

Hay House Live Podcast

Enjoy a selection of insightful and inspiring lectures from Hay House Live, an exciting event series that features Hay House authors and leading experts in the fields of alternative health, nutrition, intuitive medicine, success, and more! Feel the electricity of our authors engaging with a live audience, and get motivated to live your best life possible!

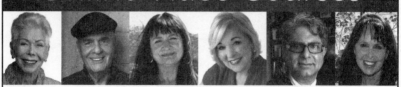

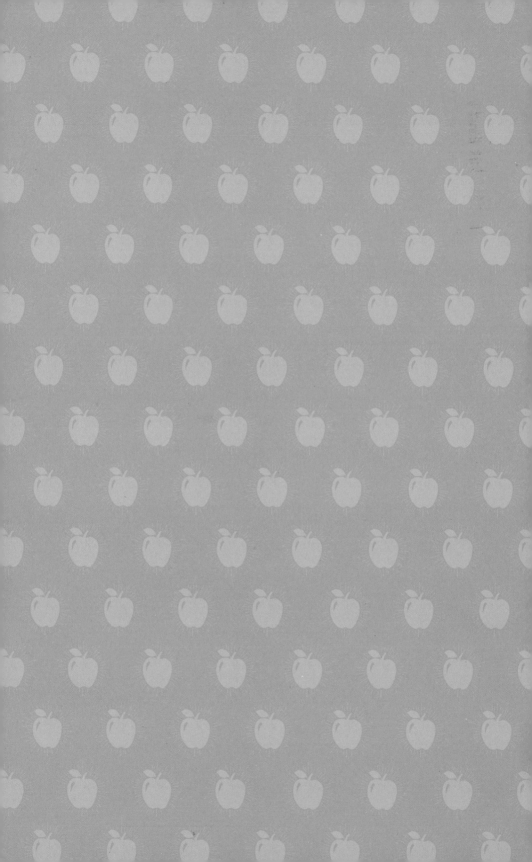

Nation on the Take

BOOKS BY WENDELL POTTER

Deadly Spin: An Insurance Company Insider Speaks Out on How Corporate PR Is Killing Health Care and Deceiving Americans

Obamacare: What's in It for Me?

Nation on the Take

*How Big Money Corrupts Our Democracy and
What We Can Do About It*

WENDELL POTTER AND
NICK PENNIMAN

BLOOMSBURY PRESS

NEW YORK · LONDON · OXFORD · NEW DELHI · SYDNEY

Bloomsbury Press
An imprint of Bloomsbury Publishing Plc

1385 Broadway	50 Bedford Square
New York	London
NY 10018	WC1B 3DP
USA	UK

www.bloomsbury.com

BLOOMSBURY and the Diana logo are trademarks of Bloomsbury Publishing Plc

First published 2016

ISBN: HB: 978-1-63286-109-2
        ePub: 978-1-63286-110-8

Library of Congress Cataloging-in-Publication Data has been applied for.

2 4 6 8 10 9 7 5 3 1

Typeset by RefineCatch Limited, Bungay, Suffolk
Printed and bound in USA by Berryville Graphics Inc., Berryville, Virginia

To find out more about our authors and books visit www.bloomsbury.com. Here you will
find extracts, author interviews, details of forthcoming events and the option to sign up for
our newsletters.

Bloomsbury books may be purchased for business or promotional use. For information on
bulk purchases please contact Macmillan Corporate and Premium Sales Department at
specialmarkets@macmillan.com.

To our dear families, and the country we all love.
And in loving memory of Emily Jacqueline Potter.

Contents

Preface

We were drawn to collaborate on this book out of a common sense of love and heartbreak. Love for our country, heartbreak for what is happening to it. We suspect that most people feel the same way, perhaps many for the same reasons.

Our grand 240-year-old project of self-government has been derailed, replaced by a coin-operated system that mainly favors those who can pay to play.

This is not what our American predecessors bled for, not just during the Revolution but during other wars, as well as during many moments of protest and resistance.

We hope *Nation on the Take* will be seen as the most comprehensive guide to this critical issue for years to come. Part 1 presents the big picture and traces the history of the problem. Part 2 connects the dots to show how the hijacking of policy and politics has significant downstream effects on us all. Then part 3 discusses solutions and how to encourage a new kind of movement to get those solutions passed into laws.

Throughout, we provide graphs and charts and believe that we've written in a way that avoids esoteric references. We have set out to explain and expose this crucial problem in straightforward terms, to revive our imaginations about what our democratic republic can be, and to describe how we can all come together to renew it. In this era of intense political polarization, doing so may serve to bring us together in surprisingly powerful ways.

Both of us have reported on government and politics at different times in our careers. As a young reporter in Washington, D.C., during the 1970s, Wendell covered national politics when Gerald Ford and Jimmy Carter were in the White House and congressional leaders included Senate Minority Leader Howard Baker from Wendell's home state of Tennessee. It was a time when there were far fewer lobbyists on Capitol Hill and when the vast majority of campaign contributions came from people who could actually vote for the candidates they supported. Political Action Committees existed but played relatively minor roles. There was no such thing as a super PAC. Corporations were not considered people, and millionaires and billionaires contributed relatively little to campaigns.

Wendell's longer career, after he left Scripps-Howard's Washington bureau, was in corporate public affairs. Among his responsibilities at Cigna, where he served as head of corporate communications until he left in 2008, was administering the company's PAC and coordinating efforts with the industry's lobbyists. He had firsthand knowledge of how huge corporations had become political power brokers and how they were able to deploy cash very strategically to influence both elections and public policy with the goals of rigging the rules for their own self-interests.

When Wendell left his job after a crisis of conscience, which was described in his first book, *Deadly Spin*, he played a key role in the debate to reform the U.S. health care system, testifying before several congressional committees. During one hearing he told lawmakers that if they caved to pressure from insurance industry lobbyists they might as well call their bill, "The Health Insurance Industry Profit Protection and Enhancement Act."

It turned out to be a prescient warning. As Wendell has written in his columns for numerous media outlets, among the biggest winners after the reform dust had settled were insurance companies. The share prices of the largest investor-owned insurers have more than tripled—and in some cases have more than quadrupled—since President Obama signed the Affordable Care Act into law in 2010.

It's not that the sponsors of the reform law wanted to kowtow to the special interests. They had no choice. Legislators knew that even modest reforms could not be enacted unless they had first made certain that their bill would get a thumbs-up from the corporate and trade-association lobbyists.

That remarkable ability for a small group of people to bend the levers of power is what drew Nick to this cause, too. For more than a decade, working as a journalist and magazine publisher in D.C., Nick saw how great ideas never got a hearing, not because they lacked public support, but because they lacked the support of well-financed special interests. We, the people, he concluded, know how to fix many of the problems before us; we just don't have the power to do what we know.

Most recently, he helped launch an investigative reporting project that focused on the aftermath of the financial meltdown and the battle inside Washington to rein in Wall Street. Witnessing the failed attempts by good people to create a stable and sane financial system was akin to the profound frustration that many recovering stroke victims must feel: the ideas and desires are in the head, but it's nearly impossible to move the mouth or limbs.

It's time to end the paralysis, not just for the sake of legislating solutions, but also for the sake of reviving our faith in this remarkable country.

We believe we have written a book grounded in common sense and fueled by a sense of patriotism. We hope you'll find it not just useful but energizing.

PART 1

INTRODUCTION

America is a dream.
The poet says it was promises.
The people say it is promises—that will come true.
—LANGSTON HUGHES, "FREEDOM'S PLOW"

Our country is indeed a dream—a dream created during a period of time known as the American Enlightenment, which came to a focal point during the American Revolution and lasted until the early nineteenth century.

The leading political thinkers of the day were the ones we know so well: Thomas Jefferson, John Adams, James Madison, Thomas Paine, George Mason, Alexander Hamilton, Benjamin Franklin. Their dream was to create a democratic republic, in which ultimate power rested with the citizens. Just after the Declaration of Independence asserts the unalienable rights to "life, liberty and the pursuit of happiness," it states:

> That to secure these rights, governments are instituted among
> Men, deriving their just powers from the consent of the governed,
> That whenever any Form of Government becomes destructive of
> these ends, it is the Right of the People to alter or to abolish it,
> and to institute new Government, laying its foundation on such

principles and organizing its powers in such form, as to them
shall seem most likely to effect their Safety and Happiness.

They knew that self-government would be messy and inefficient at times,
but they had faith that common ground would be regularly found and
that people would slowly but surely build a better nation together. As
Jefferson said: "Sometimes it is said that man cannot be trusted with the
government of himself. Can he, then, be trusted with the government of
others? Or have we found angels in the form of kings to govern him? Let
history answer this question."

In addition to the Declaration of Independence, the Constitution of
the Commonwealth of Massachusetts is a shining example of the idealism
that defined the era. Ratified in 1780, it is thought to be the world's oldest
still-functioning written constitution. Drafted in part by John Adams, it
inspired and informed the U.S. Constitution, forged seven years later.
Part I, Article VII, of the Massachusetts charter reads: "Government is
instituted for the common good; for the protection, safety, prosperity,
and happiness of the people; and not for the profit, honor, or private
interest of any one man, family, or class of men; therefore, the people
alone have an incontestable, unalienable, and indefeasible right to institute government; and to reform, alter, or totally change the same, when
their protection, safety, prosperity, and happiness require it."

Government for the common good, not for the "profit, honor, or
private interest of any one man, family, or class of men."

Those words don't seem to ring true today. Not just for those who
follow politics, but for all of us. A profound shift has occurred—one that,
perhaps because it has occurred slowly, has yet to fully register as the
serious crisis it is. But it has by no means gone unnoticed.

A few years ago, CBS News conducted a poll about Americans' percep-
tion of government. The headline of the resulting story they published:
ALIENATED NATION: AMERICANS COMPLAIN OF GOVERNMENT DISCON-
NECT. The first sentence reads: "Americans see their leaders in Washington
as overpaid agents of wealthy individuals and corporations who are
largely disconnected from the concerns of average Americans."

We, the people, are losing our faith in the dream of democracy. As our
collective power is increasingly eclipsed by a rigged system of politics and
governance dominated by a handful of billionaires and a phalanx of well-
financed special interests, we are growing skeptical that the promises will
come true.

Right now there is no credible outside threat to our American way of life. No other nation is sounding the death knell of ours. But the rapid proliferation of a system akin to oligarchy—within our own country—threatens to cripple our march forward.

It's a threat the Founding Fathers knew we would always have to guard against. In the summer of 1787, when delegates to the Constitutional Convention were in the heat of their debates, they were obsessed with bribery, influence, and corruption. James Madison, who kept meticulous notes, recorded the word "corruption" fifty-four times. To them, the notion of corruption was both the corruption of the individual and the corruption of the system of governance. They were less obsessed with corrupt individuals—with bad apples—than with the system itself, with the orchard. The rotting of the fruit of liberty was seen as the dominance of private interests over the public interest. It was the bending of governing priorities away from the common good—a process that would, over time, fatally damage the whole project of a democratic republic—of "We, the people," of the "consent of the governed."

Seen in this light, government is us. Or it should be. We give our government our money, in the form of taxes. Then we hire its executives, through elections. Then we imbue it with directions and instructions, in the form of legislation. If all goes well, our politicians utilize our tax dollars to manifest our brightest ideas. The most exquisite dynamic is achieved when the common good is served while individual liberty is protected. No kings, no dictators. Us, in charge of ourselves, leveraging our resources behind our highest hopes, while protecting each other's freedoms, shaping our country, forever working to form "a more perfect union."

Yes, of course: there were—and always will be—bad people and bad pieces of legislation. The factions and special interests will fight for their legislative handouts and carve-outs, and politicians will lose their virtue. Corrupt moments in our future are inevitable.

And, of course, for centuries, women, people of color, and nonland-owners were legally excluded from voting and running for office. But powerful, popular grassroots movements like suffrage, abolition, and civil rights—fueled by the early American Enlightenment's dreams of liberation and equality—forced profound course corrections that are among this country's greatest accomplishments, not just for United States citizens but for humankind.

Today we all seem to feel as if we need another such profound course correction, one that is focused on reclaiming our right to self-government and renewing our hope in the American dream. Correctly, we suspect that the system is rigged, our government has become coin-operated, and that we've been sidelined.

Obviously, money's dominance of politics and governing isn't the only factor behind the dysfunction of our democracy. Gerrymandered congressional districts, presidential elections entirely focused on a handful of states, low voter-turnout rates, petty and polarized political parties, superficial and partisan media, and an increasingly rude public arena all contribute to the breakdown of our ability to govern together. But Big Money makes a lot of these factors worse, and it's time for the political class—which has grown way too cozy with the status quo—to step out of its elite bubble and recognize that the crisis we are in is eating away at the country.

In 1998, the total amount of money spent on federal elections was $1.6 billion. By 2012, it had nearly quadrupled to $6.2 billion.

The Supreme Court's 2010 *Citizens United* ruling was akin to crop-spraying gasoline onto a wildfire. In a narrow 5–4 decision, the majority of justices asserted that corporate spending in politics is an act of free

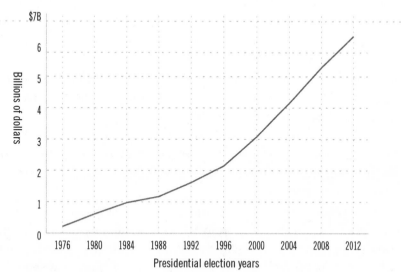

Increasing Cost of Elections
Sources: Federal Election Commission, Center for Responsive Politics, Campaign Finance Institute
Methodology: *Nominal dollars. Includes spending by presidential, Senate and House candidates, political party spending, outside groups' independent expenditures.

speech and should therefore be unlimited. Subsequent lower court rulings have expanded that rationale to reduce some limits on political campaign contributions, which has put the chase for political money on steroids.

At times, the news seems almost surreal. Take for instance, how a single family—the Kochs—which owns Koch Industries, has forged a small but very wealthy network of donors who have pledged to spend nearly $900 million influencing the outcome of the 2016 elections. That's $500 million more than the Republican National Committee spent in 2012.

WHERE THE MONEY IS SPENT

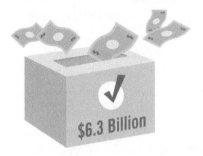

Total Spending in 2012 Election **$6,285,557,223**

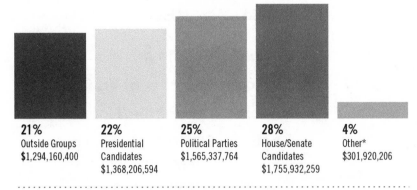

21%	22%	25%	28%	4%
Outside Groups	Presidential	Political Parties	House/Senate	Other*
$1,294,160,400	Candidates	$1,565,337,764	Candidates	$301,920,206
	$1,368,206,594		$1,755,932,259	

Source: Center for Responsive Politics (opensecrets.org)
Methodology: *FEC convention outlays, delegate candidate spending, etc.

Where the Money is Spent
Source: Center for Responsive Politics (opensecrets.org)
Methodology: *Nominal dollars. Category spending in graphic doesn't equal total election spending because political conventions, PAC overhead money left out.

On the other side of the Big Money equation—the fundraising side—
the nonstop scramble for campaign cash is distracting and exhausting
our elected officials as never before, and perpetually repelling good people
from office. Members of Congress simply don't spend as much time
thinking about us as they once did. They spend most of their time
thinking about how to get enough money from wealthy individuals,
lobbyists, and political action committees to get reelected—it's what
political operatives refer to as a "permanent campaign" mentality.

In January 2013, newly elected Democrats in the House of Representatives
were being given an orientation session by the Democratic Congressional
Campaign Committee about how they should spend their time serving in
the House—what was once referred to as the "People's House." Among the
materials they were presented with was a "model daily schedule." That
schedule provided for four hours of "call time," one to two hours of
"constituent visits," two hours of committee hearings or floor votes, one
hour of "strategic outreach," and one hour of "recharge time." You have no
doubt already guessed what "call time" and "strategic outreach" are: fundraising. Which means that new representatives are expected to spend half
of their time either dialing for dollars or attending fundraising events.

Who are they calling? Probably not you. Certainly not us. Mostly, very
wealthy donors in the richest cities in America. And who's throwing the

MODEL DAILY SCHEDULE - DC

- ☑ **4 hours** **Call Time**
- ☑ **1-2 hours** **Constituent Visits**
- ☑ **2 hours*** **Committee/Floor**
- ☑ **1 hour** **Strategic Outreach**
  Breakfasts, Meet & Greets, Press
- ☑ **1 hour** **Recharge Time**

*How Members Spend their Time: How House Democrats were told they should
spend their time in Washington*
Source: PowerPoint delivered by the House Democrats' campaign committee,
2013, obtained by the *Huffington Post*.

daily fundraisers for them? Often, the very industries they are supposed to be regulating, based on their congressional committee assignments. The Finance Committee members rake in contributions from the bankers and their lobbyists, the Natural Resources Committee members from the oil and coal executives and their lobbyists. That's why these types of committees on Capitol Hill are referred to as "cash committees." In 2014, for instance, the top industries contributing to members of the House Financial Services Committee, formerly known as the Banking Committee, were finance, insurance, and real estate. Individuals and PACs from those sectors collectively chipped $30 million dollars into the committee members' coffers.

As Ray Plank, the former founder and chairman of the Apache Corporation, told the conservative journalist Peter Schweizer, whose book *Extortion* was later turned into a *60 Minutes* episode, campaign cash and corporate contracts with well-connected lobbying firms are "protection money. It's what you expect from the mafia."

Yet, in Washington and the state capitals, such activity is not seen as mafia-like. It's run-of-the-mill. It's the way things get done. Anyone who questions it, or wants to change it, is deemed naïve or—even worse!— idealistic.

And it's done in broad daylight. Although an estimated 5 to 10 percent of money in the political system is what's called "dark money," which is much harder to trace, all of the direct contributions to politicians' campaigns, all of the PAC and superPAC money, and the large checks to the political parties are disclosed. They're not disclosed in real time, which is one of the commonsense reforms that need to be passed. But otherwise you can track 95 percent of the money in the system and pretty easily deduce who's likely feeling beholden to whom.

One of the many pernicious effects of this endless extraction of campaign cash from lobbyists and wealthy individuals is that politicians have little time to form strong relationships with one another, particularly across the aisle. For all of the newspaper editorials and Press Club forums about gridlock, partisanship, and polarization in Washington, and all the appeals to politicians to get along, too little attention is paid to whether they have time to get along. When announcing in early 2013 that he wouldn't be seeking reelection in 2014, Senator Tom Harkin (D-IA) remarked, "The time is so consumed with raising money now, these campaigns, that you don't have the time for the kind of personal relationships [between lawmakers] that so many of us built up over time."

Our legislators—our employees, remember—also have less time to draft, study, or pass legislation. The more than nine thousand registered lobbyists in D.C. are keenly aware of this vulnerability, and they are poised to take advantage of it. Collectively, they annually disclose more than $3 billion in expenses—including the many events they hold for members of Congress. The nonprofit transparency group the Sunlight Foundation tracks categories of influence peddling. One category is called "Hill coverage," which is defined as the "average percentage of incumbent members of Congress receiving contributions from the organization over the course of the 2008, 2010 and 2012 election cycles." AT&T, for instance, has 88 percent Hill coverage—meaning that 88 percent of members of Congress have received contributions from AT&T sources. Honeywell International also has 88 percent coverage. United Parcel Service has 87 percent. Lockheed Martin has 80 percent. Comcast, General Electric, Boeing, and Verizon all have around 70 percent.

How much coverage do you have? How much coverage do we, the people, have? How much do Main Street businesspeople have? How much attention do people who have little or no money get in such a system? We know that the banks wield enormous power over politics and policy decisions in D.C. But who's representing the families facing foreclosure? As Bob Dole once famously quipped: "There is no poor people's political action committee."

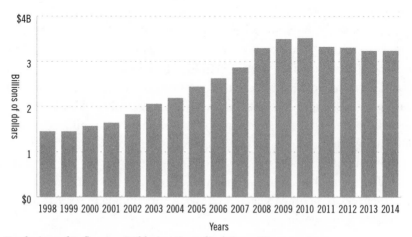

Explosion of Influence: Lobbying Spending Over Time
Source: Source: Center for Responsive Politics (opensecrets.org)
Methodology: *Nominal dollars. Includes federal spending data only.

There are also few members of Congress who, upon leaving the Hill, have any interest in starting a poor people's political action committee. In 1974, around 3 percent of former members became lobbyists. Now, half of them pass through Washington's "revolving door" and stroll from the Hill down to K Street, many of them to lobby for the industries they once oversaw, based on their congressional committee assignments. Served on the Finance Committee? Become a bank lobbyist. As the *New York Times*'s Mark Leibovich observed: "In some sense, [they are] living proof of the thing that most voters loathe about Washington: the notion that membership in its political class guarantees a win-for-life lottery ticket."

Throughout this book, we will talk about both lobbying and campaign contributions and expenditures. Big Money is both. And well-financed special and corporate interests deploy both as a means of bending the apparatus in Washington and the state capitals to their will. It's worth pointing out early in the book that large corporations—along with wealthy corporate executives and the lobbyists the corporations hire—really dominate the game. Yes, unions play the game, and any meaningful reforms of the system should include them. Just look at the inability to accomplish meaningful education reforms. But in 2014, as an example, business interests outspent union interests 15 to 1.[1]

It's also important to point out early on that lobbying in its purest form is not bad. Making arguments to members of Congress is part of the democratic process. Sharing information and expertise is a good thing. It's a form of free speech, and a healthy democracy should have plenty of lobbying going on, as long as it is occurring on behalf of *all* sides of an issue. Our concerns about lobbying involve the relationship between lobbying and political cash, the lobbyists who have little or no fealty to the broader public interest, and those politicians or Hill staffers who see public office as a pathway to a lucrative influence-peddling career. We are also disgusted by lobbying groups that knowingly leverage millions of dollars into false and misleading communications campaigns, which destroy the possibility of having a thoughtful, genuine debate about weighty policy ideas.

Stanley Collender, who has had extensive experience on Capitol Hill and in the private sector, is widely considered to be one of the leading experts on U.S. budget policy. He remembers when the lightbulb went on for corporate lobbyists. In a piece titled "How Big Money Corrupts the Budget," published by the *Democracy Journal*, he chronicles one of the most crucial moments in the saga of American politics and money.

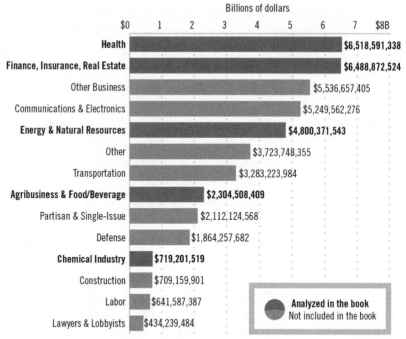

Where the Money Comes From: Lobbying Expenditures
Source: Center for Responsive Politics (opensecrets. org), authors' analysis (1998 to first quarter 2015).

In 1975, the Democratic Senate Budget Committee chairman, Ed Muskie, from Maine, successfully led a charge against a defense authorization bill. At the time, Collender was an intern for the committee. It was customary for defense authorization bills coming out of the powerful Armed Services Committee to become law without being challenged. But Muskie saw an opportunity to bring more scrutiny to the budget process. According to Collender,

> That was the moment when lobbyists discovered the congressional budget process. It was also the moment when budget committee decisions free of lobbyist influence ended and action on the deficit, debt and federal priorities started to be determined more by those who could devote resources to getting what they wanted than by national need and appropriate fiscal policy.

Let's pause for a moment on that last part of that sentence: *more by those who could devote resources to getting what they wanted than by national need and appropriate fiscal policy*. If it is functioning well, our country's project in self-government would be mainly driven by, among other virtuous objectives, *national need* and *appropriate fiscal policy*. We would not only know the right policies to enact—we would also enact them. But when government is coin operated—when America becomes a nation on the take—the nation's needs get shoved aside like neglected children.

Which brings up another crucial link that isn't discussed often enough: Although the system creates special economic benefits for those who can pay to play, the overall well-being of the economy does not necessarily improve. For too long, campaign finance reform has been viewed as an "anti-corporate" cause. Instead, it should be seen, in part, as pro competition and anti-cronyism.

Luigi Zingales, a conservative economist at the University of Chicago Business School and author of *A Capitalism for the People*, compellingly documents how the system of lobbying and legislative favors is dangerously reducing economic competitiveness and opportunity. He writes:

> American capitalism . . . grew in a unique incubator that provided it with a distinct flavor of competitiveness, a meritocratic nature that fostered trust in markets and a faith in mobility. Lately, however, that trust has been eroded by a betrayal of our pro-business elites, whose lobbying has come to dictate the market rather than be subject to it, and this betrayal has taken place with the complicity of our intellectual class.

Who suffers from this betrayal? Consumers (you and us), small- and medium-sized business owners, big corporations whose lobbyists get beat by their competitors' lobbyists, and entrepreneurs—that is, nearly everyone. As John Arensmeyer, the founder of the group Small Business Majority, said: "With the *Citizens United* decision, the political system has become even more stacked against the interests of small firms. Small businesses end up paying the price for big money politics that allow large firms to secure special perks and advantages over their smaller, less politically connected competitors."

You see, wherever you are, and whatever you do, whether you love politics or hate politics, whether you devour news or never look at the news, whether you see yourself as an environmentalist or a business leader (or both), as a conservative or a liberal, every moment of your life is being affected by the system of Big Money.

Imagine a baby named Eve, born this morning in a hospital whose regulations—medical equipment, pharmaceuticals, staff training, and certification—were partly created by the system.

Little Eve will ride home tonight in a car that was engineered by the system as much as it was by engineers. The mileage it gets, how safe it is, the materials it's made of, what goes into the gas tank, how it's taxed, what comes out of the tailpipe.

Eve will arrive at a home built to standards established, in part, by the system. Lobbyists, trade groups, phony "citizens" groups and corporate executives have waged massive campaigns for decades that have determined the quality of every breath of air Eve draws into her new lungs.

Her mother's breast milk has already been infused with pesticides, herbicides, and hormone disruptors that chemical companies and their representatives have fought to keep on the market.

Once Eve starts eating solid food, what other chemicals will she be consuming? Spoiler alert: less than a third of the eighty thousand chemicals on the U.S. market today are regulated at all, so it's ultimately an unanswerable question. Was the food inspected, and if so, to what degree and by whom?

The banking lobby has its fingerprints all over the regulations that shape her parents' mortgage, their taxes, their medical bills, their job opportunities.

Eve can't escape the reach of the system. You can't. We can't. Government is us, and it's either working for us, or it's working for those who are trying to rig it to get what they want, sucking our employees (our legislators) into their agendas and often diverting our resources (tax dollars) into their pockets.

The middle of this book is dedicated to exploring the connections between political and policy manipulations in Washington and the price we all pay for those manipulations. We present case studies to demonstrate how the bending of—or outright obstruction of—the legislative process creates kitchen-table problems. We hope you'll see that we have to first fix our democracy and put ourselves back in the driver's seat of governing, if we want to fix the other problems we all face.

So is it fixable? Yes, if we are clear about what success means. The reformers' slogan, "Get Money Out of Politics," is misleading. We can't get money completely out of politics, but we can create a much, much higher-functioning and responsive system. It requires money to run campaigns, to hire door knockers, to print lawn signs, and to run TV, radio, and online ads (the bulk of the spending). Groups like the NRA, the Sierra Club, and the National Association of Manufacturers will always want to weigh in on key public policy debates. And they should.

What we can do is restore our power—the people's power—within the system by limiting the most egregious sources of the money, by creating new ways of financing politics that reorient politicians to their voters back home, by demanding total transparency in the giving and spending of political cash, by enacting new ethics and lobbying laws that reduce conflicts of interest and shut down the most transactional forms of political giving, and by making sure that campaign and lobbying laws are evenly and effectively enforced.

These things shouldn't seem so hard to achieve. We've won similar fights before. We're Americans, after all. We're the ones who make dramatic course corrections when things are going wrong or when new and revolutionary ideas emerge. We're not a defeatist or cynical people (although our level of cynicism is rising fast). We know that we can accomplish extraordinary things.

The reforming spirit that has fueled successful fights against Big Money was perhaps best embodied a century ago by Teddy Roosevelt. His time, just like ours, was one of unprecedented technological change when wealth and power were aggregating at the top of society. Massive corporate conglomerations—the bank, oil, railroad, and mining trusts, especially—threatened free and competitive markets. The rich were getting richer by the year. And the public felt outraged, yet exhausted, by the increasing pace of industrialized life and by the sense that their voices no longer mattered.

Roosevelt was a master at drawing battle lines:

> At many stages in the advance of humanity, this conflict between the men who possess more than they have earned and the men who have earned more than they possess is the central condition of progress. In our day it appears as the struggle of freemen to gain and hold the right of self-government as against the special interests, who twist the methods of free government into machinery for defeating the popular will.

He saw political reform as the precursor to winning other reforms—antitrust, public health, consumer safety.

As most who have read about TR know, he was not just talk. In fact, quite the opposite. In 1907, he helped ram through the first major campaign finance reform bill of the modern era, called the Tillman Act, which banned corporations from contributing directly to political campaigns.

These days, there are signs that Roosevelt's spirit might be coming back to life. As of the writing of this book, all of the Democratic presidential candidates have embraced money-in-politics reform as a central pillar of their campaigns. Many Republican candidates have acknowledged the increasing severity of the problem, although have been less clear about solutions. Love him or hate him, Donald Trump has been refreshingly blunt about what political money buys.

There are signs, too, that the Washington establishment is starting to come around. In the spring of 2015, the dean of Washington journalism, Bob Woodward, who as a young *Washington Post* reporter broke the Watergate scandal, said at a commencement address at Loyola University:

> There is a new governing crisis here and it is getting worse. It is about money in politics. It involves both political parties. I won't name names. If you follow the news at all, you know . . . It is important that the next president be able, unfettered and unbought, to find and move the country to the next stage of good.

A *governing crisis*. This is a dramatic statement for a careful wordsmith like Woodward.

Inhabiting a totally different part of the political ecosystem from Woodward's is a guy like John Feehery. Feehery was Dennis Hastert's chief of staff when Hastert was the Republican Speaker of the House in the early 2000s. He's now an executive at a big D.C. lobbying and public relations firm. Yet the same week that Woodward gave his Loyola commencement speech, Feehery wrote in the *Wall Street Journal*:

> I don't have anything against billionaires. It would be nice to have access to that kind of money. But our political system shouldn't be run by the super-rich for the super-rich's pet causes.

Run by the super-rich for the super-rich's pet causes is another way of saying *oligarchy*. America, an oligarchy. It's almost sickening to see those words next to one another. Imagine the heartbreak that John Adams and his compatriots would feel if they were alive today.

Then there are public servants of both the executive and legislative branches of government, such as John Kerry. Before he left the Hill to head the U.S. Department of State, Kerry delivered a moving speech to his colleagues from the floor of the Senate, in which he asserted:

> We should not resign ourselves ... to a distorted system that corrodes our democracy. This is what contributes to the justified anger of the American people. They know it. We know it. And yet nothing happens. The truth requires that we call the corrosion of money in politics what it is: it is a form of corruption and it muzzles more Americans than it empowers, and it is an imbalance that the world has taught us can only sow the seeds of unrest.

They know it. Indeed we do. A growing number of people, of all political stripes, are increasingly fed up. Last year, CBS News partnered with the *New York Times* on a poll, the conclusion of which was: "In a rare show of unity, Americans, regardless of their political affiliation, agree that money has too much influence on elections, the wealthy have more influence on elections, and candidates who win office promote policies that help their donors."

But it's no longer true that nothing is happening. More than at any time since Watergate, regular people are realizing that this situation has to change.

Since 2010, more than six hundred anti–*Citizens United* resolutions have been passed by cities and states. New campaign finance systems are already functioning in places including Connecticut, Arizona, and New York City. In 2014, led by the reform group Represent.Us, 67 percent of voters in Tallahassee, Florida, supported a major reform package, including lower campaign contribution limits, creation of a new, independent ethics commission, and a program to empower nonwealthy people to participate in funding politics. The coalition that was assembled to win consisted of progressives, independents, and Tea Party members.

Similar coalitions are forming around ballot measures in cities and states throughout the country. And there's the possibility for immediate progress at the federal level. Even if Congress isn't ready to legislate, the White House can act, and it should use its authority to do so. Hundreds of thousands of people have urged President Obama to sign an executive order that would require federal contractors—given that they are receiving taxpayer dollars—to disclose their political activities. If such an order were signed, 70 of the Fortune 100 companies would have to do so.

The Securities and Exchange Commission could also help. More than a million comments have been submitted to pressure the SEC to issue a rule requiring publicly traded companies to disclose the political dollars they spend on behalf of investors. Former Republican SEC Commissioner William Donaldson and former Democratic SEC Commissioner Bevis Longstreth are among the chorus calling for change.

But for these types of executive actions and state-based efforts to take root, we must immediately build a much stronger—and politically broader—citizen army. There is already a battalion of reformers working hard every day. But they are waiting for major reinforcements to arrive. That means you. And your friends. It will take you, and us, and millions of other kindred spirits to create a patriotic force powerful enough to reorient the power in this country back to "We, the people."

What are we up against? First or foremost, our own cynicism and resignation. Too many people—rich and poor, political and apolitical—have decided that we simply can't overcome the power of monied interests and have given up trying.

In fact, fixing this is *technically* remarkably simple compared to other things we need to fix—we could do it in a day with a single piece of legislation. No pipes or wires or army bases have to be moved. No new power plants need to be built or retrofitted. No cyber attacks need to be defended against. No international humanitarian missions need to be launched. No families or individuals have to change the way they eat or drive or raise their children. No new federal agency needs to be funded. No school needs to alter the way it educates our children. No hospital or health center needs to amend the way it cares for patients or bills insurance companies. No trade agreements need to be nullified. No workers need to be retrained. Those things—transportation, education, public health, national security, good jobs—are complicated. And, by the way, most of them are harder to fix because of the influence of money in politics. This, though—how money flows in and around our political system and our government—should be something we routinely clean up, like making sure the gutters on our homes are clear of leaves.

After all, what are we up against? There are maybe a hundred thousand political power brokers in this country who are truly invested in the perpetuation of a coin-operated government. They see no problem with it. They are unabashed about their participation in it. They figure that's how the world works. Money buys access. More money—and fundraising events and favors and nice trips—engender a sense of obligation between politicians, political donors, and lobbyists. So be it. Such people will say that spending money is an act of free speech. And some who say that genuinely believe it.

A few specific foes of reform: Senator Mitch McConnell (R-KY), although he used to be less antagonistic. The U.S. Chamber of Commerce has attacked most attempts to improve the system. More inside-the-Beltway Republicans are opposed to major reforms than Democrats, although that dynamic is changing. Outside the Beltway, more than a decade of public opinion polling shows that regular Republicans feel just as disturbed about the problem as do Democrats and independents. Many people who work on K Street—Ground Zero of the lobbying community in D.C.—like the system the way it is, although they will never say so publicly. Others on K Street would be happy if they didn't have to make campaign contributions and constantly attend political fundraisers.

It's possible that a hundred thousand might be too high a number. But, for the sake of argument, let's stick with it. That's 0.03 percent of the United States' population. We, the other 99.97 percent, have to push aside our cynicism and exhaustion and join with others from all walks of life to create a new, surprising, mighty reform moment in history.

Just as we won our right to self-government by fighting the British monarchy more than 240 years ago, we will lose it if we fail to fight to reclaim it now.

Imagine what would happen if we don't. Can any one of us truly claim that we will be able to revitalize our country as long as this problem worsens? Does anyone believe fixing our democracy is optional? Who among us would surrender ourselves, our children, our communities, to an oligarchy?

America is indeed a dream.

The poets are right: it is promises.

Once again it's time to prove that the people are also right: it is promises—that will come true.

CHAPTER 1

How We Got Here

I hope we shall take warning from the example and crush in its birth the aristocracy of our monied corporations which dare already to challenge our government to a trial of strength, and bid defiance to the laws of their country.

—THOMAS JEFFERSON, LETTER TO GEORGE LOGAN, 1816[1]

Money has a long history in American politics. Not even George Washington was immune. Before he earned a spot in every history book, on every map, and in every wallet across America, Washington was a victim of unchecked campaign spending. He lost his first race—for the House of Burgesses in 1755—by an enormous margin after his opponent supplied would-be voters with an admirably large and diverse selection of liquor. Not to be bested twice, Washington fought back with a vengeance three years later, coasting to a commanding victory after supplying voters with his own stash of booze.[2]

Washington's behavior was not out of the ordinary. Landed, wealthy men had the vote, and they were the ones who typically ran for office, largely funding their own campaigns. Back then, phrases like "campaign finance reform" or "money in politics" didn't exist—the Founders could not have imagined the scope and scale of today's political races, nor the massive buildup of the lobbying industry. Back then, campaigns were local and fundraising was minimal.

But larger questions about the role of wealth in the republic were in the air. In 1816, for instance, Thomas Jefferson had been out of office for seven years, having served two successful terms as president. Like many of the luminaries of his generation, he wrote extensively about politics. In a letter to his friend and colleague, the former senator George Logan of Pennsylvania, he expressed concern about the threat posed to the national interest by the growing influence of corporate wealth. He—and his contemporaries—were beginning to see trends emerge that could threaten the system of government they had bled for in the Revolution, helped construct at the Constitutional Convention, and worked to implement as elected officials.

Some of what they predicted—those "monied corporations which dare already to challenge our government to a trial of strength"—emerged full force in the middle of the nineteenth century, as the nation's economy modernized and industrialized at a breathtaking pace. With the manufacturing boom—and the shift away from what we today call "family farming"—came the rise of the transnational corporation. The men behind these powerful businesses have been woven into the fabric of the American story—Rockefeller, Carnegie, Morgan.

Americans were unsettled by the breakneck changes they were experiencing. They saw how a handful of aggressive businessmen could control swaths of the economic landscape. As the big corporations grew richer, they began to exert greater control over the political realm, too. History has shown that when wealth aggregates, it has a tendency to assert its power in order to protect itself.

Expanding voting, first to men without property, and then, over time, to nonwhite men after the Fifteenth Amendment in 1870, broadened the electorate. This process diluted to some extent the political power of the wealthy, who had once exclusively controlled the right to vote. But a populist groundswell was also brewing, built in opposition to the corporate titans of the era. As industrialization and corporate consolidation filled their coffers, elites sought to counter the forces opposing their continued political dominance through political contributions. If they couldn't be in power themselves, they could fund those who would be.

Senator William Chandler of New Hampshire, who had been one of the founders of the Republican Party as a young man in the mid-1850s, understood the public's concerns. In a 1904 letter to Wisconsin governor

Robert La Follette, Chandler gave voice to the zeitgeist at the turn of the century: "When corporations can furnish money to carry elections from corporate treasuries, individualism in government is gone.... When the custom grows broad enough the whole character of government is changed, and corporations rule, not men."[3]

Chandler echoes Jefferson. The Founders thought intensely about the character of the government they were creating, grappling with notions of individual and systemic corruption. As we discuss throughout this book, the distinction between the two is crucial for analyzing the state of the American political system. As the Founders saw it, the Fordham University law professor Zephyr Teachout writes, "corruption—writ large—is the rotting of positive ideals of civic virtue and public integrity."[4] This isn't the much-maligned, Jack Abramoff–style quid pro quo corruption—this kind of systemic rot goes much deeper than bribery. When citizens lose faith in their government, the government has been corrupted, and this can bring down even the mightiest democracy. In the late 1800s, the rise of the corporate economy brought with it the rise of the corporate campaign—and some Americans worried that the character of their government *had* been changed. As the historian Doris Kearns Goodwin quotes in *The Bully Pulpit*, Republican president Teddy Roosevelt saw the same problem during the Gilded Age, later noting, "the power of the mighty industrial overlords of the country had increased with giant strides, while the methods of controlling them, or checking abuses by them on the part of the people, through the Government, remained archaic and therefore practically impotent."[5]

The First Corporate-Funded Campaign

The election of 1896 might be considered the first modern presidential contest, thanks largely to the efforts of Marcus Alonzo Hanna. Hanna was a successful businessman, running a prosperous coal and iron business in his home state of Ohio. He also had an interest in politics—which, combined with his deep pockets, landed him a position as a fundraiser for the Republican National Committee. Hanna used his checkbook to wield massive influence in the party primary, bankrolling his friend William McKinley's campaign almost entirely with his own money.

Hanna's big innovation was to travel to New York to solicit contributions from the big banks and trusts that operated there—essentially seeking money in exchange for assurance that government policies would favor their interests. The business community would fare better, he argued, if McKinley were elected president.[6] This strategy was unprecedented: in previous cycles, candidates had dedicated a percentage of their salaries to fund their campaigns. But such novel ideas often end up working. Big business responded to Hanna by opening its collective wallet, hoping to shield its growing fortunes. McKinley raked in $96 million in today's dollars using the new approach, including the equivalent of $6.9 million from Standard Oil. The contest kicked off a pattern of rising campaign costs that would come to define American elections.

The election of 1896 was truly a watershed moment. As a percentage of GDP, no election before or since has seen spending levels as high.[7] The rise of outside contributions triggered fundamental questions about politics and elections in the minds of many Americans.

As the historian Robert Mutch, author of *Buying the Vote*, argues, questions of campaign finance are fundamentally inseparable from broader questions of democracy, and the era's economic inequality and powerful corporations brought this discussion into focus. He writes:

> [It] opened a new phase of the old debate about how our democracy should work, turning it into a question about money as well as votes. Like earlier differences about how far to extend the suffrage, the debate over where campaign funds should come from is part of the constitutional issue of deciding who should govern.[8]

Much as they do today, people had begun to worry that a handful of wealthy men had co-opted the political system. Indeed, as Hanna famously said, "There are two things that are important in politics. The first is money and I can't remember what the second one is."[9] By the turn of the century, big business had established itself as a force to be reckoned with in the political system.

Teddy and Pitchfork Ben

When the irascible Teddy Roosevelt took over after McKinley was assassinated by the anarchist Leon Czolgosz in 1901, he would prove to be an entirely different type of leader. As president, he would pursue campaign finance reform—the first president to take up the cause—as one of many means of fighting the monopolistic corporations.

In 1903, two years after taking office, Roosevelt was in full trust-busting mode. The previous year, he had invoked the all-but-ignored Sherman Antitrust Act of 1890 to take on J. P. Morgan's behemoth railroad holding company.[10] The case, *Northern Securities Co. v. United States*, would eventually result in a landmark Supreme Court decision restricting corporate consolidation.[11] Roosevelt commended the decision, but he realized the need for additional change. In a lengthy speech delivered at the State Fair in Syracuse, New York, in 1903, he railed against monopolistic power:

> The death-knell of the republic had rung as soon as the active power became lodged in the hands of those who sought, not to do justice to all citizens, rich and poor alike, but to stand for one special class and for its interests as opposed to the interests of others.[12]

Roosevelt's opposition to corporate consolidation and his reputation for independence, along with a strong stance on foreign policy, helped him breeze through the 1904 election to win a second term.[13] But that year's campaign also hit a strong note of irony. Soon after the election, the press reported that his campaign had received possibly nefarious corporate contributions, including an alleged $100,000 donation from John D. Rockefeller's Standard Oil Company.[14] The *New York Times* attacked with a scathing editorial, mercilessly headlined THE ROOT OF ALL EVIL, that is worth quoting extensively from here:

> Certainly the virus has penetrated deeply and has wrought subtly when a man of Mr. Roosevelt's native scorn for corruption can be the willing, the eager beneficiary of funds paid into the campaign chest through his former secretary and former Cabinet officer with the undisguised hope that it will be repaid in favors to the subscribers . . . When we make Governmental action a source of private profit we invite, we compel, large numbers of men to seek to influence that action for their own advancement or defense. And since such action depends on the party in control of the government, the first effort of those who would influence it is toward the success of the party that will favor them. Thus we have not merely the class of eager, aggressive, sometimes unscrupulous business men who depend on the policy of the government and on the party control of the Government, but we have also the

vast number of politicians and place holders all animated by the same interest, all pursuing practically the same end, combining, plotting, working together to bend the minds of those responsible for public action away from the general and common good and toward their own private advantage. No more potent force, or complex of forces, tending toward substantial corruption has ever been known in political history.[15]

Roosevelt was quick to call for the complete prohibition of corporate donations to campaigns. In his 1905 message to Congress, he proclaimed, "All contributions by corporations to any political committee or for any political purpose should be forbidden by law."[16] Taking the lead in fulfilling this mandate was Senator Benjamin Tillman of South Carolina.

Tillman, a Democrat, may not have been the likeliest choice to help push Roosevelt's agenda, given the checkered history between them. The two had begun clashing when the notoriously fiery "Pitchfork Ben," as he was known, got into a fistfight with another senator on the Senate floor. Roosevelt, who thought such behavior unbecoming of a senator, had rescinded Tillman's invitation to an upcoming state dinner. Tillman was terribly offended and had resolved to be a thorn in Roosevelt's side.

Thanks to some political gamesmanship, however, Roosevelt's proposed ban on corporate campaign contributions bore Tillman's name. Though the Tillman Act passed the Senate with ease, the House proved a tougher crowd—but Roosevelt, beloved for his tenacity, did not falter. The first item on the agenda in his 1906 message to Congress: admonishing the House for their failure to pass the bill. Roosevelt left no room for misunderstanding of his position. "Let individuals contribute as they desire," he proclaimed, "but let us prohibit in effective fashion all corporations from making contributions for any political purpose, directly or indirectly."[17] The House passed the bill shortly thereafter, and Roosevelt signed it into law in early 1907. With the Tillman Act, America had passed its first major campaign finance law.

As the 1908 election loomed, big donations still weighed heavily on the public's collective conscience. Both major candidates—William Jennings Bryan and William Howard Taft—committed to disclosing their donors, in part because of the embarrassing revelations Roosevelt had suffered in the wake of his 1904 election. Taft, the Republican, looked beyond big business in New York to a larger web of smaller donors, and he translated that broader support into a winning campaign.

In 1910, congressional Republicans passed additional campaign finance laws, which restricted House campaign spending and required political parties to report their expenditures and donations, but only after the election had occurred. A coalition of Republicans and Northern Democrats amended the law in 1911 to mandate pre-election disclosure by candidates as well as parties for primary and general election campaigns, and they extended the spending limits to Senate candidates.[18]

In 1925, Congress amended the 1910 law again—this time to remove the disclosure mandate for primary elections and require political committees to report contributions that were made between election cycles.[19]

Going After the Unions

All was relatively quiet on the reform front until the late 1930s, when the Hatch Act—which officially bore the rather grandiose title of "An Act to Prevent Pernicious Political Activities"[20]—gained momentum. Introduced by New Mexico senator Carl Hatch, the legislation was a response to reports of New Deal relief workers doubling as campaign operatives. The Hatch Act, still in effect today, explicitly banned the intimidation or bribery of voters and restricted political campaign activities by federal employees.

By the early 1940s, both parties had cemented their main donor bases, with Republicans relying on big business and Democrats relying on organized labor. Just as corporate contributions at the turn of the century spurred Democrats to call for reform, conservatives moved to check the rising union power that had lifted FDR into the White House.

In 1943, when the United Mine Workers union broke its promise not to go on strike during the war, congressional Republicans mobilized to pass the Smith-Connally Act, which allowed the federal government to seize striking industries involved in the war effort and banned union contributions to federal campaigns. The Congress of Industrial Organizations (CIO) responded with a campaign finance innovation that survives to this day—the political action committee, or PAC. Rather than drawing from its treasury to contribute directly to campaigns, the union set up a PAC that was able to raise donations from members. It was a work-around of sorts—the unions were no longer making contributions to political campaigns, the PACs were. It's worth noting that unions could still make direct political *expenditures*—just not campaign contributions.[21]

Corporations had been engaging in similar practices—*strongly recommending* that employees vote for certain candidates and donate to specific campaigns—to work around their own ban on direct campaign contributions. Congress reacted to the CIO PAC by moving to end such a stratagem, including a provision in the anti-union Taft-Hartley bill that would ban both corporations and unions from *directly* spending money on politics.[22] The *indirect* spending, though, through PACs, was just beginning.

The bill enjoyed conservative support in the newly elected 80th Congress, which inaugurated in January of 1947, where Republicans controlled both the House and the Senate for the first time in fifteen years. Northern Democrats were less enthused; the vote on the bill split cleanly along partisan lines. President Harry Truman, a Democrat, sided with his party. He vetoed the bill on June 20, pulling no punches in his accompanying message to Congress:

> I would have signed a bill with some doubtful features if, taken as a whole, it had been a good bill . . . But the Taft-Hartley bill is a shocking piece of legislation. . . . Under no circumstances could I have signed this bill . . . The restrictions that this bill places on our workers go far beyond what our people have been led to believe. This is no innocent bill.[23]

Unions didn't take the new restriction lying down; the CIO immediately challenged the constitutionality of the expenditure ban. *United States v. Congress of Industrial Organizations* has provided precedent for campaign finance law ever since. As the government wrote in its brief, corporate and union contributions and expenditures could be classified and banned together, since Congress had passed the laws to "control the power represented by the aggregate wealth of entities, organized primarily for nonpolitical purposes . . . in a position to exercise a disproportionate influence on federal elections."[24] The "aggregate wealth" argument was powerful. The law stood, and the classification of corporations and unions as similar aggregators of wealth for federal campaign finance restrictions has largely remained intact to this day.

For practical purposes, though, the laws on the books remained largely ineffective. Beginning with the Tillman Act, the enforcement of which Robert Mutch has called "a legal and practical impossibility,"[25] campaign finance laws in the first half of the twentieth century were rife with loopholes and widely ignored by political players.

Taft-Hartley ushered in a decades-long lull in reform efforts. There was little policy action to speak of until 1971, when President Richard Nixon signed the Federal Election Campaign Act into law. FECA was designed to join the separate, weaker campaign finance laws of previous decades into a strong, centralized piece of legislation. Taking full effect in April 1972, FECA required the complete reporting of campaign contributions and expenditures.[26] Along with the 1971 Revenue Act, it also instituted the first federal financing system for presidential campaigns. Ronald Reagan took advantage of the program for his winning bid in 1980, and all major party presidential candidates since then utilized matching funds in the general election, if not in the primary, until Barack Obama in 2008.[27]

The Revenue Act may have been intended to make sweeping changes to the system of campaign finance—but, like so many laws before it, it did not include sufficient means for administration or enforcement. After the 1972 election, more than seven thousand cases were referred to the Justice Department, which was able to prosecute just a few of them.[28] Campaign finance reform groups used FECA reporting requirements to bring more disclosure into the public view.

Money Becomes Speech

It took the Watergate scandal and the end of a presidency to make real progress with regard to enforcement. The revelation of the Nixon administration's wide-ranging abuse of power, including campaign violations and slush funds of illegal contributions shook Americans' faith in their government. Once again, crisis would sow the seeds of change.

Out of the ashes of the scandal rose a means of enforcing the laws on the books. In 1975, Congress created the Federal Election Commission to oversee all aspects of the campaign administration and finance process. The FEC consolidated the administrative responsibilities and enforcement authority that, up to that point, had been split between agencies.[29] Everything about the group's operation is bipartisan by design. Of its six commissioners, three must be Democrats and three Republicans; in

FEC (established 1975) with a mission to administer and enforce:

- Public disclosure of funds raised and spent to influence federal elections

- Restrictions on contributions and expenditures made to influence federal elections

- The public financing of presidential campaigns

Basic Federal Campaign Finance Laws:

- Contributions to candidates limited to $2,700 from individuals and $5,000 from PACs.

- Contributions to candidates banned from corporations, labor unions, government contractors and foreign nationals

- Super PACs can raise and spend unlimited amounts of money. Such spending is not supposed to be coordinated with candidates or their committees.

Federal Election Commission (FEC)
Source: Federal Election Commission (fec.gov)

order for it to take action, at least four of the members must agree.[30] In theory, this system prevents partisan abuses. In practice, it has resulted in profound inefficiency and crippling deadlock, making meaningful enforcement difficult.

Perhaps the late 1970s' most significant legacy came not from government agencies or legislation, but from the courts. As the reform movement pushed for more and better controls on campaign contributions, those in favor of maintaining the status quo crafted a powerful, lasting rebuttal. As the historian Robert Mutch puts it, campaign-finance-reform foes "developed a First Amendment doctrine that so closely linked campaign speech with campaign money that it would have made any regulation of that money unconstitutional."[31] This is the intellectual wellspring of *Citizens United*: since campaign spending is a form of political expression, limits on it are impermissible. Armed with this line of thinking, anti-reformers challenged FECA.

In 1976, the Supreme Court handed down its landmark decision in *Buckley v. Valeo*. James L. Buckley, a first-term senator from New York and then a member of the newly minted Conservative Party, boasted an impressive conservative pedigree. His younger brother, William F. Buckley, was the founder of the *National Review*. Before James's election to the Senate, both brothers ran long-shot campaigns for Congress just to ensure that their ideas made it into the conversation.

Despite Buckley's often partisan ways, the lawsuit that bore his name was remarkably bipartisan. His rather unlikely bedfellow was former senator Eugene McCarthy of Minnesota—the liberal who had sought and lost the Democratic nomination for president just a few years earlier. The lawsuit aimed to overturn the post-Watergate reforms that limited the amount of money federal candidates could receive from an individual donor, as well as how much of their own money they could spend.

Many years later, Buckley would describe the case's outcome to the *Wall Street Journal* as "50/50." The Court ruled that a cap on individual campaign spending violated the First Amendment right to free speech. They also decided, however, that campaign contributions should be limited so as to avoid corruption, or the appearance thereof.[32] And they affirmed the need for disclosure and upheld the presidential public financing system—important tools for the reform efforts of today and tomorrow.

The idea that money is speech is by no means a universally held belief by the courts, though. In a 2000 case, the Supreme Court held that *Buckley*'s contribution limit principles apply to contribution limits in state elections. As Justice John Paul Stevens wrote in his concurring opinion, political money is protected, but not at the same level as speech:

> In response to [Justice Anthony Kennedy's] call for a new begin-ning, therefore, I make one simple point. Money is property; it is not speech ... The right to use one's own money to hire gladiators, or to fund "speech by proxy," certainly merits signifi-cant constitutional protection. These property rights, however, are not entitled to the same protection as the right to say what one pleases.[33]

Stevens's line of thinking—that money is property—is an important alternative constitutional reading. But *Buckley v. Valeo*'s precedent, that political spending is an act of speech, has informed many of the major Supreme Court campaign finance decisions of the last four decades.

The Advent and Explosion of Soft Money

Corporations, unions, and political parties took advantage of the Court's decision. The money began to pile up, fast.

"Soft" money, which was unrestricted and raised for nebulous "party building" activities, came into vogue in the 1990s. In contrast to the tightly regulated, disclosed "hard" money contributed directly to candidates' campaigns, soft money was tough to track and control. Parties built up massive war chests, exploiting the spotty federal regulatory apparatus and more generous state laws, and rewarded their big-money donors. In one egregious example, major Democratic donors were offered sleepovers in the Lincoln bedroom of the Clinton White House.[34]

The 2000 election was another leap forward for Big Money. George W. Bush declined to avail himself of the presidential public financing option in the primary election—primarily out of fear that the billionaire Steve Forbes would self-finance his way to a victory—and, to everyone's surprise, raised $100 million just for the primary. He then used the public financing system in the general election. According to Doug Weber of the Center for Responsive Politics, no one in Washington thought a candidate could rake in that much cash—conventional wisdom had dictated that presidential campaigns would raise some campaign money and then use public federal funds to boost their totals.[35]

Bush's bypassing of the presidential public financing system in the primary, plus the amount of "soft money" the political parties were pumping into the elections, led to another major wake-up call. It was the "extraordinary amount of soft money in the 2000 election that marked what many political scientists saw as the final collapse of FECA," Mutch writes.[36] Americans were unsettled by the soft-money explosion, and good-government groups agitated for change. Reform came two years later, with the Bipartisan Campaign Reform Act (BCRA) of 2002. This act is often called "McCain-Feingold" after its bipartisan duo of sponsors: Senators John McCain (R-AZ) and Russ Feingold (D-WI). McCain-Feingold extended pre-existing statutes prohibiting corporations from using company funds to broadcast advertisements advocating for or against a candidate for federal office within a certain period before elections. It also prohibited soft money (unlimited) contributions to national political parties.[37]

Analyses of McCain-Feingold are remarkably similar to those of the Tillman Act. Proponents of McCain-Feingold argued that with soft money contributions no longer allowed, smaller donations would replace the large sums that corporations had been able to donate.[38] Compare that with a June 1906 New York Times article about the Tillman Act, which at the time had not yet passed the House. A Republican

Hill staffer quoted in the item, after expressing sympathy for the corporations that had suffered "extortion" at the hands of the political parties, added:

> Parties will be put to it to fill their coffers by really voluntary contributions. These will be smaller than the old ones, but they will answer all legitimate needs for the simple reason that needs which they do not satisfy will cease to seem legitimate.[39]

Both efforts aimed to revitalize the grassroots of the political parties by forcing them to rely on a high volume of small donations instead of a low volume of large ones.

Critics, meanwhile, warned that McCain-Feingold's soft-money ban and transparency measures would simply reroute gargantuan donations to outside groups, many of which operate in a largely unregulated, uncontrolled Wild West–style system. Those fears would come to fruition to a greater extent than anyone imagined.

In 2004, "527" organizations, so named for the section of the tax code they are registered under, boomed in popularity. The groups are not bound by contribution limits, but they must disclose their donors. Most of the 527s in 2004 leaned left, with Republican groups making up only fifteen of the top fifty organizations. Americans Coming Together, a 527 created to boost John Kerry's unsuccessful campaign, pooled multi-million-dollar donations from wealthy Democrats including George Soros, Peter Lewis, and Stephen Bing.[40]

When Barack Obama ran for president in 2008, he became the first major-party candidate to bypass the presidential public financing system in both the primary and general elections. Jimmy Carter, Ronald Reagan, George H. W. Bush, Bill Clinton, and George W. Bush were all elected with public funds. (Their challengers also received public funds.) The money for the program is furnished by taxpayers who check the voluntary-contribution box on their tax forms. Had Obama opted into the program, as John McCain did, he would have received about $85 million for the general election but would have had to forgo the small-donor and major-donor fundraising that his campaign was quickly mastering. In the end, Obama raised $750 million in 2008, which is more than all of the presidential candidates collectively spent in 2004. His lack of participation in the program—combined with the suddenly enormous sums of money people now believe are necessary to run for president—has left the system in limbo. Neither Mitt Romney nor Barack Obama utilized it in 2012, and there is no indication that anyone will in 2016. Reviving the program, in a way that offers presidential candidates enough money to run robust campaigns, would be a valuable goal for near-term policy reforms.

Hillary: The Movie That Created Super PACs

In 2010, the Supreme Court ruled in *Citizens United v. Federal Election Commission* that corporations' and unions' efforts to publicly communicate their support for—or opposition to—political candidates by means of the spending of money should be protected as speech under the First Amendment. Ever since then, *Citizens United* has become a shorthand way of referring to Big Money in politics.

Two years before the ruling, in 2008, the plaintiff in the case, a conservative nonprofit organization called Citizens United was blocked from advertising and broadcasting (as a cable TV video-on-demand selection) a film called *Hillary: The Movie* just as the Democratic primaries were about to start. A federal court in Washington ruled that airing the film, which was strongly biased against Hillary Clinton, would violate a provision of the 2002 McCain-Feingold campaign finance law that prohibited certain kinds of groups from spending money on "electioneering communications" thirty days prior to a primary election and sixty days prior to a general election. The rationale behind that piece of the law was to create an opportunity in the final days of an election for voters to hear more from the candidates' campaigns and less from outside groups.

Citizens United hired James Bopp, a lawyer from Terre Haute, Indiana, to bring suit against the FEC. Bopp had built a reputation for successfully peeling back other campaign finance restrictions, arguing they violated constitutional protections of free speech.[41] He compared his client's film to CBS's *60 Minutes* broadcasts and said that banning it violated the group's First Amendment rights.

In a 5–4 decision, the Court ruled that spending money on communications is an act of speech and therefore should not be restricted, as long as the money spent was independent from (not coordinated with) the candidates' campaigns. Justice Anthony Kennedy laid out the rationale: "Because speech is an essential mechanism of democracy—it is the means to hold officials accountable to the people—political speech must prevail against laws that would suppress it by design or inadvertence."[42] He later expanded on the reasoning, to touch on an argument that is really more about freedom of the press than freedom of speech: "Premised on mistrust of governmental power, the First Amendment stands against attempts to disfavor certain subjects or viewpoints or to distinguish among different speakers, which may be a means to control content."[43]

That's the most laudable aspect of the decision. There are all kinds of corporations—from global media conglomerates to one-person start-ups—that pump out content and ideas about politics and politicians in the context of elections. Trying to distinguish among the sources is fraught. In the wrong hands, it could potentially lead to outright partisan censorship on behalf of the government—something that should scare any American.

Fifty years ago—even fifteen years ago—it was easier to tell the difference between "the press" and others. The press was, for the most part, people who had the money to buy presses, radio towers, and TV stations. But in the age of the Internet, where publishing is essentially free, where can the lines be drawn? It's all a mixed-up mess of content and opinion. What's the difference between a Fox News special report that's critical of Hillary and a Citizens United movie that's critical of her? Should one be allowed, under the rules of McCain-Feingold, and one banned? What about a negative video about Donald Trump, sponsored by a progressive organization (a nonprofit corporation), and a negative piece about him on MSNBC (a subsidiary of a for-profit corporation)?

Michael McConnell is a senior fellow at Stanford University's Hoover Institution and the director of Stanford's Constitutional Law Center. Formerly, he served as a federal judge, nominated by George W. Bush. It was rumored that he was eyed by Bush as a potential Supreme Court nominee. He's no liberal. Writing in the *Yale Law Journal*, McConnell praises, for lack of a better term, the "free press" piece of the *Citizens United* decision:

> It is not constitutional for the government to punish the dissemination of such a documentary by a media corporation, and it therefore follows that it cannot be constitutional to punish its dissemination by a non-media corporation like Citizens United unless the freedom of the press is confined to the institutional

media. Precedent, history, and pragmatics all refute the idea that freedom of the press is so confined.[44]

But then he takes to task the rest of what Justice Kennedy wrote:

> The opinion is overly long and unfocused. It seems to stretch for unnecessarily broad interpretations of free speech law, beyond what the parties argued or what the facts demanded ... The opinion itself was written with a broad brush, turning its back on several plausible narrower grounds for decision. But the most important flaw—a flaw to which the parties and the lower courts contributed—was to analyze the case under the wrong clause of the First Amendment. If the Court had analyzed the case under the Press Clause, it could have avoided muddying the waters of campaign finance law governing contributions, which presents different constitutional considerations, and it would have side-stepped the controversy over whether for-profit corporations, in general, have constitutional rights.[45]

Justice John Paul Stevens, who penned the dissent for the four liberal justices, was so angered by the ruling that he made the rare move of reading his dissent aloud from the bench. His criticism, like McConnell's, includes a broadside against the reckless overreach of the majority:

> Today's decision is backwards in many senses. It elevates the majority's agenda over the litigants' submissions, facial attacks over as-applied claims, broad constitutional theories over narrow statutory grounds, individual dissenting opinions over precedential holdings, assertion over tradition, absolutism over empiricism, rhetoric over reality.[46]

Stevens goes a step further, asserting that the decision could at some point unleash gushers of corporate cash into the political debate that could drown out the marketplace of ideas and create a monopoly of opinion. He additionally argues, as some of the Founders might have, that such extensive—and expensive—political activity could have such a dominating effect on elected officials that it could corrupt the government: "At bottom, the Court's opinion is thus a rejection of the common sense of the American people."[47]

Stevens was correct about the common sense of the American people. A 2014 poll showed that 80 percent of Americans opposed the *Citizens United* decision. Only 18 percent supported it. The breakdown of opposition is hardly partisan: Republicans, 72 percent; Democrats, 82 percent; independents, 84 percent.[48]

On the potentially corrupting influence of the decision, we turn to Norm Ornstein, a resident scholar at the American Enterprise Institute, who is one of the most respected observers of the ways of Washington:

> Ask almost any lobbyist. I hear the same story there over and over—the lobbyist met with a lawmaker to discuss a matter for a client, and before he gets back to the office, the cell phone rings and the lawmaker is asking for money. The connections between policy actions or inactions and fundraising are no longer indirect or subtle. Now comes [another] component. As one Senator said to me, "We have all had experiences like the following: A lobbyist or interest representative will be in my office. He or she will say, 'You know, Americans for a Better America really, really want this amendment passed. And they have more money than God. I don't know what they will do with their money if they don't get what they want. But they are capable of spending a fortune to make anybody who disappoints them regret it.'" No money has to be spent to get the desired outcome . . . This is what Citizens United hath wrought. It is thoroughly corrupting.[49]

This kind of deep understanding of how money and politics interact is something that Ornstein has developed after decades of examining Washington up close. Notice, the senator who spoke to Ornstein didn't say: "Well, because Americans for A Better America is an independent-expenditure group, they have no effect on my thinking or behavior." And notice that there is no quid pro quo—no specific exchange of campaign contributions for legislative favors. As Ornstein notes, "no money has to be spent to get the desired outcome."

But the Supreme Court justices inhabit such a rarefied intellectual bubble that they don't understand how money works its way on the political system. Sandra Day O'Connor was the last justice to have held elected office. Their naïve assumption that "independent expenditures" have no potentially corrupting effect on the behavior of politicians is the most glaring example of such a blind spot.

FOR   **AGAINST**

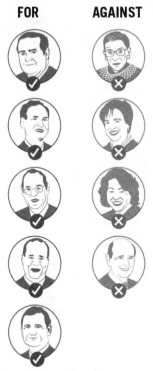

Corporations and unions can now spend on ads advocating a candidate's election or defeat, without restriction.

Individuals can make unlimited contributions to super PACs.

Of the $1 billion spent in federal elections by super PACs in the five years following the ruling, almost 60 percent came from 195 individuals and their spouses, according to the Brennan Center for Justice.

What Citizens United Changed.

"The two most abrupt breaks with the historical meaning of corruption—*Buckley* and *Citizens United*—have occurred when no politicians were on the [Supreme] Court," writes Fordham University law professor Zephyr Teachout in her book *Corruption in America*. "While lower courts and state courts have consistently expanded the scope of corruption laws, an opposite movement has happened on high. The [Supreme] Court has become populated by academics and appellate court justices, and not by people with experience of power and politics, who understand the ways in which real problems of money and influence manifest themselves."[50] Teachout argues that the court has too narrowly defined corruption as quid-pro-quo corruption—the direct exchange of money for specific legislative favors or outcomes. This form of corruption is basically already forbidden by law. It's called bribery. And, as we stated earlier in the book, it's not the kind of corruption the Founding Fathers were most worried about. They were concerned with preventing systemic corruption, or the bending of the government away from the public good and toward private gain.

That's why Kennedy's massive overreach in the scope of the case was so dangerous—if you're going to go off trail and bushwhack in the dark, you'd better know the terrain—in this case, the terrain of money in politics. Justice Ruth Bader Ginsburg, who joined in Stevens's dissent, said in a 2014 interview: "I think the notion that we have all the democracy that money can buy strays so far from what our democracy is supposed to be . . . Members of the legislature, people who have to run for office, know the connection between money and influence on what laws get passed."[51]

The Supreme Court didn't stop with *Citizens United*, either. The money-as-speech argument spawned another case, in 2014: *McCutcheon v. FEC*. In a 5–4 decision, the Court struck down aggregate contribution limits—the caps on total donations to candidates and party committees in a given election cycle—on the grounds that if contributions are considered political speech, limiting the number of those contributions is unconstitutional. Now a wealthy donor can cut a $2,700 check, for both the primary and general elections, for every candidate in the country. *Citizens United* continues to metastasize.

Bipartisan Angst Over *Citizens United*

Members of Congress are speaking out about what the Court has wrought. Nearly every Democrat in both the House and Senate has condemned *Citizens United*. In a symbolic moment before the 2014 midterm elections, Senate Democrats staged a debate about amending the Constitution to reverse the ruling. And it's not just Democrats. The nonprofit group Free Speech for People has identified more than 150 Republican leaders— from former Bush and Reagan White House officials to governors and members of Congress—who have been critical of the decision.

In the summer of 2015, former Republican senator John Danforth of Missouri, a man widely respected by members of both parties, said: "The Supreme Court's decision in *Citizens United* undermines our republican form of government and should not stand . . . [It has] further separated candidates and voters by inserting interlopers between the two. These interlopers are well-heeled individuals and corporations that pour massive amounts of money into supposedly independent campaigns."[52] His statement was especially powerful given that he shepherded Justice Clarence Thomas's confirmation through the Senate. Thomas stood with the majority in *Citizens United*.

One technical point: The pouring of "massive amounts of money into supposedly independent campaigns" is actually not a direct result of *Citizens United*. It's the progeny of a case called *SpeechNow.org v. FEC*. In its March 2010 decision, the D.C. Circuit Court of Appeals ruled, based on the logic of *Citizens United*, that if *spending* by independent groups (organizations not directly affiliated with politicians' campaigns) should be unlimited, then *giving* to such independent groups should be unlimited, too. Super PACs were born of this *SpeechNow.org* decision. It sanctioned unlimited contributions to independent groups capable of spending unlimited amounts of money to elect or defeat candidates.

These types of rulings have sped up the decline of self-government, both because they have "further separated candidates and voters" and because they have created a political arena so dominated by colossal forces that nearly everyone, other than an elite group of politically motivated billionaires and special interest groups, is feeling irrelevant in our democracy.

A March 2015 Rasmussen poll found that 58 percent of Americans think most members of Congress will sell their vote for cash or campaign contributions, while 63 percent believe most incumbents are reelected because election rules unfairly benefit them.[53]

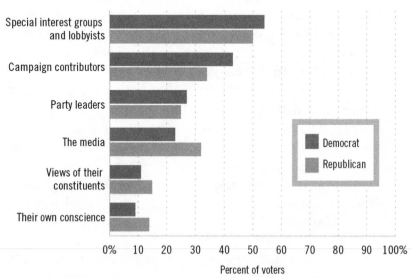

Who Does Congress Listen To? Constituents rank themselves near the bottom of the list
Source: Democracy Corps and Every Voice (everyvoice.org), 2014.

Another recent poll asked voters who has the most influence on how members of Congress vote. Fifty-four percent of Democrats and half of Republicans said "special interests and lobbyists." Coming in second were "campaign contributors." At the bottom of the list were "constituents," who 11 percent of Democrats and 15 percent of Republicans said were most influential.[54]

Ellen Miller has started three enduring good-government groups in the last thirty years—the Center for Responsive Politics, Public Campaign (now called Every Voice), and the Sunlight Foundation. She was the first to make campaign finance data more accessible to the public, back in the 1980s. When we asked her about the current movement, and about what she has witnessed with the rise of Big Money over politics in the last three decades, she was blunt: "I couldn't have imagined that it would get this bad. To suggest the situation is dire would be a vast understatement. Our electoral democracy has been steadily and effectively taken away from American people. Money has practically become the sole determinant of who runs for office, who wins, and what they say and do. It's a true American tragedy."

Looking back at the full span of our history, it becomes clear that we once again stand at a crossroads. We have to grapple with the role of money and power in our democratic republic. Campaigns, and campaign finance, have come a long way since landed aristocrats enticed voters with booze. But Jefferson's worries—about monied interests challenging "our government to a trial of strength"—are as valid today as ever.

CHAPTER 2

Rigged

"I won't dispute for one second the problems of a system that demands [an] immense amount of fund-raisers by its legislators," said Representative Jim Himes, a third-term Democrat of Connecticut, who supported the recent industry-backed bills and leads the party's fund-raising effort in the House. A member of the Financial Services Committee and a former banker at Goldman Sachs, he is one of the top recipients of Wall Street donations. "It's appalling, it's disgusting, it's wasteful and it opens the possibility of conflicts of interest and corruption. It's unfortunately the world we live in."

—"BANKS' LOBBYISTS HELP IN DRAFTING FINANCIAL BILLS,"
NEW YORK TIMES, MAY 23, 2013

It's unfortunately the world we live in.

Let's spend more time exploring the world our elected representatives live in. Although, as countless polls have shown, nearly all Americans believe money dominates politics, not many actually know the details, even fewer know how bad it's gotten, and too many think it's mostly attributable to *Citizens United*.

Make no mistake about it: as we stated a few pages ago, *Citizens United* was a bad decision that has created a great deal of reckless political behavior since it was handed down six years ago, especially among some billionaire political donors. But the role of money in politics, and its contribution to the decline of self-government in America, has been in the making for decades.

In 1998, the total amount of money spent on federal elections was $1.6 billion. By 2012, it had nearly quadrupled to $6.2 billion. In 1998, the average winning House candidate spent $650,000 and the average winning Senate candidate spent $5.2 million. In 2014 those numbers were $1.45 million and $10.6 million, respectively.

Spending by the influence industry in Washington to shape the decisions of policy makers has also increased exponentially in recent decades. In 1960, when John F. Kennedy was elected president, 289 lobbying groups spent a grand total of $30.4 million (in today's dollars) on lobbying activities.[1] The highest-spending group that year was the AFL-CIO, which shelled out the equivalent of just over $1 million. A report on the year's lobbying noted that a new power player, the American Petroleum Institute, had emerged. Adjusting for inflation, the API had spent $722,000.[2] In 1975, total revenue for Washington lobbyists was about $100 million. In 2014, lobbying spending reached $3.23 *billion*, more than a hundred times the 1960 total.[3] The biggest spender, the U.S. Chamber of Commerce, paid a staggering $124 million to a bevy of firms

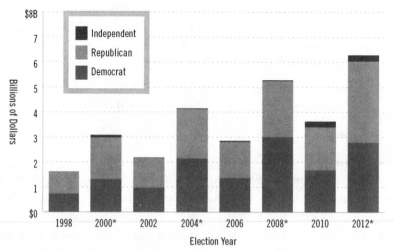

Total Cost of U.S. Elections by Party
Source: Center for Responsive Politics (opensecrets.org)
Methodology: *Presidential election cycle.

and a small army of lobbyists.[4] The top five sectors spending lobbying money in 2014 were health insurance ($533 million); finance, insurance, and real estate ($497 million); health industries ($488 million); communications and electronics ($379 million); and energy and natural resources ($346 million).

"Influence" is now the third-largest industry in D.C., behind government itself and tourism. According to Lee Drutman, a political scientist and author of the book *The Business of America Is Lobbying*, businesses spend more money lobbying Congress than we taxpayers spend funding the salaries, benefits and expenses of all members of Congress and their staffers. Yes, that's right: more is spent each year in Washington lobbying the people who work for Congress than is spent paying and supporting the work of all those members of Congress and congressional staffers.

Drutman's book traces the rise of the influence industry:

> Starting in the early 1970s, corporate America began to devote attention and meaningful resources to politics. The current spending levels merely mark the latest moving capstone in a 40-year period of nearly continuous expansion of corporate political activity . . . Corporate lobbying expenditures now dwarf the comparable investments of unions and "diffuse interest" groups (my preferred term for what others more commonly call "public interest groups" or "citizen groups").

The gap in resources between corporate lobbyists and union and public interest group lobbyists is enormous. For every dollar spent by the unions and public interest groups, corporations and corporate trade groups spent $34 in 2012.

Once a sleepy and rather dowdy city, the nation's capital has been transformed into an expensive, nonstop influence-peddling battleground, full of restaurants that are happy to charge $40 for steaks and spas that will ease the difficulties of digesting those steaks with $150 massages. So much money has been pumped into the Beltway in recent years that, according to the Bureau of Labor Statistics, it is now the most expensive American city to live in. Yes: more expensive than even New York City.

Stroll around Capitol Hill in Washington and you can see the physical manifestations of the confluence of campaign donations and lobbying.

Just a few blocks east of the Capitol dome are street after street of stately townhouses that real families used to call home. Today, many of them house not families but comfortable spaces where members of Congress spend much of their time. Several of the townhouses are occupied by lobbyists, others by trade associations and big corporations. According to a 2010 analysis by the nonprofit Sunlight Foundation, 126 townhouses and offices around the Capitol are used for fundraisers. Seventy percent of those venues are run or owned by lobbyists or groups that hire lobbyists. FedEx and UPS have "homes" on the Hill now, as does the U.S.

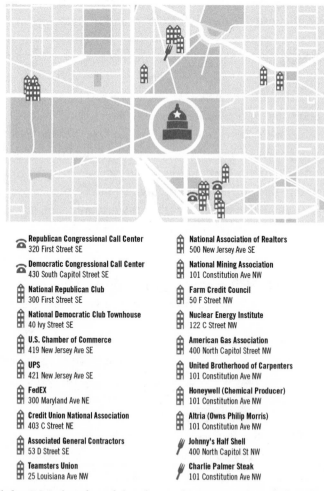

Republican Congressional Call Center
320 First Street SE

Democratic Congressional Call Center
430 South Capitol Street SE

National Republican Club
300 First Street SE

National Democratic Club Townhouse
40 Ivy Street SE

U.S. Chamber of Commerce
419 New Jersey Ave SE

UPS
421 New Jersey Ave SE

FedEX
300 Maryland Ave NE

Credit Union National Association
403 C Street NE

Associated General Contractors
53 D Street SE

Teamsters Union
25 Louisiana Ave NW

National Association of Realtors
500 New Jersey Ave SE

National Mining Association
101 Constitution Ave NW

Farm Credit Council
50 F Street NW

Nuclear Energy Institute
122 C Street NW

American Gas Association
400 North Capitol Street NW

United Brotherhood of Carpenters
101 Constitution Ave NW

Honeywell (Chemical Producer)
101 Constitution Ave NW

Altria (Owns Philip Morris)
101 Constitution Ave NW

Johnny's Half Shell
400 North Capitol St NW

Charlie Palmer Steak
101 Constitution Ave NW

Around the Capitol: A few of the places where money is raised and politicians are influenced.

Chamber of Commerce. Then there are groups with typical D.C. names such as Associated General Contractors, the National Association of Realtors, the National Automobile Dealers Association, and the National Pork Producers Council. About five hundred yards north of the Capitol is the headquarters of the Teamsters Union.

These townhouses have become especially valuable properties because they are a short walk from politicians' offices. Members of Congress are routinely whisked by their staffers to those houses for receptions at which—or after which—checks will be written. Many of the roughly nine thousand registered lobbyists in Washington provide much of the cash at such events.

An increasing number of those lobbyists are former members of Congress themselves. A study by the watchdog group Public Citizen found that around half of House and Senate members—and their staffs— went directly from being public servants to working as lobbyists.

It used to be that politicians would leave Congress and run quasi-public institutions such as colleges and universities and think tanks. Or they would return home and take up their former professions—lawyers, businesspeople. But lobbying is so lucrative. Take, for instance, former congressman Steve Bartlett (R-TX), who was making roughly $150,000 a year when he left the House of Representatives in 1999. While in Congress, he served on the House Banking Committee. The year he left, he was named the head of the Financial Services Roundtable, one of Wall Street's largest lobbying and advocacy groups. When he left the Roundtable, in 2011, he was making $2 million a year.

The members need such lobbyists for campaign cash, and they all but command their presence at fundraisers. Peter Schweizer, president of the Government Accountability Institute and a Republican political adviser, writes in his book *Extortion* that those lobbyists and political donors who want to play the game have to pay the toll. "If you are invited, you are expected to be there. There is an implicit aspect of the request that makes that clear. And when you get there, you better show up with a check," former Shell Oil president John Hofmeister told Schweizer.[5] "I feel extorted," he said.

D.C.'s Sweatshops

Not too far from the Capitol Hill townhouses are the call centers that both Democrats and Republicans use to dial for dollars. Endlessly.

This is how Senator Dick Durbin, Democrat of Illinois, described it: "We sit at these desks with stacks of names in front of us and short bios and histories of giving . . . and we make calls to our faithful friends and ask them to give money or host a fundraiser."[6]

National Public Radio tried to get access to the call centers for a story on fundraising in 2012 but got no further than a description of them from members of Congress.

Former representative Dennis Cardoza, a California Democrat, compared his party's call center to a sweatshop with thirty-inch-wide cubicles set up for the sole purpose of begging for money. He said the need for constant fundraising helped push him into retirement.

Peter DeFazio, a Democrat from Oregon, told NPR, "If you walked in there, you would say, 'Boy, this is about the worst looking, most abusive looking call center situation I've seen in my life.' These people don't have any workspace, the other person is virtually touching them."

Members of both parties say the time they have to spend in the cramped call centers is humiliating. Representative John Larson, Democrat of Connecticut, likened it to "putting bamboo shoots under my finger-nails." One female member of the House told us that, probably because she's a woman, when she makes her fundraising phone calls the donors are much more casual with her than she would expect—or hope. She recounted a call she made to a Hollywood mogul's home. The wife answered the phone. After the congresswoman introduced herself, "The wife launched into a tirade about some new curtains that had just arrived at her house, which were the wrong color of yellow. I had to sit and politely, sympathetically, listen to her so that I could get to the point of asking her for a twenty-five-hundred-dollar contribution to my campaign."

How much time do our elected representatives spend trying to collect money from wealthy people? Roughly 50 percent. One former congressman, Tom Perriello (D-VA), told reporter Ryan Grim at the *Huffington Post* that even that may be "low-balling the figure so as not to scare the new members too much."[7]

This feverish fundraising begins even before a freshman gets sworn in. After former representative Walt Minnick, a conservative Democrat from Iowa, won his first election to Congress in 2008, he took just five days off before heading back to the phones. He needed to raise $10,000 to $15,000 a day because his district is considered competitive and he knew he would face a tough reelection. Many freshman members get right to the townhouse circuit before they even move into a Washington apartment.

The constant need for campaign cash not only greases the wheels in Congress for the well-financed special interests but also reduces the amount of time our legislators spend considering or crafting legislation.

Dan Glickman (D-KS) has seen it all, from all angles. He served in the House for eighteen years, representing the people of Wichita, Kansas, then headed the Department of Agriculture for six years, during Bill Clinton's presidency, then became head of the Motion Picture Association of America, Hollywood's lobbying and advocacy arm in D.C. According to Glickman,

> The sad truth is that given the frenetic search for money in federal congressional elections, there simply isn't enough time in the day to stay competitive in campaign finance and do the actual job of policy making . . . I remember when I was first elected to Congress, I and many other House members would often go down to the floor of the House of Representatives and just listen to the debate. I may not have had an amendment to the bill or a particular interest in the issue but I always felt that watching policy discussions and witnessing the crafting of laws was an important part of my day. It gave me the chance to educate myself and interact with members of Congress on both sides of the aisle. Today most lawmakers would tell you that any free moment not used raising dollars is time wasted.[8]

This theme of members of Congress not being able to commit time to doing the increasingly complicated job of examining and deeply understanding legislation comes up over and over again. It's not just driving them nuts, it's also driving many of them out of office, and it's deterring good people from even thinking about running.

Senator George Voinovich, an Ohio Republican, left the U.S. Senate in 2010. At the press conference announcing his retirement, he said that it would be impossible to be an effective legislator while also meeting the fundraising demands of running for another term. "You can't do both of them," he said. "You're either going to do the job or you're going to be out there raising money."[9]

Of course, not all the fundraising occurs in dreary call center cubicles and trade-association-owned townhouses in D.C. As the *New York Times* investigative reporter Eric Lipton chronicled in 2014, "destination events" have become all the rage. Republicans join lobbyists and business executives for spa weekends in Las Vegas and ski trips at the Four Seasons resort in Vail. Democrats join lobbyists and business executives on the Ritz-Carlton's private beach in Puerto Rico and on quail hunts in Georgia.

Such trips are often sponsored by political campaigns or political action committees, which are funded, in part, by . . . you guessed it: the lobbyists and corporate executives who are attending the festivities, and who have business interests they think the members of Congress might be able to help them with.

As Lipton reported, among those attending a Vail event in January of 2014 were:

> Representative Edward Whitfield, Republican of Kentucky, and Katie Ott, a lobbyist for PPL Corporation, the single biggest contributor to Mr. Whitfield.
>
> Mr. Whitfield is chairman of the Energy and Commerce subcommittee that regulates energy utilities, making him one of the most important players in Congress for the industry. Only days after the Vail trip, he introduced legislation that would allow utilities like PPL to build new coal-burning power plants, overriding environmental restrictions recently imposed by the Obama administration.

Super PAC Attack

Much of this type of activity—the endless fundraising phone calls, the in-person fundraising, the resort retreats—has been intensifying for years. Newer to the scene, though, are super PACs, which, as we discussed in the last chapter, are the progeny of *Citizens United*. One of the many things the five Supreme Court justices failed to envision was how closely super PACs would align with candidates' campaigns—how these allegedly "independent expenditure" entities are not really independent from the candidates at all. Through skilled lawyers, operating in the dim light of an under-resourced and dysfunctional FEC, the candidates have, for all practical purposes, been able to treat these "independent" groups as extensions of their own campaigns.

Presciently, Harvard Law School professor Lawrence Lessig, in a September 2010 commentary for the *Boston Review*, wrote, "No doubt, as corporations exercise this new right, candidates will become skilled in the dance necessary to get enormous corporate wealth spent for their political benefit."[10]

It was widely reported in the spring and summer of 2015 that former Florida governor Jeb Bush was working closely with Right to Rise, a super PAC backing his bid for the 2016 Republican nomination. The group, with Bush's direct help, raised $114 million in the first six months of its existence. Bush was able to coordinate with the group because he had not yet *officially* declared his candidacy. The rationale is laughably adolescent: if Jeb hasn't officially filed paperwork for his campaign, then he's not a candidate for office, so there's no question that Right to Rise is "independent" of his campaign, because there's no campaign to speak of. Kind of like a junior in high school saying to his parents, "I wasn't in Jimmy's basement when the cops broke up the party down there—I was in the kitchen."

Watchdog groups led by the Campaign Legal Center and Democracy 21 filed complaints with the FEC, calling out not only Bush but also fellow Republicans Scott Walker and Rick Santorum and Democrat Martin O'Malley for flouting the law.[11] "These 2016 presidential contenders must take the American people for fools—flying repeatedly to Iowa and New Hampshire to meet with party leaders and voters, hiring campaign staff, and raising millions of dollars from deep-pocketed mega donors, all the while denying that they are even 'testing the waters' of a presidential campaign," said Paul S. Ryan, senior counsel for the Campaign Legal Center, adding that all four "appear to be violating federal law."

In the spring of 2015, Bush's team was reportedly hatching a plan to use his super PAC in an unprecedented way. It would take on tasks that a more accountable, traditional campaign would normally handle: setting up and running phone banks, arranging television advertising, and managing get-out-the-vote operations.[12]

Richard L. Hasen, professor of law and political science at the University of California, Irvine, School of Law and author of *Plutocrats United: Campaign Money, the Supreme Court, and the Distortion of American Elections*, wrote for *Slate*, "By signaling that Right to Rise is his campaign arm, Jeb Bush has broken down the wall between his super PAC and his campaign committee in the eyes of donors."[13]

Outside spending on congressional races doubled from 2010 to 2014, when it reached a staggering $486 million, much of which went undisclosed. In 2004, the Center for Responsive Politics estimated about $5.8 million in dark money (undisclosed) spending. That's a hundredfold increase over the course of ten years.

Money Goes Dark

Super PAC money is disclosed. So when journalists and political pundits talk about "dark money," don't think of super PACs. Think of 501(c)(4) organizations, many of which appear to be set up principally to engage in politics.

Dubbed "social welfare organizations" by the IRS, 501(c)(4)s are tax-exempt groups that aren't required to disclose where their money comes from—a significant fact when you consider that some of the more powerful groups spend tens of millions of dollars each election cycle to advance a single issue or candidate.

In 1956, Alabama Attorney General John Patterson tried to compel the NAACP to disclose the names and addresses of its members in a blatant intimidation effort that would essentially shut down the organization's income. When the NAACP refused, the issue went all the way to the Supreme Court, which unanimously ruled that the organization did not have to disclose the names of its donors, arguing that "compelled disclosure of affiliation with groups engaged in advocacy" could lead to an effective "restraint on freedom" in the form of persecution or retaliation.

In recent years, political operatives have taken advantage of this exemption from disclosure—combined with inaction on regulating 501(c)(4)s by the FEC and IRS—to turn the groups into stealth political bombers. As Matea Gold reported in the *Washington Post* in the summer of 2015, "These tax-exempt groups—which can keep their donors secret even as they sponsor hard-hitting ads—are being increasingly embraced by campaign operatives looking for new ways to influence the political environment."

Groups like Priorities USA, founded by former Barack Obama staffers, and Americans for Prosperity, begun by the Koch brothers, have firmly taken root. The Republican political operative Karl Rove has run tens of millions of dollars through his (c)(4), called Crossroads GPS. New ones, with unmemorable names, are positioning themselves to play significant roles in 2016.

According to the Center for Responsive Politics, "spending by organizations that do not disclose their donors has increased from less than

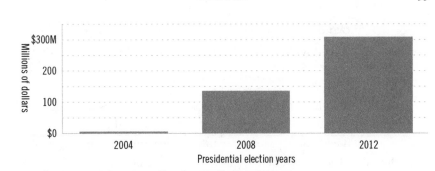

Dark Money Rising: Spending by Undisclosed Donors
Source: Center for Responsive Politics (opensecrets.org)
Methodology: Spending by 501(c)(4) organizations. Numbers are estimated because 501(c)(4) organizations are not required to disclose their donors.

$5.2 million in 2006 to well over $300 million in the 2012 presidential cycle and more than $174 million in the 2014 midterms." The *New York Times* editorial page noted, mournfully, that the 2014 midterm elections were affected by "the greatest wave of secret, special-interest money ever raised in a congressional election."

Although such dark money is a growing problem—an extra shot of poison in an already poisonous mixture—it constituted just 4.6 percent of all campaign spending in 2014.

No Help on the Hill

The Supreme Court is, of course, not solely to blame for problems associated with Big Money. Congress has passed up opportunities to enact commonsense laws for decades. Lawmakers have even failed to pass a bill that would require the funders of groups placing political ads on television to be identified in the ads so that we citizens can know who is trying to influence our votes. Congressional Democrats have introduced such a bill several times since the *Citizens United* decision, but Republicans have consistently blocked it, primarily because of Senator Mitch McConnell (R-KY), who claimed in 2010 that Democrats were behind the bill solely to *look* like reformers.[14] It's hard to tell if that's a fair criticism, but it seems the Democrats aren't taking passage of the bill terribly seriously. The House version of the legislation is called the KOCH Act—Keep Our Campaigns Honest—a personal jab at the wealthy Koch brothers, which shows the lack of seriousness of the effort.

For nearly two decades, Mitch McConnell has been a staunch opponent of campaign finance rules. In 1999, the *New York Times* opened a
story about McConnell with this:

> A bill to overhaul the nation's campaign finance laws is being
> debated on the floor of the Senate. Its advocates and their many
> allies on the editorial pages are in full cry, demanding change for
> the sake of a cleaner, better, more democratic politics. And the
> senior Senator from Kentucky, Mitch McConnell, is doing his
> best to block the bill.
>
> So it went last week: Cheerfully, with conviction, with no apol-
> ogies, Mr. McConnell stood in the well of the Senate, hour after
> hour, swatting back arguments that the system is corrupt, that it
> breeds cynicism, that it shuts out the little guy for the moneyed
> special interests.
>
> "I have sort of been the designated spear catcher on this issue,"
> Mr. McConnell said, somewhat proudly.

McConnell has been more than a spear catcher on the issue; he's been
jamming spears through the skulls of bills that could fix the problem,
including the DISCLOSE Act, despite the fact that, as evidenced by the
2015 *New York Times*/CBS News poll, 76 percent of Republicans support
disclosure of all campaign contributors to outside political groups.

In addition to obstructing legislation, McConnell has engaged in other
forms of spear catching. He brought a lawsuit challenging the McCain-
Feingold law the day Congress passed it in 2002, arguing that it violated
the First Amendment. The Supreme Court in 2006 ruled against him, but
he mushed on nonetheless, praising *Citizens United* when it came down
and filing amicus briefs on behalf of others seeking to weaken campaign
finance laws.

Why he turned so spitefully against reform is unclear.

Interestingly, he was not originally opposed to campaign finance
reform. He supported disclosure for decades.[15] As a Republican Party
county chairman in Louisville in 1973, he even advocated campaign
spending limits and praised public financing efforts.[16] In 1987, McConnell
said he would support a constitutional amendment to allow Congress to
regulate independent expenditures.[17] In 1989, he sponsored a bill, with
Senator Harry Reid (D-NV), that would have required outside groups to
disclose their donors.

President Obama hasn't exactly been a champion of reform, either. Despite some of his strong rhetoric—for instance, his statement at a White House press conference in 2013 that "There aren't a lot of functioning democracies around the world that work this way, where you can basically have millionaires and billionaires bankrolling whoever they want, however they want, in some cases undisclosed"—he has failed to champion the cause. For instance, despite repeated requests from Common Cause and more than fifty other organizations, President Obama (as of the writing of this book) has been unwilling to sign an executive order requiring that all companies receiving federal contracts disclose their political spending.[18]

Other government entities that could help with some of the problems we discuss in this book never seem to get their act together. The Federal Election Commission is the most wretched of examples. The six members of the commission—three Democrats and three Republicans—must be approved by the Senate. As the atmosphere in Washington has become increasingly partisan, the FEC has, for all practical purposes, become paralyzed. A 2013 analysis by the Sunlight Foundation showed a sharp decrease in the dollar amount of fines levied against violators of campaign finance laws as well as a sharp decline in the number of cases commissioners could even agree to make a decision on.[19] "It is dysfunctional," a remarkably blunt Ann Ravel, the 2015 FEC chairwoman, told the *New York Times*. "The likelihood of the laws being enforced is slim."[20]

One of the main duties of the FEC, which was created by Congress in 1975 in the wake of Watergate, is to collect and disclose campaign finance information. Yet in recent years, Republicans and Democrats on the commission haven't been able to agree on how to do that.

Ironically—or perhaps we should say pathetically—members of both parties did unite on at least one issue: letting wealthy people donate more to political parties. Late in 2014, the offices of Harry Reid (who was still Senate majority leader) and House Speaker John Boehner feverishly negotiated the specifics of a $1.1 trillion spending bill. At the very end of their chess game, they agreed to slip in language allowing people to give $1.5 million to the national parties per election. The move was seen as an attempt to strengthen the political parties, which have been overshadowed and outspent by outside funding. CNN called the measure "the latest in a string of setbacks for restrictions on money in politics." House Minority Leader Nancy Pelosi, a Democrat, said it "would work to drown out the voices of the American people." Boehner countered that it and other provisions were "worked out in a bipartisan, bicameral fashion or they wouldn't be in the bill."

Big Money Goes Local

We wish we could claim that coin-operated government exists only at the national level. Sadly, that's not the case. Just as the influence industry has mushroomed in Washington in the last two decades, influence peddlers and political operatives have sought new ways to accomplish their agendas at the state and local levels. You will read, in future chapters, about specific ways in which money and influence place pressure on state and local legislators and regulators, but we want to flag the trend here:

> Four years after the Supreme Court ruled that Congress cannot restrict spending by political groups not directly affiliated with candidates, the "Super PACs" and other spending committees that [have] sprung up in the wake of that decision are becoming a fixture in races farther down on ballot sheets, where their money can have a greater impact.
>
> In some cases, they are looking to bypass a gridlocked Washington . . . In other cases, local operators are adopting tactics first developed at the national level.

That's from a Reuters report, published in October 2014. Journalist Nicholas Confessore wrote the initial "trend piece" about this phenomenon in the *New York Times* earlier that year. In it he quoted the Republican strategist Ed Gillespie: "People who want to see policies enacted, and see things tried, are moving their activity to the states, and away from Washington. There is a sense that you can get things done."

Another Ed—Ed Bender, who directs a watchdog group called the National Institute on Money in State Politics—called the migration of Big Money to the state and local level logical, but unfortunate. "It is less expensive than playing politics at the federal level and the odds of success are often way better," Bender told us. Paul Ryan, a senior attorney at the nonpartisan watchdog group Campaign Legal Center, concurred: "It's often the way things work in money and politics: practices are developed at the national and federal level, and those that work are replicated at the state and municipal level."

An investigation by the Center for Public Integrity found that just fifty individuals and organizations—from former New York City mayor Michael Bloomberg to the Democratic Governors Association—steered $440 million to state candidates and parties in 2014. Eighty-five percent of candidates who got donations from one of those fifty donors won.[21]

Giving directly to state candidates, who raked in $1.2 billion in 2011–2012, is often easier than giving to federal candidates, who can face tougher donation limits.[22] Six states allow limitless giving directly to candidates, and another six have only slight restrictions. Data show that in states like California, Georgia, and South Carolina, all of which have high contribution limits, elections are less competitive. By contrast, elections in Maine, Arizona, and Minnesota, all of which have some form of public financing, are typically much more competitive.[23]

State and local ballot measures attract some of the most deep-pocketed out-of-state business interests and individuals. In 2012, the amount that groups backing or opposing ballot measures raised approached $1 billion, an all-time high.[24] In 2014, a mere fifty donors pumped $266 million into such efforts. More than three quarters of the donors were corporations.[25]

Groups that represent well-financed business have been tilling the fields at the state level for quite some time. The American Legislative Exchange Council (ALEC) has promoted the causes of business interests who pay to be a part of its network for more than forty years. ALEC, which has been described as a "corporate bill mill," connects business lobbyists and state legislators at posh retreats and conferences. It helps the lobbyists build connections with state legislators, then furnishes the legislators with model legislation, often drafted by the corporate lobbyists, to file in the form of actual bills. Regrettably, the legislators, many of whom can't afford to travel to such resorts, and most of whom only work for the public part time, are more than happy to embrace the largesse of ALEC, as a reporter at a Savannah, Georgia, television station discovered while sitting at the bar at an ALEC retreat:

> When I asked the state representative how he pays for a trip like this, he told me that ALEC picks up the hotel room and $350 in expenses directly. He has to come up with the rest, or tap into his ALEC state reimbursement fund. "This is where you would come in, ma'am," he said, turning toward the lobbyist. "I'm the state chair of ALEC, and I look for financial supporters, lobbyists and

the like such as yourself, to send us a couple thousand bucks
every so often."

Super PACs are also getting involved in city council and even school
board elections across the country. A super PAC called the Committee
for Economic Growth and Social Justice filed papers in Washington and
promptly sent more than $150,000, funded largely by the bail bond
industry, to unseat several members of a school board in Elizabeth, New
Jersey. The PAC reportedly was launched by a state senator who wanted
to kick his longtime rivals off the board.[26]

An ally of the losing candidates was shocked. "We've never experienced
or expected that outside interest groups would come in and invest this
kind of money into a local school board race," school board president
Tony Monteiro told *USA Today*. "It boggles the mind . . . The whole landscape has changed."[27]

As the CNN reporter Teddy Schleifer, who covers money in politics,
put it, "A century ago, party bosses ruled cities. Today, super PACs are in
charge. Elections in the nation's cities are increasingly the territory of
deep-pocketed donors who are finding that a dollar spent in a low-cost
municipal race can easily put an ally in power."[28]

Weighting the Scales of Justice

Of the major trends that Ed Bender is watching carefully, efforts by political groups to elect state supreme court justices is at the top of his list—
among all varieties of state races, judicial elections have seen the biggest
percentage increase in independent-money expenditures over the past
decade.

We Americans elect judges in thirty-nine states, including state
supreme court justices. Between 2000 and 2014, these judges—the people
we trust to be the fairest in our society—raised $275 million, according
to *Politico*.[29] That means many judges are making the kinds of solicita-
tions and phone calls to well-financed individuals and interests that
our lawmakers make in Capitol Hill call centers. In the 2012 election
cycle, outside spending in judicial races almost doubled from the
previous cycle.

The nonprofit group Justice at Stake, which focuses on reducing the
role of moneyed interests in judicial elections, asserts that "Since 2000,
elected Supreme Courts have been Ground Zero of an unprecedented

money war, in which competing groups have spent tens of millions on negative ads, in an attempt to pack courts with judges friendly to their agendas."

George W. Bush's former U.S. solicitor general, Ted Olson, has stated, "The improper appearance created by money in judicial elections is one of the most important issues facing our judicial system today." Olson should know. He once represented a man named Hugh Caperton. In 1998, Caperton, who owned a small coal company in West Virginia, filed a lawsuit against the Massey Coal Company. The suit stated that Massey illegally violated a contract to force Caperton's company out of business. When the case went to court, a jury ordered Massey to pay $50 million in damages.[30]

Soon after, Massey's then CEO, Don Blankenship, gave $3 million to help a judicial candidate named Brett Benjamin gain a seat on the West Virginia supreme court. When Massey's appeal came before his court, Benjamin overturned the $50 million ruling against the company.

Caperton took the case all the way to the U.S. Supreme Court, arguing that he hadn't had a fair trial because Judge Benjamin, although entangled in potential conflicts of interest with Blankenship, refused to recuse himself from the appeal. In July 2009, the high court agreed with Caperton in a 5–4 ruling.

After the campaign finance connections to the judge were exposed, Massey was found culpable in a tragic 2010 mine accident at its Upper Big Branch Mine resulting in the death of twenty-nine miners. The mine explosion resulted from excessive buildup of flammable coal dust gas. In its report to the governor, the investigating commission stated: "What is factual and well-documented is that Massey Energy CEO Donald Blankenship had a long history of wielding or attempting to wield influence in the state's seats of government." After $10.8 million in fines, the company was sold to Alpha Natural resources for more than $7 billion, and in 2014 Blankenship was indicted by a federal grand jury on four counts, including one of conspiracy with intent to circumvent mine safety regulations.

Caperton v. Massey, with Ted Olson's help, brought national attention to the issue of money in judicial elections. The other true champion of this cause is former U.S. Supreme Court Justice Sandra Day O'Connor, who was nominated by Ronald Reagan. She advocates replacing judicial elections—which she says have become "political prizefights"—with bipartisan judicial selection commissions.[31] "When you enter one of these courtrooms, the last thing you want to worry about is whether the judge is more accountable to a campaign contributor or an ideological group than to the law," she says. The public agrees: Justice at Stake cites a poll in which 93 percent of respondents said judges should not hear cases involving major campaign supporters.

A variation on that insight rings true for the whole of our democratic republic: the last thing we, or the Founders, would want is for our public servants—judges, elected representatives, government officials—to feel more accountable to a campaign contributor than to all of us.

CHAPTER 3

Oligarchy, Gridlock, Cronyism

Money is poisoning our political system. The people who matter most to a representative democracy—the ordinary voters in whose interests elected politicians are supposed to act—feel as though they've become an afterthought in the political process. The tidal wave of money washing over our elections, with no end in sight, is causing Americans to lose faith in the system. In that way, the course we're on threatens the core values and principles that define us as a nation.

—LEE HAMILTON, FORMER CONGRESSMAN AND
VICE CHAIRMAN OF THE 9/11 COMMISSION[1]

When reporters write about money in politics they often do so with a focus on the most wealthy political players—which super PAC is gearing up to back which candidate—or they focus on who's out-fundraising whom. Those reporters who are given the time by their editors to do more enterprising work—increasingly few—will sometimes try to connect the dots between Big Money players, specific legislative battles in D.C., and distorted policy outcomes. The middle section of this book is dedicated to such dot connecting. And we take it a step farther, showing how specific people are affected by those policy outcomes.

But here we want to dwell for a moment on other big-picture effects of the problem—specifically, the dominance of the wealthiest over policy making, intensified political polarization, and the rise of cronyism within our economy. We do so because we believe it's important to understand that money's influence isn't limited to just the financing of political campaigns or the influence of a few powerful industries over pieces of legislation. It has additional spillover effects as well that pose existential threats to the maintenance of vibrant political parties, bipartisan legislating, and a meritocratic economy.

"An Oligarchy"

Trevor Potter, who has served as the Republican chairman of the Federal Elections Commission, chief counsel to Senator John McCain, and chief political sidekick to Stephen Colbert, was being interviewed by a German television reporter early last year. Toward the end of the interview, the journalist said to Potter, "Tell us more about the oligarchs." Potter politely responded that he wasn't a specialist on Russia or Eastern Europe. The journalist responded, "No, the American oligarchs." As Potter told us, "It was like an out-of-body moment of awareness in which I realized that that's how people in other countries are starting to view our system of government."

Of all of the money-in-politics trends in the wake of *Citizens United*, the most alarming is the rapid and often brazen rise of the billionaire donor class. Reporter Dave Gilson calculated last year in *Mother Jones* magazine that between 1980 and 2012, the share of campaign contributions coming from the top 0.01 percent of political donors nearly tripled.

The sheer number of million-dollar contributions is reflective of this surge in political spending by wealthy Americans. According to the Sunlight Foundation, in 2010, fourteen people contributed $500,000 or more, while eight gave $1 million or more. By 2014, the number of donors who gave $500,000 had mushroomed to 134, while the number of $1-million-plus donors jumped to 63. That same year, according to *Politico*'s Ken Vogel, the one hundred largest campaign contributors donated $323 million. Compare that with the $356 million given by the 4.75 million people who donated $200 or less.[2]

The casino magnate Sheldon Adelson is a prime example of the dominance that a ballroom full of centimillionaires and billionaires now have over the system and the resulting fawning attention they receive from our most powerful elected officials. Chairman and CEO of the Las Vegas

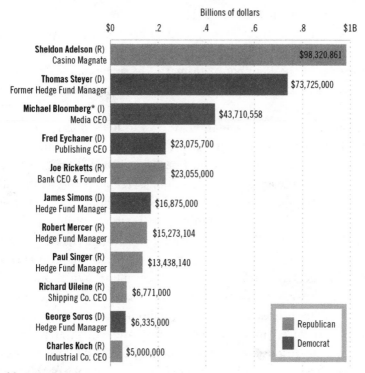

Billions of dollars

	$0	.2	.4	.6	.8	$1B

Sheldon Adelson (R) Casino Magnate — $98,320,861

Thomas Steyer (D) Former Hedge Fund Manager — $73,725,000

Michael Bloomberg* (I) Media CEO — $43,710,558

Fred Eychaner (D) Publishing CEO — $23,075,700

Joe Ricketts (R) Bank CEO & Founder — $23,055,000

James Simons (D) Hedge Fund Manager — $16,875,000

Robert Mercer (R) Hedge Fund Manager — $15,273,104

Paul Singer (R) Hedge Fund Manager — $13,438,140

Richard Uileine (R) Shipping Co. CEO — $6,771,000

George Soros (D) Hedge Fund Manager — $6,335,000

Charles Koch (R) Industrial Co. CEO — $5,000,000

■ Republican
■ Democrat

Notable Mega Donors
Source: Center for Responsive Politics (opensecrets.org)
Methodology: Totals include contributions by donors' wives.
* Bloomberg, an Independent who was previously a Democrat and then a Republican, has contributed primarily to super PACs supporting Democrats.

Sands Corporation and, according to *Forbes*, the eighteenth-richest man in the world, he hosts gatherings that attract not just wealthy political donors but also most of the leading contenders for the Republican presidential nomination.

Multiple GOP hopefuls flocked to an event held in 2014 at Adelson's Venetian Hotel and Casino in Las Vegas, including former Florida governor Jeb Bush and current governors Chris Christie of New Jersey and Scott Walker of Wisconsin. He invited all of them to meet with him privately so he could determine "what makes them tick," the *Washington Post* reported.[3,4]

Who would say no to the man with an estimated net worth of $27 billion and who spent a reported $100 million to influence the 2012 campaigns? The following year, additional presidential hopefuls, including Senator Ted Cruz of Texas and Governors Mike Pence of Indiana and Rick Perry of Texas, went to Las Vegas to have coffee and Diet Cokes with Adelson.[5] Whoever gets his financial support has a huge leg up in the Republican primary. He single-handedly made his favorite 2012 candidate, Newt Gingrich, a serious contender for several months.

Adelson is not merely a man who loves to meet politicians. He has several key economic interests to protect. Most important, he wants Congress to ban most forms of Internet gambling, for the sake of protecting his brick-and-mortar operations. He told *Forbes* he is "willing to spend whatever it takes" to do so.[6] Some of his money has been used to launch a group called the Coalition to Stop Internet Gambling.

Charles and David Koch, like Adelson, also host exclusive gatherings for wealthy conservative donors and candidates. *Forbes* estimates that the two brothers are *each* worth about $40 billion. Which means that, combined, they're worth more than Bill Gates, the richest man on earth. Koch Industries is a private conglomerate of paper mills and companies involved in fossil-fuel refining and chemical production. Together, their various enterprises spend millions of dollars on lobbying every year.[7] The Koch brothers vehemently deny that they or their representatives engage in any kind of rent-seeking behavior. They present themselves as free-market conservatives who lean more toward economic libertarianism. In a 2011 op-ed in the *Wall Street Journal*, Charles Koch ranted about businesses that "have successfully lobbied for special favors and treatment."

Among the estimated 450 who attended their "Freedom Partners" get-together in Palm Springs in January 2015 were Republican senators Marco Rubio of Florida, Rand Paul of Kentucky, Ted Cruz of Arizona and Governor Scott Walker of Arizona. The gatherings typically include a seminar at which the donors pledge large sums of money to finance one or more of the many groups in the Kochs' network.[8] At the Palm Springs get-together, the announced goal was to raise a total of $900 million to influence the 2016 elections.[9]

While there may not be comparably rich kingmakers vetting candidates on the Democratic side, there are several Democrats who spend big in elections. Tom Steyer is the largest. A hedge fund manager worth about $1.5 billion, he spent $74 million on the 2014 midterm elections, focused mainly on defeating foes of climate change legislation—Republican foes—and electing champions of the cause. Most of the races he engaged in lost. He says that his operation, NextGen Climate (which includes a super PAC), is in it for the long haul. "This is about consequences," he said in 2013. "If you have a pattern of voting for subsidies for oil and gas and voting against renewables and all this other stuff . . . there have to be consequences. That's the whole point of this exercise."[10]

Steyer is close to Hillary Clinton, opening up his home for a Clinton fundraiser early in her campaign. Soon after, one of his former aides had taken a job on her campaign team.[11] His super PAC dollars have often gone toward ads attacking the proposed Keystone XL oil pipeline from Canada's tar sands region in Alberta.

If you combine the amount of political money the Koch network, Steyer, and Adelson have spent in the last two election cycles, combined with what they are pledging to spend in 2016, it will likely outstrip the total cost of the entire 1998 election cycle. Let's repeat that: political spending from the networks of three American families is on track to eclipse the entire amount spent in 1998 to elect 435 members of the House and 34 members of the United States Senate (remember that only one third of the Senate is up for election every two years).

Even some long-term players within the political system are reacting with disgust to what they see happening at the top of the political giving pyramid.[12] John Feehery, who, as we mentioned earlier in the book, served as Republican Dennis Hastert's communications director when Hastert was speaker of the House of Representatives, is now head of public relations for the D.C. lobbying firm QGA Public Affairs. He wrote an op-ed in the *Wall Street Journal* in 2015 in which he asserted: "The campaign finance system is now completely in control of the super-wealthy on both the left and the right."

Mark McKinnon, who served for years as George W. Bush's communications director, has similarly written, "Let's call the system that *Citizens United* and other rulings and laws have created what it is: an oligarchy. The system is controlled by a handful of ultra-wealthy people, most of whom got rich from the system and who will get richer from the system."

Other political insiders—both Republican and Democrat—worry about the encroachment of oligarchy. Take, for instance, Rob Stein, who has a long résumé as a political insider. He served as a strategic adviser to the Democratic National Committee, chief of staff to the Clinton-Gore transition team, chief of staff at the Department of Commerce, and cofounder of the Democracy Alliance, a millionaire-billionaire liberal-donor network.

Late in 2014, Stein penned a piece in the *Huffington Post* titled "Voters, Billionaires and Elections for Whom?" In it, he lays out his concerns:

> The combination, on the one hand, of parties with diminished resources with which to support their candidates, and, on the other hand, of wealthy individuals able to create their own electoral machinery (1) is weakening the party as a mediating influence, (2) is contributing to the fracturing of each party into competing wings, (3) may eventually lead to three, four or more parties, and (4) is empowering super wealthy individuals to build their own electoral apparatus to promote their own personal messages and underwrite their preferred candidates.

Stein admitted that he can't predict what, specifically, the future will look like if these trends continue. But, in conversations with us, he was clear about the potential effects: "In this not so brave, unequal and dysfunctional new world of twenty-first-century politics, inequalities not just of income and wealth, but of democratic participation, political influence and economic and civic opportunity will be greatly exacerbated. The wealthy will not simply get wealthier, they will accumulate more and more political power and relegate America to a less inclusive, equitable and just country."

Stein's, McKinnon's, and Feehery's deep concerns about the wealthy accumulating more power are fortified by economic and political science studies that demonstrate that elected officials pay more attention to the concerns of the rich than to the concerns of the rest of us. Research by Martin Gilens and Benjamin I. Page, political scientists at Princeton and Northwestern Universities, explored whether it was empirically true that policy making bends toward the interests of the wealthy. In a much-lauded 2014 study titled "Testing Theories of American Politics: Elites, Interest Groups, and Average Citizens," the two professors examined decades of public opinion polls about policy preferences. They then compared public opinion with the policy preferences of elites, and then measured the two against which policy ideas actually became laws. What they discovered is that when the wealthy support a policy idea, it has a 45 percent chance of becoming law. When the wealthy oppose a given measure, even if it has majority support among the general public, its probability of becoming a law is 18 percent. Their conclusion:

Majorities of the American public actually have little influence over the policies our government adopts ... Americans do enjoy many features central to democratic governance, such as regular elections, freedom of speech and association, and a widespread (if still contested) franchise. But we believe that if policymaking is dominated by powerful business organizations and a small number of affluent Americans, then America's claims to being a democratic society are seriously threatened.

A study by Jesse H. Rhodes and Brian F. Schaffner at the Massachusetts Institute of Technology expresses similar findings. Relying on data from a firm that specializes in microtargeting voters, they found that millionaires do indeed get more representation from their elected officials. In districts where millionaires comprise about 5 percent of the population and the poor about half the population, millionaires got "about twice as much representation."[13]

The hugely successful investor Warren Buffett didn't need to conduct an academic study to come to a similar conclusion. When asked in the spring of 2015 by CNN reporter Poppy Harlow if the wealth divide in America would continue to worsen, Buffett bluntly stated: "With *Citizens United* and other decisions that enable the rich to contribute really unlimited amounts, that actually tilts the balance even more toward the ultra-rich ... The unlimited giving to parties, to candidates, really pushes us more toward a plutocracy. They say it's free speech, but somebody can speak twenty or thirty million times and my cleaning lady can't speak at all."

Polarization and Gridlock

The 112th Congress, which served from January 2011 to January 2013, was the least productive in modern history, passing just 283 laws in two years, a third of which were ceremonial acts such as naming buildings or issuing commemorative coins. The 113th Congress would have tied the 112th had it not managed to pass thirteen more laws.

To put this into historical perspective, the 112th Congress was less productive than the notorious "Do-Nothing Congress" of 1946 and 1947, which for decades had been the poster child for congressional inaction. President Truman used the lack of progress made during the 80th Congress as a main platform for his reelection campaign. And it worked.

Almost seventy years later, the need for action in our nation's capital has never been so great. The national debt has reached a staggering $18 trillion and the economy has not sustained consistent growth in the wake of the Great Recession. Income inequality is at the highest level since the Great Depression and racial tensions continue to rise in the wake of police brutality. The national student loan burden is $1.2 trillion and climbing, while the unemployment rate for recent college graduates in 2014 was more than 12 percent.[14] And those are just some of the domestic issues our elected officials have on their plate. If ever there was a time for our leaders to step up and lead, it's now.

Yet Congress is more divided today than at any time since Reconstruction; moderate politicians are an endangered species. So is the public. A 2014 Pew Research Center poll found that the number of people with "consistently conservative or consistently liberal opinions" has more than doubled over the past twenty years, jumping from 10 percent to 21 percent. Whereas in previous years there was some ideological overlap between people who were expressly Democrat or Republican, now 92 percent of Republicans find themselves to the right of moderate Democrats, and 94 percent of Democrats find themselves to the left of moderate Republicans.

Many members of Congress blame gerrymandering for the increasing levels of partisanship and polarization. Republican Aaron Schock, who represented Illinois' Eighteenth Congressional District until he resigned in 2015 after questions were raised about his use of federal funds for personal use, said this was his one major complaint about Congress.[15] "You know, if I had a magic wand, one thing I would love to change— which you can't do unless you're king—is the redistricting process by which our boundaries are drawn. Because what has happened over the decades is he who controls the mapmaking process, you know, creates hyper-partisan districts." Indeed, the 2014 Cook Political Report Partisan Voter Index found that after the 2012 elections, only one in four House districts was truly competitive—meaning that the makeup of the district was diverse enough that Republicans and Democrats each had a real shot at taking the seat.

Both parties are culpable, having been involved in redistricting to their own advantage for decades. Take Maryland's Third Congressional District, which one federal judge said was "reminiscent of a broken-winged pterodactyl, lying prostrate across the center of the state." For the past five years, Democratic officials in the state have taken every opportunity to redraw districts so they favor liberal candidates, slicing and dicing existing maps to reallocate Democrat voters where it would benefit the party most. In 1995, the state's congressional delegation was evenly split between Republicans and Democrats. Today, Democrats hold all but one of Maryland's eight congressional seats.

All of that said, Big Money—specifically super PACs and 501(c)(4) "dark money" groups—is also contributing to a more hostile political climate. Senator Sheldon Whitehouse of Rhode Island, a Democrat, had this to say about the phenomenon:

> If you're just a plain conservative Republican and not an extreme Tea Partyite, you are very anxious about the combination of the Koch brothers producing a candidate who has untold millions of dollars in outside money coming in for him, in your primary . . . And the next thing you know, you're all done. And it's not the merits of their ideas, it is not the appeal of their personalities—it is the raw political weight of *Citizens United* money.

President Obama has also expressed frustration with the polarizing effects of Big Money. During a particular high-water mark for extreme gridlock—the government shutdown of 2013—he said: "I've continued to believe that *Citizens United* contributed to some of the problems we're having in Washington right now. You have some ideological extremist who has a big bankroll, and they can entirely skew our politics." He added, "There are a whole bunch of members of Congress right now who privately will tell you, 'I know our positions are unreasonable, but we're scared that if we don't go along with the tea party agenda, or the—some particularly extremist agenda, that we'll be challenged from the right.' And the threats are very explicit. And so they toe the line."[16]

Many super PACs and "dark money" groups are here today, gone tomorrow. They have no brands to protect, no historical rootedness in Washington or the state capitals, no other institutional relationships to maintain. They come out of nowhere, with vague names like United for a Stronger America, put a few false or misleading attack ads on the air, and then vanish. It's easier to be extreme today in such an environment than it was when the groups doing the spending were more accountable—like the political parties—and the money was traceable.

Liberal *Washington Post* columnist E. J. Dionne picked up on this trend in the 2014 elections: "Structural changes in our politics are making campaigns more mean and personal than ever," he said. "Outside groups empowered by the Supreme Court's *Citizens United* decision are using mass media in ways that turn Americans off to democracy, aggravate divisions between the political parties, and heighten animosities among citizens of differing views."

We can always hope that, despite these extreme, unaccountable groups, politicians are able to forge meaningful relationships across the political aisle and get the work of the country done. But what if they have no time to forge such bonds? When Iowa senator Tom Harkin, an Ohio Democrat, announced he was retiring in 2013, he told the *Washington Post*:

> We used to have a Senate Dining Room that was only for senators. We'd go down there and sit around there, and Joe Biden and Fritz Hollings and Dale Bumpers and Ted Stevens and Strom Thurmond and a bunch of us—Democrats and Republicans. We'd have lunch and joke and tell stories, a great camaraderie. That dining room doesn't exist any longer because people quit going there. Why did they quit going? Well, we're not there on Monday, and we're not there on Friday. Tuesday we have our party caucuses. That leaves Wednesday and Thursday—and guess what people are doing then? They're out raising money.[17]

Creeping Cronyism

Throughout this book, we've described particularly egregious examples of how money in politics influences the bread-and-butter issues of the American people. It's tempting to chalk these case studies up to bad apples. The problem, though, is that the crisis facing the American public is not one of bad apples but of a diseased orchard.

All markets are formed in response to the demand and supply for goods and services. From the floors of the world's great stock exchanges to the hidden bazaars of ancient nations, markets have both informal and formal rules. In the words of the Nobel laureate Joseph Stiglitz, "Rules matter and power matters."[18] The problem, Stiglitz argues, is that in America today, the powerful are writing the rules—and for their own benefit. Their actions not only undermine the forces of competition that characterize real capitalism, they move us further and further away from the widespread prosperity of the post–World War II years.

By pressuring elected officials and regulatory agencies to bend the rules—or to rewrite them entirely—big businesses are opting out of the competitive marketplace. This practice not only limits competitiveness and innovation, it undermines our fundamental beliefs in an economy distinguished by a level playing field.

The net result: two entirely different sets of economic arrangements—one in which companies that have successfully manipulated Congress are insulated from competition, and another in which smaller firms with less capital are left to pick up the scraps left by their larger, more powerful counterparts.

David Stockman, who served as the director of the Office of Management and Budget in the Reagan administration and is a former Republican member of Congress from Michigan, expresses similar concerns. In his book *The Great Deformation: The Corruption of Capitalism in America*, he points out that the market system is anything but "free." Instead, he argues, "Crony capitalism is about the aggressive and proactive use of political resources ... to gain something from the governmental process that wouldn't otherwise be achievable in the market." He extrapolates from this hypothesis, reasoning that the sweetheart deals offered to big businesses fly in the face of democratic norms. In his words, "We pay for [crony capitalism] in the loss of political equality ... Money dominates politics and as a result we have neither capitalism nor democracy."[19]

When a progressive Nobel laureate like Stiglitz finds himself in the same camp as a Reagan Republican on this issue, it's obvious that opposition to crony capitalism has neither partisan affiliation nor ideological bent. Ours is a time when Tea Party Patriots and Occupy Wall Street share a belief that the game is rigged against the average American, that the individual's ability to chart their own course in the business world is constrained by forces beyond his or her control.

Luigi Zingales, a professor from the traditionally conservative Booth Business School at the University of Chicago, speaks passionately of the America that once was, and the America that now is, in his book *A Capitalism for the People*. Zingales was born in Italy, a land where networks of patronage and favors meant everything. He came to the United States for his graduate studies, lured by our country's meritocratic ideals and the promise of a graduate fellowship in Boston. Zingales describes the vision he had of "the land of opportunity":

> In contrast to the rest of the world, where capitalism is too often the
> creature of a rich elite who saw an opportunity to become richer,
> America's brand of capitalism has survived and thrived because of
> a unique set of circumstances: a government attentive to the inter-
> ests of ordinary people, a set of values that have made accumula-
> tion of wealth a moral responsibility rather than an end in itself,
> and a belief that the system provides opportunities for all.[20]

Rather than pursuing government allies to buy up their products, Americans invented new technologies that met the market's needs. Instead of familial nepotism, Americans rose to higher positions largely by their ability to put new ideas out into the world and work hard.

For many years, indeed for pivotal years, Zingales's ideal accurately described the American economy. During the post–World War II era, the United States presided over a period of unmatched economic growth and stability. The economy throve, and more Americans were able to share in that prosperity.

As we all know from so many newspaper headlines and books in recent years, that economy has vanished. We now live in a time of wage stagna-tion for the majority of working families, of pronounced inequities and limited access to opportunity.

Over the past several decades, it's become the new normal for a handful of companies to dominate each major industry. Desmond Lachman, a senior fellow with the right-of-center American Enterprise Institute and former International Monetary Fund director, reports, "The gross profits of the 200 largest US corporations as a percentage of gross profits in the economy has risen steadily from 15 percent in the early 1950s to 30 percent by the early 2000s."[21] The goal of too many inventors and start-up founders is no longer to make it big through competition in the market-place but to be bought up—to be subsumed by global giants.

As Zingales points out, this tendency to aggressively acquire small upstarts rather than develop new programs in-house is also characteristic of some corporations' political strategies. He writes, "[These] incumbent large firms [many of them tech companies] are politically powerful but not necessarily the most efficient ... they have a strong incentive to manipulate the power of the state to preserve their market power through political means."[22] He has additionally stated: "Traditionally, corporations used to lobby to get the government off their backs. As they grew more skillful, their efforts went from reactive to proactive, and toward getting government in their pockets to obtain unique privileges."

While consolidating market power, many industries also work on rigging the tax code so that they can shield their income. In the introduction to this book, we mentioned the farewell address that John Kerry delivered to his Senate colleagues before he headed over to the Department of State. Lamenting the dominance of money over politics, he said, "The insidious intention of that money is to set the agenda, change the agenda, block the agenda, define the agenda of Washington. How else could we possibly have a U.S. tax code of some 76,000 pages? Ask yourself, how many Americans have their own page, their own tax break, their own special deal?"

There are a myriad of opinions about what taxes the government should levy, who should pay what, and how that money should be spent. But there is overwhelming agreement on one thing: our tax code—which was just twenty-seven pages long in 1913—is needlessly complex. There are tax breaks on everything from private jets to cat food and luxurious vacation homes. In 2012, the *New York Times* reported that loopholes in the tax code could have cost anywhere from $700 billion to $1 trillion the previous year.[23] Yet after years of debates to address what Senator Ron Wyden, chairman of the Senate Finance Committee, called the "dysfunctional, rotting mess of a carcass that we call the tax code," tax reform remains dead in the water because of the gridlock caused by wealthy special interests.

The poster child for tax preferences is something called "carried interest." This is the portion of income earned by a hedge fund manager's investments above a certain threshold. It is taxed at the current capital gains rate of 20 percent rather than at the upper bracket income rate of 39.6 percent.

The Real Estate Roundtable estimates that the revenue loss to the United States as a result of the carried-interest tax loophole is $13 billion annually. That's not just $13 billion that could go into deficit reduction or rebuilding the nation's crumbling infrastructure; that's 13 billion extra dollars—each year—that are going into the pockets of people who are already astonishingly rich.

Lynn Forester de Rothschild is the chief executive of EL Rothschild, a family-owned investment company. As you can imagine, she's a very wealthy woman who likely knows a lot of hedge fund managers. But in 2013 she wrote an op-ed in the *New York Times* stating:

> Of the many injustices that permeate America's byzantine tax code, few are as outrageous as the tax rate on 'carried interest' ... This

state of affairs denies our Treasury much-needed revenue; fuels public cynicism in government; and is evidence of the 'crony capitalism' that favors some economic sectors over others. When plutocrats join with both parties to protect their own vested interests, the result is a corrosion of confidence in the free-market system.

As Warren Buffett once quipped, the loophole allows him to pay a lower tax rate than his secretary.

There have been multiple attempts to close the sweetheart tax deal down. In 2007, a bill to do so was introduced by Representative Sander Levin (D-MI). But the hedge fund industry blocked him. In 2010, there was another attempt in the Senate to remove the "carried interest" from the tax code. Lobbyists representing some of the most powerful hedge funds unleashed their dogs. Take just one of them—Blackstone. Working on its behalf were Drew Maloney, formerly a staffer for Representative Tom DeLay, and Moses Mercado, who used to work for Representative Dick Gephardt. They were joined by dozens of other Republican and Democratic lobbyists who were aligned in their desire to keep the loophole open. When the provision made its way to a vote, every single Republican voted against the change, joined by one Democrat, Senator Ben Nelson (D-NE). The bill failed to advance.

For our fellow Americans, the case of "carried interest" produces two entirely different sets of economic arrangements—one in which hedge fund managers who've successfully lobbied Congress are given an economic advantage with no economic justification, and another in which regular people are required to play by the normal rules.

Tim Carney is a reporter who writes for the Republican-leaning *Washington Examiner* and a fellow at the American Enterprise Institute. He is obsessed with these sweetheart deals and unfair advantages. He promotes the idea of "libertarian populism" and believes that "the game is rigged in America today, government is rigging it in in favor of the well connected, and that free and open markets are the way to unrig the game, and help the middle class."[24] In his book *The Big Ripoff*, he argues that big government and big business go hand in hand—the two operate in a mutually beneficial relationship that marginalizes small enterprises.[25]

In Carney's eyes, this is not an issue that is exclusively tied to Democrats or Republicans—both parties are at fault. In a 2013 article, he provides a laundry list of examples of corporate cronyism, spanning the latter Bush and early Obama years: ethanol, incandescent lightbulb bans, the automotive industry and Wall Street bailouts, the economic stimulus deals for green tech companies, and multiple provisions of the Affordable Care Act, or Obamacare.

You will read about more specific examples of cronyism later in this book. But the point we want to leave you with here is that a growing number of prominent thinkers—left, right, and center—are beginning to conclude that our increasingly rigged political system is leading to an increasingly rigged economy.

The combination of the two threatens the very promise of what America, and other Western democracies, offered to the world in the latter half of the twentieth century—a model in which "liberal" democracy and market-based, merit-based capitalism were seen as the only viable model for societies.

In 1989, the neoconservative writer and thinker Francis Fukuyama published his breakthrough essay "The End of History," in which he declared: "What we are witnessing is not just the end of the cold war, or a passing of a particular period of postwar history, but the end of history as such: that is, the end point of mankind's ideological evolution and the universalisation of western liberal democracy as the final form of human government."

In 2013, Fukuyama published an essay that can be seen as a course correction, or perhaps a lament, titled "The Decay of American Political Institutions." The first reason he cites for such decay is the lack of power within the executive branch to administer the government. The second:

> The accretion of interest group and lobbying influences has distorted democratic processes and eroded the ability of the government to operate effectively . . . Interest groups, having lost their pre–Pendleton Act ability to directly corrupt legislatures through bribery and the feeding of clientelistic machines, have found new, perfectly legal means of capturing and controlling legislators. These interest groups distort both taxes and spending, and raise overall deficit levels through their ability to manipulate the budget in their favor.

Crony capitalism can be fought only if we first regain our right to self-government. If we don't, it will be harder for us to recreate an economy that works for everyone, not just those who can afford to put coins in the machine.

PART 2

CHAPTER 4

Too Big to Beat

Let's take you back to early September 2008. The federal government had just done something previously unthinkable—committing nearly $200 billion of taxpayers' money in an emergency takeover of the troubled mortgage giants known as Fannie Mae and Freddie Mac.[1]

A week later, on Sunday, September 14, 2008, one of the country's most prestigious brokerage houses, Merrill Lynch, mired in billions of dollars of toxic assets nobody wanted and in danger of collapsing, agreed to sell itself to Bank of America.[2] On the same day, Lehman Brothers, another big Wall Street firm, collapsed. The following day, one of the world's largest insurance companies, AIG, accepted an $85 billion federal bailout, the largest of a private company in U.S. history.[3]

On Wednesday, September 24, with credit markets frozen and banks refusing to lend money, Republican presidential nominee John McCain suspended his campaign and called on Barack Obama to do the same. (Obama ignored the suggestion.) Then came the biggest bank failure in American history, when Washington Mutual was seized by federal regulators and sold, in part, to JP Morgan Chase. Other bankers were terrified, fearing that their institutions would go belly up, too. Many wanted capital from the government because, they said, that's what would let them start lending again.

Americans were anxious, and many already were suffering. Six in ten people polled worried that a depression was likely.[4] Unemployment rose to the highest levels since 1994. One in ten homeowners were either behind on their mortgage payments or facing foreclosure.[5]

The federal government soon did come to the rescue, of course. The recovery for the banks was so complete that within a few years after the bailout they were posting near-record profits[6]—$40 billion in the second quarter of 2014 alone. The stock market has surged. The Dow Jones Industrial Average, in fact, has nearly tripled from its low point in 2009. In 2015, it hit an all-time high, going above 18,000 for the first time.[7] In 2013, corporate profits reached their highest levels in eighty-five years.[8]

The recovery has been much less swift for regular folks, certainly for the millions of people who lost their jobs and in many cases their homes. Growth in real wages has been stagnant since 2009—near zero since the depths of the recession.[9] In 2015, nearly three fourths of those polled by the Pew Research Center said they believed government policies had done little or nothing to help the middle class. Nearly one third said the recession had had a major effect on their finances and that they still had not recovered.[10]

Washington's response to the financial crisis, which almost led to the collapse of the U.S. and global economies, is our starting point for part 2 of this book. That crisis was perhaps our lawmakers' most important moment to take big action, to correct the practices of an industry that had brought us to the brink of financial collapse. But important reforms to keep our economy safe did not make it out of Congress, and they remain undone today.

The major congressional response to the crisis, the 2010 legislation known as Dodd-Frank (its lead sponsors were Christopher Dodd of Connecticut in the Senate and Barney Frank of Massachusetts in the House), has brought some needed transparency to the banking industry and contains important consumer protections, but almost no one believes it will prevent another crisis in the years ahead. And that is precisely because of the undue influence of the financial sector, which we will detail in this chapter. It goes without saying that action that should have been taken years earlier that could have prevented the crisis and resulting recession didn't happen, either. That's because lawmakers and regulators have long been more focused on helping the banks than on protecting you and me from reckless lending practices.

In part 2, we will show how the unbridled power and influence of numerous industries affects our government, our economy, and by extension, all of us. And, as you read in part 1, that power and influence have only grown in recent years as the cost of elections has skyrocketed, drawing elected officials ever closer to the donors they need in order to get reelected. It is a self-perpetuating system that benefits a few at the expense of the many.

In this section, we offer glimpses into how Big Money manipulates much of our government and affects our daily lives: our financial security and the roofs over our heads; the medications many of us rely on to stay alive; the quality of the air we breathe, the water we drink, and the food we eat; and the sickening toxins we can't avoid because of their pervasiveness in thousands of products, from flooring to pesticides to hair spray.

When it became clear that the $200 billion takeover of Fannie Mae and Freddie Mac, which Treasury Department officials announced on Sunday, September 7, 2008, would not be sufficient to steer the nation's economy away from the cliff, the Bush administration began putting together what would be called the Troubled Asset Relief Program (TARP), a $700 billion government investment in banks, insurers, and automakers.

The proposed plan sparked a full-on blitz by lobbyists, who knew they had only a short time to shape the program to their liking. "This is not following any normal process," the then chief executive of the American Bankers Association (ABA), Ed Yingling, told the *New York Times*. "It's like a big Category 4 hurricane coming through."[11]

The interest groups had the resources to meet their goals. The ABA alone had a roster of nearly a hundred hired lobbyists.[12] Pressure also came from groups such as the U.S. Chamber of Commerce, the biggest lobbying kingpin in Washington, which spent $92 million in 2008 alone.[13] In all, financial, insurance, and real estate interests dropped more than $450 million lobbying Washington that year to make sure the bailout package met their needs.[14,15]

According to Yingling, the ABA had never wanted TARP, which was unveiled on September 19. But it was clear "we had to help it pass" because, as he wrote in an email, "its defeat would cause a huge market panic." He added, "We did have some success in keeping it clean as it went through Congress."

The legislation, which essentially would make the government the owner, at least temporarily, of billions of dollars in toxic assets, did not sail smoothly through Congress, however. On September 29, 2008, after a contentious debate, the House stunned Wall Street when it rejected the bailout. The Dow Jones dropped 778 points that day— the largest ever single-day fall.[16] That was not the only record set that day: $1.2 trillion in market value had vanished on Wall Street by the time the markets closed. Days later, a spooked Congress finally passed the bill.

What was not in the bailout plan: any tax on financial institutions to finance it. Nor did it include a provision, opposed by the banks, that would allow judges to renegotiate mortgage terms to help homeowners facing foreclosure. And as a result of lobbying by the U.S. Chamber of Commerce, it did not contain the limits on executive compensation that many lawmakers felt were warranted.

Banks Benefited When Democrats Turned Right

This crisis, of course, didn't happen in a vacuum. In the decades leading up to the Great Recession, Wall Street's power over Washington had grown steadily. A major reason for that was a change in attitude among Democratic lawmakers and candidates. Many Democrats, who had some-times stood up to the big banks in Congress, had become as close to Wall Street as many Republicans. That's understandable when you consider that the financial sector has become the biggest source of reelection dollars. Since 1990, it has fed $3.89 billion in contributions to federal candidates and super PACs, far more than any other industry.[17] And of the one hundred firms that have contributed the most to federal campaigns since 1989, there are more financial companies than energy, healthcare, defense, and telecom companies combined.[18]

Democrats in Congress had once often served as a check against the bank lobbyists' efforts to loosen regulations, including their goal of weak-ening or even repealing the Glass-Steagall Act of 1933, which prohibited commercial banks from participating in the investment banking busi-ness. When commercial banks pushed for a repeal in the early 1980s, for example, congressional Democrats helped block it.[19] Later, when the Federal Reserve ruled that banks could, in effect, dedicate small percent-ages of their revenues to investment banking, a Democratic-led House and Senate passed a bill declaring a moratorium on the Fed's approvals of banks' applications to deal in securities.[20]

But a slow shift began during the Reagan administration. One of the factors leading to the shift was the emergence of the Democratic Leadership Council, formed in response to Ronald Reagan's 1984 landslide victory over Walter Mondale. The DLC sought to move Democrats more to the right, especially in the South, as a way to win more seats. Another reason was the fact that the Democratic National Committee was deep in the red at the time.

The DLC was formed in 1985 by a political operative named Al From, who felt the party should be more business-friendly and centrist. Two of its early devotees were Bill Clinton of Arkansas and Al Gore of Tennessee. The group's goal was to turn the Democratic Party away from activists, labor unions, and hot-button social issues and toward fiscal restraint, smaller government, and a free-market outlook, as Robert Dreyfuss reported in the *American Prospect* in 2001.[21] If Democrats had to look beyond labor unions for funding, banking was a more palatable business than, say, coal. The "New Democrats," as the DLC members called themselves, raised money by bringing wealthy donors into the same room as elected officials. By 2000, the group was raising about $5.5 million per year for like-minded candidates.[22]

With many New Democrats befriending Wall Street just as much as Republicans did, the financial industry poured more and more money into congressional coffers throughout the 1990s. Political contributions from the finance, real estate, and insurance sectors have skyrocketed since then, from $62 million in 1990 to $320 million in 2000 to nearly $675 million in 2012, according to the Center for Responsive Politics.[23]

Taking a Page from the GOP's Money-Raising Playbook

The Democrats' desire for new and bigger sources of reelection cash contributed to a turn toward a number of policies favorable to Wall Street. In terms of fundraising, the Democrats were getting slaughtered by the GOP, whose three big national committees had nearly five times as much revenue as the Democrats by 1986, as documented in the book *Winner-Take-All Politics* by the political scientists Jacob S. Hacker and Paul Pierson.[24]

That also began to change in the early 1980s, when Representative Tony Coelho of California was appointed chair of the Democratic Congressional Campaign Committee. Coelho was a much more aggressive fundraiser than his predecessors at the DCCC, developing a reputation as "the guy who sucked up all the PAC money in the world,"[25] as the *Los Angeles Times* reported.[26] Coelho tripled the DCCC's fundraising by 1986.[27]

As Marjorie Williams wrote in the *Washington Post* in a postmortem about Coelho's time at the DCCC:

> The positive way of summarizing what Coelho accomplished is to say that he placed a limit on the GOP realignment, preserving the House as a seat of Democratic resistance to Reagan's realignment all through the '80s. Less generous accounts conclude that Coelho sold the party's soul in the process, by vastly expanding the contributions of business political action committees—and the expectations those contributors felt in return . . .
>
> The crux of Coelho's appeal to businessmen was the unsubtle reminder that Democrats already controlled the House. He went to business and said, in effect, "You might not like us, but we've got our hands on the levers right now; you have to give to us." . . . He also started the "Speaker's Club," which offered business PACs, for a contribution of $15,000, the chance to "serve as trusted, informal advisers to the Democratic Members of Congress."

In a similar piece in the *New Republic* in 1995, Ruth Shalit wrote of Coelho that he

> aggressively marketed the once pro-labor Democratic Party as increasingly pro-business, often during candidate forums for corporate PAC managers. The contradictions of policy or philosophy never slowed him down. During these forums—nicknamed meat markets or cattle calls—Coelho forced candidates to stand behind tables, each with a name card and a place to display his or her literature.

Among the industries Coelho embraced most: finance. Specifically, the savings and loan industry, where Coelho cultivated deep relationships with unsavory—but very wealthy—characters, some of whom ended up going to jail in the wake of the savings and loan collapse in the late 1980s and early 1990s. Some of his fundraising adventures were well chronicled by the *Wall Street Journal* reporter Brooks Jackson in his book *Honest*

Graft. Here is Williams's summary of what Jackson and other journalists uncovered:

> Most damningly, Jackson and other reporters also exposed Coelho as he stepped blindly into bed with the savings and loan industry. He appointed as the DCCC finance cochairman one Dallas multimillionaire, Thomas Gaubert, who was eventually convicted of S&L fraud and barred from the Texas thrift business by federal regulators. Another major DCCC donor was Donald Dixon, later convicted of looting Texas's Vernon Savings & Loan, which ultimately cost U.S. taxpayers $1.3 billion. Coelho was given the use of Vernon corporate aircraft and a luxury yacht, the *High Spirits*, for travel and party fund-raising; when this was reported, he was forced to reimburse almost $50,000—more than half of it from his personal campaign committee—to Vernon, which was by then run by federally appointed conservators. Speaker of the House Jim Wright tried to intercede with federal regulators on behalf of both Gaubert and Dixon—in the latter case, at Coelho's direct urging. And in 1987, Coelho also helped S&L owners by scaling back a bill authorizing funds that bank regulators desperately needed to stay on top of the exploding crisis.

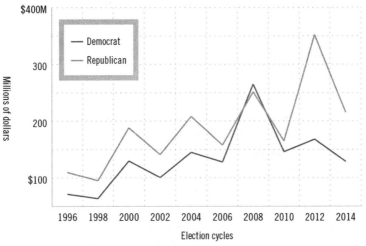

Financial Sector Donations to Each Party
Source: Center for Responsive Politics (opensecrets.org)
Methodology: Donations to federal candidates and parties from financial, insurance, and real estate interests.

In 1989, Coelho resigned from Congress after the exposure of a personal financial scandal in which he failed to disclose a financial transaction with an investment company that Coelho had helped while in office.[28] He was never charged with any specific crime. Soon after resigning, he became an investment banker for a New York firm.[29]

But the trend that Coelho started—aligning the Democratic Party with industries that, throughout most of the twentieth century, it had approached with greater caution—certainly continued. In 2008, for instance, during the height of the financial crisis and the Obama-McCain presidential race, the Democratic Senatorial Campaign Committee (led by New York senator Chuck Schumer) raised about three times more from Wall Street than the Republican Senatorial Campaign Committee did.[30]

The Cash Committee

The number of members serving on the House Financial Services Committee has increased significantly in recent years—from fifty members in 1995 to sixty in 2015—not so much because of its importance to the nation's financial well-being but because of its importance to the political parties' financial well-being. If party leaders think a rank-and-file member in a competitive district might need a big campaign war chest to get reelected, he or she stands a good chance of getting appointed to the committee, which the *Huffington Post*'s Ryan Grim and Arthur Delaney dubbed the "Cash Committee."[31]

The Cash Committee members are especially reliant on Wall Street money. Of all the contributions to House Financial Services Committee members, the money they received from finance, insurance, and real estate interests increased from 26 percent in 1999–2000 to 35 percent in 2013–2014, according to the Center for Responsive Politics. They're also very likely to be poached by lobbying firms offering them much higher salaries than the government can, which is another incentive for the members to be viewed as helpful to the financial sector.

"Traditionally, the money committees as a whole have always been the most valuable places to jump from the Hill to K Street," Ivan Adler of the headhunting firm the McCormick Group told the *Huffington Post*.[32] The *Huffington Post* looked at the staffers who have left the House Financial Services Committee between 2000 and 2009. Of the 126 people identified, 62 went on to register as lobbyists.[33] It works the other way, too.

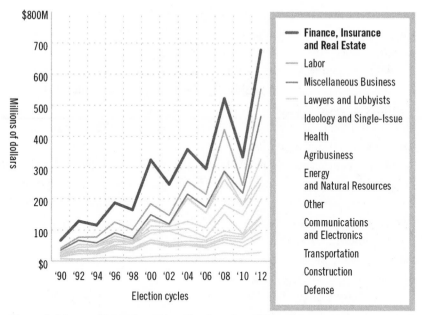

Financial Sector Campaign Contributions Dominate
Source: Center for Responsive Politics (opensecrets.org)

In 2009, 18 percent of the Financial Services Committee aides had worked on K Street before getting to a job on the Hill.[34] This all leads to tight collaboration between the overseers and the overseen.

Members of Congress, Tear Down This Wall!

By the late 1990s, with Democrats now fully on board with Wall Street, the stage was set for what would become a tragedy for millions of Americans a few years later. A deregulatory fever had taken hold in Washington.

The Financial Crisis Inquiry Commission, which was commissioned by Congress to look into the origins of the crisis, began its January 27, 2011, final report with these words: "We conclude that this financial crisis was avoidable."[35]

One of the key reasons, the FCIC concluded, was the failure of regulators to police the industry. "More than 30 years of deregulation and reliance on self-regulation by financial institutions, championed by former Federal Reserve chairman Alan Greenspan and others, supported by successive administrations and Congresses, and actively pushed by the powerful financial industry at every turn, had stripped away key safeguards, which could have helped avoid catastrophe."[36]

Glass-Steagall was the biggest of those safeguards. And it did not fall in one fell swoop. The banking lobby had been chipping away at it for years, resulting in Federal Reserve Board regulatory changes in the 1980s that allowed federally insured banks to earn a percentage of their profits from investment banking activities.

As noted earlier, Glass-Steagall was enacted in the midst of the Great Depression. It forced banks to choose between being either a commercial bank that could make loans to borrowers, or an underwriter of stocks and bonds. In essence, it erected a firewall between commercial and investment banking. That law also created the Federal Deposit Insurance Corporation, providing government insurance of bank deposits (a part of Glass-Steagall that, fortunately, remains intact).

On the floor of the U.S. Senate on November 5, 1999, just before the Senate was about to vote to repeal Glass-Steagall, Senator Byron Dorgan, a North Dakota Democrat and one of the few congressional opponents of its repeal, warned of the consequences: "I think we will look back in 10 years' time and say we should not have done this but we did because we forgot the lessons of the past, and that that which is true in the 1930s is true in 2010."[37]

Another opponent of the repeal measure was Democratic senator Paul Wellstone of Minnesota, who, as reported by the *New York Times*, said that Congress "seemed determined to unlearn the lessons from our past mistakes." He added: "Scores of banks failed in the Great Depression as a result of unsound banking practices, and their failure only deepened the crisis. Glass-Steagall was intended to protect our financial system by insulating commercial banking from other forms of risk. It was one of several stabilizers designed to keep a similar tragedy from recurring. Now Congress is about to repeal that economic stabilizer without putting any comparable safeguard in its place."[38]

Dorgan and Wellstone were among just eight senators to vote against repeal. Ninety of their colleagues voted for it.

After the House voted that same night, 362 to 57, to repeal Glass-Steagall, the bill was on its way to the White House, where President Clinton signed it a week later. Among the biggest cheerleaders of the repeal bill had been Clinton's Treasury secretary, Lawrence H. Summers.

Enter Sandy Weill

Glass-Steagall might still be in place had it not been for the influence of a Wall Street executive with close ties to the Clinton administration: Sandy Weill, a big fundraiser for the Democratic Party who was the CEO of Travelers Group. In 1998, Weill and John Reed, the CEO of Citicorp, announced that their two companies would merge to form the world's largest financial services company, which would be called Citigroup Inc. Although the merger would have been in violation of Glass-Steagall, Weill and Reed were able to complete the deal—the biggest corporate merger in history—by agreeing that the new company would divest itself of its insurance business in two years.

In the weeks leading up to the merger announcement, Weill made calls to the president, Treasury Secretary Robert Rubin, and Federal Reserve chairman and former JP Morgan director Alan Greenspan, who ultimately approved the merger under existing precedent giving corporations two to five years to divest before officially violating Glass-Steagall.[39]

After the merger was announced, Citigroup and other financial lobbyists pushed to remove the parts of Glass-Steagall that would force them to spin off the insurance industry. They had strong partners in the White House's two pro–Wall Street regulators—Rubin and Summers (who at the time reported to Rubin as deputy secretary of the Treasury)—and in GOP senator Phil Gramm of Texas, who guided the legislation through the Senate. From 1989 to 2002, Gramm received more campaign contributions from commercial banks than any other senator.[40] (After retiring in 2002, he was hired as a lobbyist for Swiss Bank UBS, earning an undisclosed sum, and was still a consultant there in 2015.)

Citigroup had upped its political game to help make sure the repeal vote would succeed. Just look at its flow of money over the course of less than a decade: In the 1992 election, Citicorp contributed about $1.5 million to federal candidates and political parties.[41] By the 1999–2000 election cycle, its contributions had increased to more than $4 million.[42] It spent another $16.5 million in lobbying expenses from 1998 to 2000, more than any other bank.[43]

In all, according to the *New York Times,* the financial sector devoted more than $300 million to lobbying and campaign contributions in 1997 and 1998 as part of its effort to get rid of Glass-Steagall.[44]

Good Fixes Proposed, but Never Passed

The too-big-to-fail banks that had to be bailed out because of their reck-less practices were certainly not the only financial institutions that caused the near meltdown of the U.S. economy. In fact, the loosely regulated mortgage lending companies that began to proliferate in the 1990s and early 2000s may have contributed more to the dire straits many Americans found themselves in than the Wall Street companies.

Many of those companies granted subprime loans to people who would likely have difficulty making repayment; in exchange for the added risk, lenders charged higher interest rates. In 2006, at the height of the subprime bubble, the nonpartisan Center for Responsible Lending projected that 2.2 million of the 14 million subprime loans made between 1998 and 2006 would end in foreclosure, destroying as much as $164 billion of wealth.[45]

These lending companies included big names like Countrywide and Ameriquest. Ameriquest's political action committee and its employees and their relatives dispensed more than $20 million to state and federal political groups from 2002 to 2006, according to the *Wall Street Journal*, and they played a big role in weakening existing lending laws in the states, Georgia and New Jersey in particular.[46] As Countrywide dived deeper into subprime lending, it bought Washington protection, increasing its lobbying budget from $60,000 in 1998 to more than $1.5 million seven years later.[47]

In the early 2000s, several state legislatures passed laws to protect their citizens against predatory lenders. Georgia passed one of the toughest in 2002. But lobbyists for surging mortgage lending companies—led by Countrywide and Ameriquest—flocked to the states to persuade legisla-tors to relax the new laws, and Georgia's law was soon clawed back.[48] Lobbyists for big banks, some of which also originated subprime loans in the mid-2000s, also argued against state laws curbing predatory lending.[49]

Members of Congress had many opportunities to rein in the subprime bonanza but always turned the other way. Former Maryland Democratic senator Paul Sarbanes, who chaired the Senate Banking, Housing and Urban Affairs Committee, introduced the Predatory Lending Consumer Protection Act in 2000 and again in 2002, but the bill was never enacted because of industry opposition. One of the most outspoken critics of Sarbanes's bill was the top Republican on the committee—once again, Senator Phil Gramm.

The money was always stacked against Sarbanes and other advocates of fair lending. Though Sarbanes's bill was endorsed by more than a dozen civil rights and consumer groups in 2002, most had little if any money to spend on lobbying, and only two—AARP and the Leadership Conference on Civil Rights—had a lobbying budget above $300,000.

The ultimate authority to curb subprime lenders lay with the Federal Reserve Bank, which is charged with the responsibility for the "safety and soundness" of our financial system and "protecting the credit rights of consumers." But under former chairman Alan Greenspan's leadership, the Fed didn't show much interest in what was happening in the mortgage business, despite calls from housing advocates to take action.[50] It wasn't until Greenspan left the chairmanship that the Fed, in 2007, finally proposed a rule prohibiting lenders from making mortgage loans without considering borrowers' ability to repay them.[51]

"We Are Not Represented in This Melee"

The 2010 Wall Street Reform and Consumer Protection Act, better known as Dodd-Frank, was our best chance to address the fundamental flaws in the U.S. financial services industry and prevent another crisis from developing. The legislation made serious strides despite Wall Street opposition—including the creation of the Consumer Financial Protection Bureau, greater oversight of payday lenders, more transparency into derivatives markets, and the reserve requirement, which has shored up the capital of lending institutions. But, regrettably, the law did not sufficiently address the underlying causes of the crisis.

As a consequence, it may be only a matter of time before we find ourselves at the brink of another financial meltdown. When asked by the journalist Bill Moyers in 2012 whether that is likely, *New York Times* business reporter Gretchen Morgenson replied: "It will happen again, and the unfortunate fact is we did not fix the problem."[52] When asked why, she responded:

> Well, a big part of it is the money problem, that money—the big powered, moneyed institutions are in control in Washington, there's no doubt about it. You and I don't have a lobbyist and so we are not represented in this melee, call it what you will, that happens, you know, when laws are created.[53]

Former senator Ted Kaufman, a Delaware Democrat, went so far as to call the final version of Dodd-Frank a victory for the bank lobby. "Look at what their financial reports and bonuses look like since Dodd-Frank," Kaufman said, adding that the banks' change in behavior lasted "about 48 hours."

Lobbyists were hugely influential in the drafting of the Dodd-Frank law, which passed in July 2010. They were able to kill proposals that they considered especially onerous, and they were able to write the law in a way that gave regulators too-wide discretion. They were betting that their close relationships with regulators would enable them to influence the rule-writing process—which is used to create greater specificity about the intention of the legislation—and even slow down the implementation of the law. It was a safe bet.

As Congress was finalizing and implementing provisions of Dodd-Frank, financial industry lobbyists vastly outnumbered consumer lobbyists.[54] The industry and its allies also spent an estimated $1 billion on lobbying in the months leading up to the passage of the bill, and it continues to spend millions more to undo and weaken reforms, provision by provision.[55] Among the industry's well-heeled allies: the U.S. Chamber of Commerce, which spent $132 million on lobbying in 2010 on Dodd-Frank and other matters.[56] The biggest spender among groups defending Dodd-Frank, by contrast, has been the nation's largest union of public sector workers, known as AFSCME, which spent less than $3 million on lobbying that year.[57]

What the Money Buys: Face Time with Regulatory Agencies

Number of lobbyist meetings since passage of the Dodd-Frank law. July 2010-April 2013

Top 5 consumer protection groups

Americans for Financial Reform: **47**
Consumer Federation of America: **41**
Center for Responsible Lending: **15**
AFSCME: **11**
U.S. Public Interest Research Group: **2**

116

Top 5 commercial banks

Goldman Sachs: **238**
JP Morgan Chase: **222**
Morgan Stanley: **189**
Bank of America: **153**
Wells Fargo: **99**

901

Money Buys Face Time with Regulators
Source: Infographic by Tracy Loeffelholz. Research by the Investigative Fund at the Nation Institute from sunlightfoundation.com.

As we have seen, banks also rely on former congressional staffers who can leverage their relationships and expertise gained while on taxpayer-paid salaries. The financial sector, which comprises finance, real estate, and insurance firms, has had more employees go through the revolving door than any other clearly defined sector, according to the Center for Responsive Politics. The six biggest banks and their trade associations employed more than 240 former government staffers and members of Congress as lobbyists during the two years after the first bank bailout in 2008.[58] By 2014, nearly nine out of ten Citigroup lobbyists were former government staffers.[59]

The banks' lobbyists take advantage of many lawmakers' inch-deep understanding of the financial sector. When members of Congress oppose reform, industry lobbyists convince many of them that finance is too complicated to treat with simple rules and principles. "They try to make this stuff out to be way more complex than it really is," said former senator Kaufman. "It isn't."

Cramdown Goes Down, Again and Again and Again

While the financial sector has thrived since the bailout, millions of American families are still struggling to recover. As we have noted, the crisis hit many homeowners particularly hard: there were 2.3 million foreclosures in 2008, far more than in previous years. The following year saw 2.8 million more foreclosures, and the year after that, 2.9 million more.[60]

Although there have been efforts to help those affected, many have found the efforts inadequate, especially if they have had to file for bankruptcy. Consumer and civil rights advocates and some congressional Democrats promoted a bill in 2008 and 2009 that would have allowed people facing foreclosure an option to stay in their homes. It would have closed a loophole that bars judges from decreasing homeowners' mortgage payments if they file for bankruptcy on their primary residence. It's a loophole because bankruptcy judges can write down the value of nearly all other forms of debt.[61] As a presidential candidate in 2008, Senator Barack Obama called the bankruptcy exemption for mortgages "the kind of out-of-touch Washington loophole that makes no sense."[62]

Many experts think that this reform, known in Washington as "cramdown," a term that means imposing terms on creditors they had not accepted, is needed. Georgetown University law professor and Consumer Financial Protection Bureau advisory board member Adam Levitin wrote that it is the "best and least invasive method of stabilizing the housing market" and would have "little or no impact on mortgage credit cost or availability."[63] But the cramdown legislation was not approved because of opposition by the banking industry. Despite a strong push in 2009 by Dick Durbin and other members of Congress and a thumbs-up from President Obama, it was defeated 51–45 in April 2009. Twelve Democrats joined the entire Republican caucus in voting against it. "Every now and again an issue comes along that we believe would so fundamentally undermine the nature of the financial system that we have to take major efforts to oppose [it], and this is one of them," the American Bankers Association lobbyist Floyd Stoner told ProPublica.[64]

One of the most determined opponents of the bill was the Mortgage Bankers Association, a trade group that had twenty-eight lobbyists in 2009, almost three fourths of whom were former government staffers. "We led the way on [the legislation] and we are clearly responsible for defeating this for the third time in the last year," David Kittle, former chair of the Mortgage Bankers Association, told the *American News Project* following the vote. It's little wonder that Kittle's group prevailed on all three occasions. It has spent $38 million lobbying government officials and, along with mortgage bankers and brokers, has contributed nearly $68 million to federal campaigns since 1990.

The defeat of the cramdown bill forced the Obama administration to take a different tack. Early in 2009, Obama had proposed the $75 billion Home Affordable Modification Program (HAMP), which gave banks financial incentives to write down mortgages. But HAMP is entirely voluntary and has been of little help to many homeowners. Near the end of its first year, even Treasury Department officials admitted HAMP was not working well.[65] Overall, it aimed to help three or four million homeowners, but by 2014 it had resulted in only about 1.3 million loan modifications.[66]

One of the homeowners affected by HAMP's shortcomings was Lisa Douglas, a forty-seven-year-old mother of six living in the Chicago area. Years before applying for a loan modification, in 2006, Douglas and her now ex-husband were given a subprime loan with an adjustable interest rate, a common tactic of the subprime industry.

By 2009, Lisa's life had taken an unfortunate turn. Her husband was injured at work and would soon move out. She soon realized that he hadn't been paying the mortgage. The mortgage payment, including fees and insurance, was close to $1,900, an amount she couldn't afford on her own. But she believed she could pay $1,400 a month under a loan modification.

Douglas applied for a HAMP mortgage modification in 2009, hoping to get quick approval, but six years later she remains in limbo. She described the experience of trying to get approval as "hell." She said she has repeatedly sent "stacks and stacks of paper" to the bank, only to be sent more letters seeking additional documentation. At one point, she did obtain what the bank referred to as a "trial modification." She said she made all of her payments of about $1,000 a month for three months but was then turned down for a permanent loan modification.

Douglas maintains, however, that she was never informed that she hadn't been approved. She says she never received a denial letter. The first she learned of it was when she received an advertisement that her home was being auctioned in a foreclosure sale in late 2012. She fought back with the help of the Legal Assistance Foundation (LAF) in Chicago. It was worth the effort: a judge later found that the foreclosure sale was invalid because her bank's failure to send her a denial letter violated the terms of its agreement with her.

That didn't end her nightmare, however. In 2015, the company that bought her mortgage from Chase Select Portfolio Services rejected her application for yet another HAMP modification. She has not been forced out of her house, at least not yet, thanks in part to the LAF's support.

The LAF says Douglas's story is very common among their clients. It is also very common across the country. An investigation by the *Huffington Post* found dozens of homeowners with similarly frustrating stories.[67] In fact, in 2009 and 2010, 2 million homeowners seeking HAMP modifications were rejected by lenders. Of that number, most were not even granted a trial modification, and about 700,000 had their trials canceled. The most common reason for a rejection, according to ProPublica, was that banks said documents were missing.[68]

What is frustrating to Levitin and others familiar with those homeowners' plight is that cramdown could have helped many families stay in their homes. It also could have had a positive effect on neighborhoods—and housing prices—according to Kathleen Engel, a research professor specializing in mortgage finance and regulation and consumer protection at Suffolk University Law School.

"They Frankly Own the Place"

The Mortgage Bankers Association held its annual "fly-in" conference—when mortgage bankers fly to Washington from across the country to discuss issues of importance to them with members of Congress—the day before the cramdown vote. During the conference, Kittle warned that

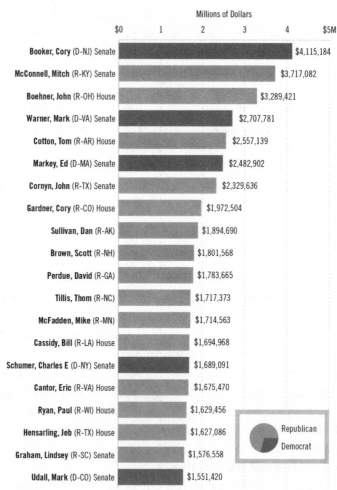

Millions of Dollars

Booker, Cory (D-NJ) Senate	$4,115,184
McConnell, Mitch (R-KY) Senate	$3,717,082
Boehner, John (R-OH) House	$3,289,421
Warner, Mark (D-VA) Senate	$2,707,781
Cotton, Tom (R-AR) House	$2,557,139
Markey, Ed (D-MA) Senate	$2,482,902
Cornyn, John (R-TX) Senate	$2,329,636
Gardner, Cory (R-CO) House	$1,972,504
Sullivan, Dan (R-AK)	$1,894,690
Brown, Scott (R-NH)	$1,801,568
Perdue, David (R-GA)	$1,783,665
Tillis, Thom (R-NC)	$1,717,373
McFadden, Mike (R-MN)	$1,714,563
Cassidy, Bill (R-LA) House	$1,694,968
Schumer, Charles E (D-NY) Senate	$1,689,091
Cantor, Eric (R-VA) House	$1,675,470
Ryan, Paul (R-WI) House	$1,629,456
Hensarling, Jeb (R-TX) House	$1,627,086
Graham, Lindsey (R-SC) Senate	$1,576,558
Udall, Mark (D-CO) Senate	$1,551,420

Republican
Democrat

Top 20 Recipients of Financial Sector Contributions
Source: Source: Center for Responsive Politics (opensecrets.org)
Methodology: The numbers above are based on contributions from PACs and individuals giving $200 or more. All donations took place during the 2013–2014 election cycle and were released by the Federal Election Commission on March 09, 2015.

even if they succeeded in killing the bill the next day, it would resurface at some time in the future. To keep their string of victories going, he said, they would need to open their checkbooks to help the MBA wage the noble fight against cramdown whenever it reappeared. "We need to keep fighting it," he told them. "We need to keep giving to the PAC. On a regular basis." He was referring, of course, to his group's political action committee, which has doled out millions of dollars in recent years to influence the outcome of elections. The PAC spent almost $1.3 million during the 2014 election cycle alone. Of the money it gave to federal candidates, 55 percent went to Republicans and 45 percent to Democrats.

It was following that May vote on the cramdown bill that, in exasperation and disgust, Durbin uttered during a radio interview what might be his most memorable quote in recent years:

> The banks—hard to believe in a time when we're facing a banking crisis that many of the banks created—are still the most powerful lobby on Capitol Hill. And they frankly own the place.

CHAPTER 5

Drugged

Bill and Faith Wildrick have never heard of Billy Tauzin, but they're paying dearly for Tauzin's tireless work for the pharmaceutical industry. So are Faith's employer and all of her co-workers. We all are. And in the future, so will our children and grandchildren.

Thanks in large part to Tauzin and Washington's infamous revolving door, the Wildricks are paying so much to fill Bill's prescriptions every month—even with their insurance—that they're barely able to make ends meet. They and most of the rest of us, including the executives and employees of MCS Industries, the Easton, Pennsylvania, company where Faith works, also have to fork over more money to health insurance companies every payday because of the deals Tauzin cut for Big Pharma.

We can also thank Tauzin and many of his friends in Washington for increases in both our taxes and the national debt. In fact, by 2023, the U.S. government's debt will likely be more than a trillion dollars higher than it otherwise would be because of the way Tauzin and other lobbyists—with the blessing of President George W. Bush and Republican leaders in Congress—wrote the Medicare drug bill in 2003.

And in large part because of Tauzin's deal making and the millions of dollars at his disposal, the Affordable Care Act—with the blessing of President Barack Obama and Democratic leaders in Congress—was written in a way that boosts drug company profits while doing little to make prescription medications more affordable for the vast majority of Americans. In fact, drug prices are going up at a faster clip than ever before.

As drug industry profits soar, millions of people—including most of our elected officials—continue to accept as gospel Big Pharma's talking points that (1) any constraint on pharmaceutical companies' ability to gouge us would "stifle" or "have a chilling effect" on innovation and (2) they have to charge Americans more because other countries won't let them gouge their citizens. For the success of this propaganda we can thank the millions of dollars in dark money the industry spends every year on deceptive PR campaigns.

Americans pay far more for their prescription medications than citizens of any other country. In fact, we pay almost 40 percent more than Canada, the next highest spender on drugs, and twice as much as many European countries, including France and Germany. In 2013 we spent exactly 100 percent more per capita on pharmaceuticals than the average of the 34 countries that comprise the Organization for Economic Cooperation and Development (OECD), of which the United States is a member. And the portion of our tax dollars that go to Medicare likely will continue to increase because Congress, under the influence of the pharmaceutical industry's cash, made it impossible for Medicare to negotiate with drug companies in order to lower costs.

In 1980, spending on health care in the United States totaled $255.8 billion. Of that total, we spent 39.3 percent on hospital care, 25.3 percent on physician/professional services, and 4.7 percent on prescription drugs. In just a little more than three decades, our total spending on health care exploded to $2.9 trillion. Between 1980 and 2013, the percentage of the total that we spent on hospital care dropped to 32.1, while spending on physician/professional services increased slightly, to 26.6 percent. Spending on prescription drugs, by contrast, almost doubled, to 9.3 percent.[1]

Partly because of that steep increase, health care spending reached 17.4 percent of the U.S. Gross Domestic Product in 2013, nearly double the average of 9.3 percent[2] of the OECD countries. Spending on health care per person in the United States reached $9,255 in 2013, compared to the $3,484 average spent on health care per person in the OECD as a whole.[3]

If you're a young, healthy person you probably can't even remember the last time you had to get a prescription filled. You may be wondering why you should even care about the rising cost of drugs and the ability of big corporations and their lobbyists to keep the status quo firmly in place.

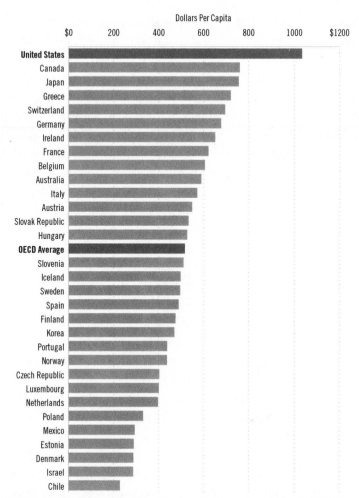

U.S. Pharmaceutical Spending, Per Capita, Compared to Other OECD Countries
Source: Organization for Economic Co-operation and Development
Methodology: Numbers are per capita for 2013 or nearest year: Data not available for New Zealand, Turkey, and the United Kingdom.

You should care because even if you're not a regular customer at the pharmacy counter, you're paying for the millions of other Americans who are, through taxes and health insurance premiums that are going up every year because drug companies have so many politicians, Democrats and Republicans alike, in their corner.

According to Express Scripts' prescription price index, a branded drug that cost $100 in 2008 had almost doubled in price six years later. This rapid increase in drug prices is one of the reasons why health insurers and employers that offer coverage to their workers are constantly raising not only the premiums we have to pay but also our out-of-pocket costs through higher deductibles and coinsurance rates.

And if you do get sick enough to need meds that aren't yet available in generic form, your insurer will make you pay much more for them than you would have just a few years ago. Since 2000, the average copayment for such drugs has doubled, according to the Kaiser Family Foundation. And coinsurance rates for people who have to pay a percentage of their prescription drug costs instead of a fixed copayment have risen even faster. The average coinsurance rate for drugs was 14 percent in 2008. The rate had jumped to 32 percent by 2013, according to the consulting firm Towers Watson.

The Cagey Cajun

It's worth taking a closer look at Tauzin's life, both to understand the power a single industry wields over Capitol Hill and to witness the ways in which Washington's revolving door works.

Born into a working-class French-speaking Cajun family in Lafourche Parish, Louisiana, Wilbert Joseph Tauzin II might have settled into the life of a construction worker—his father taught him how to wire houses and install air conditioners—had he not been bitten by the political bug even before college.

The "Cagey Cajun," as he would later be called in Washington, was audacious enough to throw his hat in the ring for student council president of Thibodaux High School when he was just a sophomore. It was the first of many political campaigns he would win.

After graduation, he enrolled in Nicholls State University, which is just two and a half miles from his high school. Not being able to count on his family for much financial support, he worked, at various times, as an electrician's helper, an oil rigger, and a pipefitter to cover his tuition.

While in college, Tauzin realized that remaining loyal to a single political party has its drawbacks. Campus politics when he was a student was dominated by a party system. At the time, Tauzin, who later would be known as a conservative lawmaker, considered himself a Liberal. But when he sought the Liberal Party's nomination for student body vice president, he came up a few votes short. Instead of supporting the Liberal candidate who beat him, however, the young Tauzin decided to stay in the race as an independent. He went on to victory.

He was a Democrat when the voters in Louisiana's Third Congressional District elected him to Congress in 1980. Within a few years he had become one of his party's assistant majority whips. He also would play a key role in bringing together a group of his conservative and moderate colleagues who came to be called Blue Dog Democrats, a name inspired by Cajun artist George Rodrigue's famous Blue Dog paintings, one of which graced a wall of the congressman's office.

But after the Gingrich Revolution of 1994, which put Republicans in charge of Congress, Representative Tauzin crossed the aisle and soon became the deputy majority whip for House Republicans. Thus he became the first member of Congress to have served in leadership positions of both parties. He's "as wily as any alligator in the swamp," former Tennessee congressman Jim Cooper, a Democrat, told the *New York Times* during the debate on what would ultimately become the Affordable Care Act.[4]

For many years, Tauzin was one of the pharmaceutical industry's most important allies in Congress, especially from 2001 to 2004, when he chaired the House Energy and Commerce Committee, which oversees the Food and Drug Administration. While he held that chairmanship, drug companies and insurance and health professionals contributed nearly $1 million to Tauzin's congressional campaigns, according to the Center for Responsive Politics.[5] That's chump change, though, compared to what the pharmaceutical industry paid him as its top lobbyist when he left Congress in 2005. His salary increased more than twelvefold—from $162,100 to $2 million—the minute he signed on as president and CEO of the Pharmaceutical Research and Manufacturers of America (PhRMA), the industry's powerful trade group.[6]

PhRMA spent $26 million on lobbying in 2009, during the debate over the Affordable Care Act, to shape the law to its satisfaction. Individual companies within the pharmaceutical and health products industry spent millions more on top of that. In fact, at $275 million, the industry's federal lobbying expenditures in 2009 stand as the greatest amount ever spent on lobbying by one industry in a single year, according to the Center for Responsive Politics.[7] The total swelled to $558 million when lobbying expenditures from hospitals, medical device manufacturers, and other health care companies and organizations were included. The industry also doled out millions of dollars in campaign contributions in 2008 and 2009, much of it to Democrats who ostensibly were in charge of writing the reform legislation.

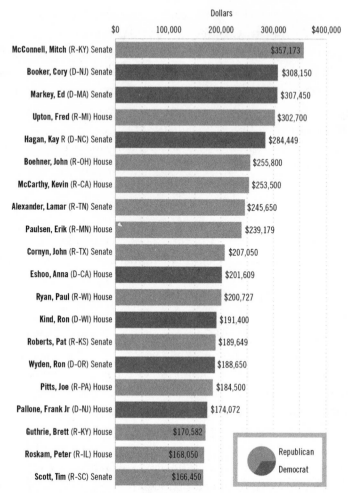

Top 20 Recipients of Pharmaceutical and Health Sector Contributions
Source: Center for Responsive Politics (opensecrets.org)
Methodology: The numbers above are based on contributions from PACs and individuals giving $200 or more. All donations took place during the 2013–2014 election cycle and were released by the Federal Election Commission on March 09, 2015.

PhRMA's ability to influence elections and public policy has made it the envy of most other corporate advocacy groups in Washington. Not only is PhRMA consistently among the top spenders on lobbying activities every year[8], it is widely considered to be the most effective. The PR and consulting firm APCO Worldwide asked hundreds of the city's movers and shakers in 2013 which of approximately fifty leading trade associations had the most clout. PhRMA came out on top, garnering the most wins in the most categories. It was voted the best at lobbying, the most effective at having a local and federal presence, and the group whose members most frequently "mobilize to contact policymakers."[9] In other words, what PhRMA wants, PhRMA is very likely to get.

PhRMA, Clinton, Bush, Obama

Although Tauzin's five-year reign at PhRMA proved extremely successful, the group has been a major force in Washington for more than twenty years. One of the industry's most important victories came in 1994, when it teamed up with lobbyists for doctors, hospitals, medical device manufacturers, and insurers to defeat President Clinton's health care reform proposal. Clinton wanted to give Medicare the ability to negotiate with drug companies and to make it legal for medications made in the United States and exported to Canada and other countries to be imported back into the States and sold at lower prices. Both of those policy changes undoubtedly would have cut into drug company profit margins. But the Clinton reform legislation never made it to the floor of either the House or Senate for a vote. Industry lobbyists were able to kill it in committee.

Lawmakers of both parties tried to put those proposals back on the table nearly ten years later, when President George W. Bush, looking to shore up his support among older voters, pledged to work with Congress to add a voluntary prescription drug benefit—which came to be known as Part D—to the Medicare program. Not wanting to risk losing generous campaign contributions from the pharmaceutical industry, however, Bush and congressional leaders, including Tauzin, who by then chaired the House Energy and Commerce Committee, Republican House Speaker Dennis Hastert of Illinois, and House Majority Leader Tom DeLay of Texas, invited drug company lobbyists to help shape what would become the Medicare Prescription Drug Improvement and Modernization Act of 2003. Also invited to the table were lobbyists for health insurers. They made certain that Medicare beneficiaries who wanted drug coverage would have to buy it from private insurers.

As Bruce Bartlett, who served as domestic policy adviser to President Ronald Reagan, wrote in the *New York Times* ten years later, enacting a new drug benefit—written by lobbyists without cost containment provisions—had Bush's full support.[10] "Looking ahead to a close reelection in

2004, he thought a new government giveaway to the elderly would increase his vote share among this group," Bartlett wrote.

As it turned out, it would take all of Tauzin's charm and wiliness as well as unprecedented flouting of House rules and procedures to pull off what Bush—and the lobbyists—wanted.

Early in the morning of Friday, November 21, 2003, just before the Thanksgiving break and after months of negotiations with drug companies and other special interests, a thousand-page bill finally landed on House members' desks. To their astonishment, they were told they would have only a few hours to review it before having to vote on it.

Many Republicans were just as angry and upset as many Democrats, not only about the unrealistically short amount of time available to read and understand the bill but also about the fact that it would add hundreds of billions of dollars to the deficit while padding drug companies' bottom lines. "The pharmaceutical lobbyists wrote the bill," a disgusted Republican Representative Walter Jones of North Carolina's Third Congressional District later told *60 Minutes* after voting against the measure.

The timing of the vote was in itself unusual. What came next, however, was something that had never happened before in the history of the country. Jones said it was the "ugliest night" he had ever witnessed in more than two decades as a member of Congress.

Tauzin, Hastert, and DeLay, who had received hundreds of thousands of dollars from drug companies during their political careers, knew it wouldn't be easy to pass the legislation without a plan to pay for the costly new entitlement other than through permanent deficit spending. But they believed they had the support they needed when they called for a vote at three A.M. on Saturday.

When asked why he thought House leaders had scheduled the vote long after most Americans had gone to bed, Representative Dan Burton (R-IN), who also voted against the bill, said "a lot of shenanigans were going on that night (that) they didn't want on national television." Among the shenanigans, reportedly sanctioned by House leaders: freezing C-SPAN cameras and allowing lobbyists on the House floor as the vote was being taken. (Lobbyists who previously served in Congress had floor privileges until the enactment of the Honest Leadership and Open Government Act of 2007, which was passed in the aftermath of the Jack Abramoff lobbying scandal.)

Despite the arm twisting, the bill was still short of the 218 votes needed for passage after the standard fifteen-minute voting period. Rather than accept defeat, however, Hastert added two minutes to the voting clock. When that wasn't enough, Hastert decided to keep the vote open indefinitely to give the pharmaceutical lobbyists more time to change minds.

Meanwhile, Thomas Scully, the former hospital industry lobbyist whom Bush had appointed to head the Centers for Medicare and Medicaid Services (CMS) and who had been the White House's lead negotiator for the bill, waited nervously for the result. Scully had a personal as well as a political stake in the outcome of the vote. A few weeks before Congress had started debate on the bill, Scully had asked for—and been granted—a federal government ethics waiver from Health and Human Services Secretary Tommy Thompson, who also had a hand in writing the legislation. The waiver allowed Scully to ignore regulations that barred him from negotiating for future employment with anyone who might be affected financially by his work at CMS.[11] It would be learned later that Scully was in talks with five firms whose financial interests would be affected by the legislation he would soon help to pass. He subsequently joined two of those firms. There were no repercussions.

As Scully knew, and as Bruce Bartlett noted in his *New York Times* op-ed, many House Republicans had said they would not vote for the Medicare drug bill if it cost taxpayers more than $400 billion over the first ten years. "Thus," Bartlett wrote, "it was a huge problem for Republicans when the chief actuary of the Medicare system, Richard S. Foster, concluded during the summer of 2003 that Part D would actually cost $530 billion over its first ten years."

It turned out not to be a problem at all, however, because Scully made sure Foster's estimate would not see the light of day before the vote. Foster later wrote that Scully "ordered me to cease responding directly to congressional requests for actuarial assistance. Instead, I was directed to provide the responses to him for his review, approval and ultimate disposition. Following several vigorous discussions, the administrator made it clear that this was a direct order and that if I failed to follow it, 'the consequences of insubordination are extremely severe.' I understood this statement to mean that I would be fired if I provided the requested information to Congress."[12] An investigation into allegations against Scully, conducted a year later by the Office of Inspector General for the Department of Health and Human Services, substantiated Foster's story and concluded that Scully had indeed threatened to sanction Foster if he released any information that Scully didn't want members of Congress to see.

If Foster's estimate—which turned out to be higher than the actual cost of Part D over the first ten years—had been made public, the bill would never have passed. In fact, it probably wouldn't have passed had House leaders not allowed drug company lobbyists to pressure members directly on the House floor for hours.

As four A.M. approached, the industry was still three votes short, but House leaders and the industry's platoon of lobbyists were not yet ready to concede. Their persistence finally paid off when Republican representative Ernest Istook of Oklahoma switched his vote. Seven other Republicans eventually followed Istook's lead. When the "yeas" reached 220 at five fifty-three A.M., almost three hours after the vote began, Hastert declared the bill passed. It was the longest electronic vote in congressional history.

Writing in the conservative *National Review* ten years later, Noah Glyn described the law as "perhaps the most prominent example of big-government Republicanism during the Bush years."[13] Norman Ornstein of the conservative American Enterprise Institute called it a "huge trophy" for the Bush reelection team.[14]

Indeed. Although his margin of victory over Senator John Kerry of Massachusetts in the 2004 general election was the slimmest in American history for an incumbent president, Bush received just enough additional votes from Medicare beneficiaries, especially in Florida with its 27 electoral votes, to make the difference.

Two days after the election, the *New York Times* reporter Robert Pear wrote that pharmaceutical and insurance company executives "were pleased and immensely relieved at the election results."[15] Bush's reelection meant the Medicare prescription drug program would be implemented as those executives—and their lobbyists—envisioned (and helped write), and that any future proposals to add profit-limiting cost containment provisions would go nowhere. Even if legislation the drug companies and insurers didn't like somehow made it through Congress, Bush could be counted on to veto it.

Also pleased and immensely relieved, with both the election and the bill Bush had signed into law, were many of the government employees, including members of Congress, who had worked on the legislation and were hoping it might lead to better-paying jobs. Within three years after Bush signed the bill into law, according to *60 Minutes*, at least fifteen members of Congress, congressional staffers, and administration officials who had played a role in the bill's passage had left office and joined the pharmaceutical industry.[16]

Among them were Tom Scully and Billy Tauzin. Ten days after Bush signed the bill, Scully signed on with Alston & Bird, a large law and lobbying firm with numerous pharmaceutical clients, and Welsh, Carson, Anderson & Stowe, a private equity firm that invests in health care and information technology companies. Both were among the potential employers Scully was able to negotiate with thanks to his ethics waiver.

Tauzin, meanwhile, had to decide whether to accept a lucrative job offer from PhRMA right away or serve out the remainder of his term and avoid a potential conflict of interest investigation. He chose to wait and continued to serve as chairman of the committee that has jurisdiction over matters pertaining to the pharmaceutical industry. His spokesman repeatedly denied that PhRMA had offered Tauzin a job while the Medicare drug benefit legislation was being considered. Regardless of when the job offer was made, PhRMA waited for him. In January 2005, within days of his retirement from the House, Tauzin started drawing his $2 million salary as the organization's CEO and chief lobbyist.

"To Trump Good Policy and the Will of the American People"

Three years later, after Democrats had regained control of both houses of Congress in the 2006 midterm elections, bills to control the cost of prescription medicines were introduced in both chambers. The House made the most progress when it passed a bill that would have permitted the reimportation of cheaper drugs. But over in the Senate, PhRMA, now led by Tauzin, was able to kill not only the reimportation bill but also the measure that would have given Medicare the ability to negotiate with drug companies. The industry's massive lobbying effort and its generous campaign contributions to senators on both sides of the political aisle had paid off yet again.

Barack Obama, who was still the junior senator from Illinois, had supported both reform proposals. After the Medicare negotiation bill failed, he took to the floor of the Senate to express contempt for the way drug companies were able to call the shots on Capitol Hill. "Once again, a minority of the Senate has allowed the power and the profits of the pharmaceutical industry to trump good policy and the will of the American people," he said. "Drug negotiation," he added, "is the smart thing to do and the right thing to do, and it is unconscionable that we were not able to take up this bill today."[17]

Obama carried those sentiments into his bid for the presidency. His campaign even ran an ad depicting Tauzin as an example of what was wrong with politics. "The pharmaceutical industry wrote into the prescription drug plan that Medicare could not negotiate with drug companies," Obama was shown telling a group of voters at a town-hall-type meeting. "And you know what, the chairman of the committee, who pushed the law through, went to work for the pharmaceutical industry making $2 million a year." That, he said, was an example of "the same old game playing in Washington." He ended the ad with this: "You know, I don't want to learn how to play the game better. I want to put an end to the game playing."[18]

That turned out to be just rhetoric, once the White House decided it would make health care reform a signature accomplishment of the Obama presidency. Obama's top aides—including his chief of staff, the former congressional representative Rahm Emanuel of Illinois, and his deputy chief of staff, Jim Messina, who had worked for Senate Finance Committee chairman Max Baucus of Montana—were tasked with making sure PhRMA was kept happy in the ramp-up to the Affordable Care Act debate, and Baucus would become PhRMA's main contact on Capitol Hill as the legislation was being crafted.[19] The industry's lobbyists made it clear to the White House that if the president was serious about enacting health care reform, drug companies and their cash could help him succeed—so long as he gave up on drug reimportation and Medicare negotiation and any other price control ideas he and congressional leaders might have in mind.

The Sunlight Foundation, a nonprofit transparency group, chronicled the deals the administration and congressional Democrats felt they had to cut to move ahead with the legislation. PhRMA dispatched 165 lobbyists—some of whom focused on the White House while the others worked the Capitol—to ensure that nothing would wind up in the legislation that drug makers couldn't live with. As the Sunlight's Paul Blumenthal wrote, many of those lobbyists, including Tauzin himself, would meet with top White House aides dozens of times "to hammer out a deal that would secure industry support for the administration's health care reform agenda in exchange for the White House abandoning key elements of the president's promises to reform the pharmaceutical industry."[20] If the White House agreed to the industry's demands, drug companies would finance a $150 million ad campaign in support of what by then was beginning to be called Obamacare. It probably didn't have to be said what would happen if the White House refused to accept the industry's terms—drug companies would spend whatever it would take to kill reform, as they had done when the Clintons were in the White House.

A few months later, Baucus and Tauzin reached an agreement that Baucus would announce in a press release. Baucus said the pharmaceutical industry had agreed to "accept" $80 billion in cost-cutting measures over ten years—primarily by providing assistance to Medicare beneficiaries who were struggling with the out-of-pocket costs associated with the Part D prescription drug program. By contrast, Medicare beneficiaries could save almost $50 billion *a year* if the government could negotiate with drug companies in the same way that some European countries do, says economist Dean Baker of the Center for Economic and Policy Research.[21] Or even the same way as the U.S. Veterans Administration, which has long had the ability to negotiate with drug companies. The VA pays an estimated 40 percent less than what Medicare pays for many of the same medications.

Much of the $80 billion Tauzin and Baucus settled on would be used to help close a big gap—called the "doughnut hole"—in the Medicare prescription drug program. One of the ways lawmakers and lobbyists were able to keep the ten-year deficit expansion figure of the Medicare Part D law below $400 billion back in 2003 was through a confusing and much-vilified gimmick to limit coverage—Part D enrollees would get coverage for the first $2,250 worth of medications, but after that they would fall into the so-called doughnut hole, as their coverage would not kick back in until they had paid a total of $3,600 out of their own pockets for their prescriptions. Under the Affordable Care Act, the gap will gradually shrink and finally disappear in 2020.

Although the *Wall Street Journal*'s editorial writers accused Tauzin of selling out PhRMA's member companies by cutting the deal with the Democrats,[22] the former congressman was betting that the drug makers would do just fine when millions of newly insured Americans under Obamacare would be finally be able to fill their prescriptions. It was a good bet.

When the details of the deal Baucus and the White House struck with PhRMA became known, it became clear to patient and consumer advocates that their hopes of getting significant relief from skyrocketing prescription drug costs had once again been dashed by politicians more beholden to drug company lobbyists than to the people who voted for them. And this time those hopes had been dashed by a Democrat in the

White House who had won many of their votes by promising to end the game playing in Washington.

One of the longtime champions of legalizing the reimportation of prescription drugs, ironically, is Senator John McCain of Arizona, the Republican presidential nominee Obama defeated in the 2008 election. In 2012, two years after Obama signed the Affordable Care Act into law, McCain and Democratic senator Sherrod Brown of Ohio teamed up as cosponsors of a new reimportation bill. When he realized the drug companies would win once again through a combination of arm twisting by their phalanx of lobbyists and their strategic campaign contributions, McCain made no attempt to hide his disgust. "What you're about to see is the reason for the cynicism that the American people have about the way we do business here in Washington," McCain said as voting was about to begin. "PhRMA, one of the most powerful lobbies in Washington, will exert its influence again at the expense of low-income Americans who will again have to choose between medication and eating."

PhRMA did indeed prevail yet again. McCain and Brown's measure failed 43–54. The Senate's Democratic leaders showed no interest in extending the voting period beyond the standard fifteen minutes to give McCain and Brown additional time to persuade some of their colleagues to switch their votes.

Public Research, Private Profits

In between these big legislative moments, PhRMA does the routine work of persuading policymakers of both parties that any proposed legislation or regulation that might hurt their bottom lines would most certainly inhibit the research and development of new drugs. People who are sick, they essentially claim, will just have to stay sick. Their talking points are carefully crafted to create a fear factor with lawmakers while also appealing to a distinctly American free market ideology.

Yet the profit margins at these companies would indicate that they have plenty of extra cash on hand for R&D. Pfizer, one of the world's largest drug companies as measured by pharmaceutical revenue, for example, recorded a profit margin of 42 percent in 2013. Even without the $10 billion the company made from the spinoff of a subsidiary, Pfizer's profit margin would still have been 24 percent that year.[23] It fell to 18.69 percent in 2014, trailing Merck's 26.98 percent and Novartis's 38.41 percent. Gilead Sciences's profit margin stood at a stunning 51.69 percent.[24]

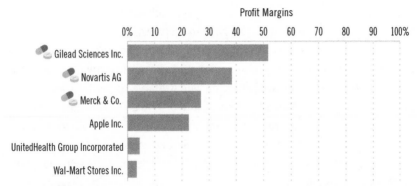

2014 *Company Profit Margins: Drug companies are among the most profitable of any sector*
Source: Yahoo! Finance

To put these numbers in perspective, the profit margin of the country's largest health insurer, UnitedHealth Group, was 4.41 percent in 2014. Walmart's was 3.32 percent, Apple's was 22.53 percent.[25]

It's also worth pointing out that much of the R&D that goes into drug development is funded by us, the taxpayers. The industry's often-cited cost for producing a drug is $1.3 billion over ten to fifteen years. But as the Harvard professor and former editor of the *New England Journal of Medicine* Marcia Angell notes in her 2004 book, *The Truth About Drug Companies*,[26] most original research is done at universities and government agencies such as the National Institutes of Health. And many "new" drugs are slight variations of existing products with patents that are about to expire. Making such "me-too" drugs is just one of the ways pharmaceutical companies are able to extend their patents, a process known as "evergreening."

Pharmaceutical companies do not disclose their exact research and development costs. Instead, they lump them in with other administrative costs that make it nearly impossible to fact-check their claims. But as Angell points out, drug makers spend far more on sales and marketing than on research.

This process—of profiting from publicly funded medical research—brings us back to the Wildricks. Gilead Sciences Inc. makes Sovaldi, the thousand-dollar-a-day hepatitis C pill that Bill Wildrick began taking in 2014. According to an analysis published in *Clinical Infectious Diseases* in January 2014, it likely costs no more than $136 to make a twelve-week course of Sovaldi.[27] That's $83,864 less than what the California-based company decided to charge for a twelve-week course in the United States.

No one else in the world pays nearly as much for Sovaldi as Americans do. In England, for example, the National Health Service was able to get the price down to $57,000—still incredibly expensive but 33 percent less than what the company was able to charge customers in the United States, including the U.S. Medicare program. The Indian government was able to negotiate an even better deal. As a result of Gilead's willingness to give deep discounts to developing countries, the price per pill in India is $10—a mere 1 percent of the cost in the United States.

Even at that price, though, the medication is beyond the reach of most of the 12 million people in India who the World Health Organization estimates have hepatitis C. Worldwide, as many as 150 million people, most of whom live in developing countries, may have hepatitis C, a chronic viral infection that often leads to cirrhosis of the liver or liver cancer.[28]

Pharmasset Inc., a Georgia-based company that grew out of a lab at Emory University, developed Sovaldi, but much of the hepatitis C research that led to the drug was actually funded by taxpayers. As *Modern Healthcare* editor Merrill Goozner wrote in May 2014, the federal government invested heavily over more than two decades in university-based scientists "to understand the genetic weak points" of hepatitis C.[29] Among the scientists the government invested in was Raymond Schinazi, the director of the Laboratory of Biochemical Pharmacology at the Emory School of Medicine who founded Pharmasset at Emory. (Emory received Pharmasset stock as partial consideration for licensing various technologies to the company.)[30] His lab received at least $7.7 million over the past twenty years from the National Institute of Allergy and Infectious Diseases, according to government filings. As Goozner put it, Pharmasset and Schinazi "hit the jackpot" when Gilead, seeing the profit potential of Sovaldi, paid $11.2 billion for the company in 2012. Schinazi reportedly walked away from the deal with $400 million.

Because there were no constraints on what Gilead could charge for the drug, Gilead and its CEO, John Martin, would also hit the jackpot. Sales of Sovaldi exceeded $10.3 billion in 2014, the first year it was on the market. Gilead's board was so pleased with the company's revenues and resulting profit—net earnings for the year totaled $12.1 billion, compared to $3.1 billion in 2013—that it awarded Martin $187.4 million in total compensation in 2014. "It's not fair to ask public and private insurers and patients through their co-pays to be the only parties at risk in the nation's search for miracle breakthroughs," wrote Goozner, author of *The $800 Million*

Pill: The Truth Behind the Cost of Drugs. "The long history of taxpayer-financed involvement in the development of Sovaldi only adds insult to the financial injury."[31]

An analysis published in February 2015 by the National Institutes of Health's National Center for Biotechnology Information confirms Goozner's assertions. It showed that more than half of the most transformative drugs—defined as pharmaceuticals that are both "innovative and have groundbreaking effects on patient care"—that were developed in recent decades had their origins in publicly funded research at nonprofit, university-affiliated centers.[32]

As many critics have noted, the $1,000 Gilead charges for every Sovaldi pill it sold in the United States seems completely arbitrary, with no bearing on either the cost to produce the drug or the overall value of it. The company maintains that in the long run, Sovaldi, in combination with other drugs, is more cost effective than previous treatments for hepatitis C, in part because patients taking Sovaldi are less likely to be hospitalized. Possibly so, but Medicare spent $4.5 billion in 2014 on expensive hepatitis C medications like Sovaldi, which was more than fifteen times the $286 million it spent the year before on older treatments for the disease, according to federal data. And a recent study published in the *Annals of Internal Medicine* suggested that only about one fourth of the money spent on the costly new hepatitis C medications would be offset by avoiding hospitalizations and other treatment costs.[33]

So why does Gilead charge us Americans so much? "The answer is because it can," Steve Miller, chief medical officer of Express Scripts, the large St. Louis–based pharmacy benefit management company, told *The Financial Times*.[34] "Other countries have come up with frameworks to make drugs affordable for people," said Miller, "whereas in the U.S. it has always been a case of what the market will bear. We think the market is no longer bearing up."

Those "frameworks" are another term for laws constructed on behalf of the common good—the kinds of laws that, because of the power of the pharmaceutical industry over Congress, we seem incapable of passing. And it is the lack of such lawmaking that forces Bill and Faith Wildrick to live paycheck to paycheck and give up many of the things they used to do that they can no longer afford.

Bill and Faith both worked at MCS Industries, which has grown since its founding in 1980 to be one of the country's largest suppliers of wall and poster frames. It has also become one of the biggest employers in

Easton, Pennsylvania, which is about sixty miles north of Philadelphia. Faith Wildrick, who packs boxes of frames to send to customers around the world, joined the company in 1993. Bill joined the company two years earlier and was there for more than twenty years, until he got so sick and weak from hepatitis C that he could no longer work.

Bill is one of an estimated 3.2 million Americans who have hepatitis C, although most of them don't know it because symptoms often don't develop until decades after infection. But the virus, which attacks the liver, can be a killer. The Centers for Disease Control and Prevention (CDC) estimates that as many as ten thousand Americans die every year from liver cancer and cirrhosis caused by hepatitis C. Bill believes he was infected in the 1970s, during a time of his life when he occasionally used drugs. The most common way to get hepatitis is by sharing needles, although some people can become infected through sexual contact. (Prior to 1992, many people also got hepatitis C through blood transfusions, but since then, all donated blood and organs are screened for the virus.) Bill said he remembers sharing a needle only one time. But one time was all it took.

It's not just Baby Boomers like Bill who are infected and facing enormous health care costs, by the way. In May 2015, the CDC reported a huge increase in rates of hepatitis C infections among people under thirty, especially in rural areas. The biggest increases were in four Appalachian states—Kentucky, Tennessee, Virginia, and West Virginia—where infection rates jumped 364 percent between 2006 and 2012. Three fourths of the new cases were the result of young people sharing needles to inject prescription drugs.

When Bill's health began to deteriorate a few years ago, he was tested for the virus and told that not only did he have it, it had already begun to damage his liver. His doctor put him on interferon, the most prevalent treatment for acute hepatitis C at the time. After six months on the drug, which is notorious for its debilitating side effects, Bill still had the virus. He was then prescribed Pegasys, another drug with similar side effects.

When tests showed that Bill still had the virus after six months on Pegasys, his doctor told him about a new drug that the FDA had approved just a few months earlier (in December 2013) and that clinical trials had shown had a 90 percent cure rate if taken every day for twelve weeks in combination with other drugs. The new drug was called Sovaldi.

Bill said his heart sank when he was told that Gilead Sciences, which owned the patent on the drug, had priced it at a thousand dollars a pill.

He would also have to take another drug, ribavirin, which would make the daily cost even higher. But he was in luck. Both he and Faith were covered under a Blue Cross health plan Faith had enrolled them in at MCS. After confirming that the policy would cover the drugs, Bill started treatment in April 2014.

Unfortunately, Bill was one of the 10 percent who still had the hepatitis C virus at the end of twelve weeks. His doctor said he needed to keep taking the drugs. Many more weeks went by. By the time his doctor said he could stop taking them, in October 2014, he had been on the medications for six months. Six months at more than a thousand dollars a day.

Although Blue Cross covered most of the costs associated with his treatment, the Wildricks still had to pay several thousand dollars out of their own pockets because they were in a high-deductible plan. Faith said their out-of-pocket costs in 2014 totaled more than $4,000 for Bill's medications alone. "Not only do I constantly worry about Bill," Faith said, "I worry every time he goes to the doctor about whether our insurance will cover it." She said she dreads checking the mail when she gets home from work because of all the bills they get from Bill's doctors and the Philadelphia hospital where he had to go on a frequent basis for testing. "Now that Bill can't work, our income has gone way down," Faith said. "So things have gotten a lot tighter. We've had to cut down on a lot of things. We used to try to go on a vacation every year, but we can't afford to do that anymore. You have to think about everything you spend. You can only stretch your paycheck so far."

Faith said she also can't help but worry about what would happen to them if she got sick and couldn't work or lost her job. "I'm the main source of income, and if I got sick, it would be devastating. I have no idea what we would do."

The Wildricks are not the only ones who are paying dearly for the high cost of Bill's medications. So is MCS. Richard Master, the company's CEO, said the amount of money MCS had to pay for drugs for the 320 employees and dependents who were enrolled in the company's health plan in 2014 was far more than in any previous year. That probably would have been the case had Bill Wildrick been the only one covered under the company health plan who was being treated for hepatitis C. Unfortunately, there were two, the other being an employee in his fifties who was on Sovaldi and ribavirin for twelve weeks. Altogether, the cost of the hepatitis C drugs the two men took in 2014 was more than $260,000. Master said that that was more than 15 percent of MCS's total health plan expenditure for the year.

MCS's experience would come as no surprise to Brian Klepper, CEO of the National Business Coalition on Health, a nonprofit organization comprising more than four thousand employers that offer health benefits to their workers. As he knows all too well, a growing number of employers across the country are experiencing similar rate increases as a result of ballooning specialty drug costs.

"The possibility of specialty drug pricing financially overwhelming business and union health plans is real," Klepper wrote in a May 28, 2015, commentary for *Employee Benefit News*. His prediction for the future of employer-sponsored health benefits was dire:

> Purchasers will be alarmed to find that their drug costs are growing much faster than other, already exorbitant health care spending. CFOs and benefits managers will watch their specialty drug spending, and calculate. To their minds, excessive specialty drug costs could capsize their plans, making it untenable to maintain good health coverage without compromising some other important health plan benefit. Just as worrisome, these costs will substantially increase their already heavy health care burdens, eating into the bottom line.

Klepper added, "Unless something changes, in just another five years we'll likely spend more on specialty than nonspecialty drugs. Or, for that matter, on doctors."

The sharp and unexpected spike in drug costs at MCS didn't go unnoticed by the company's insurer, Blue Cross, which hit MCS with a 14 percent premium increase for 2015. That was the biggest rate hike in the company's recent history. Master's insurance broker recommended that MCS switch to Cigna, which was willing to cover the company's workers at a rate that was still considerably higher than what MCS had paid Blue Cross in 2013. Even with the change, employees saw their premiums increase, and some of the hospitals that were in the Blue Cross network were not in Cigna's. That was bad news for Bill Wildrick, who was told by Cigna that if he didn't switch to a different hospital for his regular testing, he would have to pay much more out of his own pocket.

He also got more bad news in early 2015: even after six months on Sovaldi, he still had the hepatitis C virus. The good news was that Gilead had just released a new drug that might work better. The drug, Harvoni, is actually a combination of Sovaldi and the other drug that Bill had been taking, ribavirin. The catch: the wholesale price of Harvoni is $1,125 per pill. A three-month supply costs $94,500.

It's Not Just Sovaldi

Billy Tauzin's January 2005 announcement that he had decided to take PhRMA up on its two-million-dollar-a-year job offer came ten months after another big announcement from his office: he had cancer.

On March 10, 2004, the congressman's spokesman, Ken Johnson, said his boss would have surgery the following week at Johns Hopkins Hospital in Baltimore, where he had been diagnosed a few days earlier with cancer of the duodenum, a part of the small intestine. "His doctors have assured him he'll live a long, healthy and productive life," Johnson told CNN at the time. That's not at all how Tauzin later characterized what he had been told at Johns Hopkins. After the surgery, he said in a 2009 interview, "The doctor told me very frankly that I was going to die."[35]

"My doctor reviewed my options with me," Tauzin said in the interview. "I could undergo another surgery, but that would probably kill me and would be unlikely to cure the cancer. They had no approved protocol for people in my position, but there was a drug (Avastin) that had been successful in treating colon cancer but was not yet approved for duodenal adenocarcinoma. The drug works by cutting off the blood supply to tumors, which meant that the drug could either damage my healing process or kill the cancer. My wife and I decided to take the risk because we had very little to lose. It was really a choice between 'going to die'—my current situation—and 'might die'—Avastin could cure me. It's a good thing we tried Avastin because it worked like a miracle. By the end of my first round of chemotherapy, the radiologist couldn't even find the tumor on my CT scans. It was gone. I completed several courses of chemo and radiation and I've been cancer-free for over five years now."

He said it was his wife who suggested after his recovery that he take the PhRMA job. "'You know, Billy,'" he said she told him, "'you really ought to go to work for the people who saved your life.' And I thought, 'If there's a meaning in why I'm alive today, then surely it must be to use my experience to help patients like me across the world.'"

As he has told the story about his recovery, Tauzin has made no mention of how much Avastin and many other cancer drugs now cost.

There is no question that many of the products pharmaceutical companies sell save thousands of lives every day. But how long will patients—and the nation as a whole—be able to afford those products?

Like Sovaldi, Avastin, one of the most widely used cancer drugs in the world, is incredibly expensive. It's not unusual for patients—or their insurers or Medicare—to be charged $9,000 a month for Avastin. But as the *New York Times* has reported, studies have shown that for most patients, Avastin prolongs life for only a few months at best. Nevertheless, sales of Avastin, marketed by the biotech firm Genentech, reached $6.6 billion in 2013.

The next year, Genentech implemented a scheme to make even more money from the drug. In a widely criticized move, the company, which became a subsidiary of Swiss-based Roche Holding, notified U.S. hospitals in 2014 that they could no longer buy Avastin from the wholesalers they had been buying it from for years. Going forward, they would have to buy Avastin and two of the company's other cancer drugs through Genentech-approved specialty distributors.[36] That shift, as *Time* reported, meant that hospitals would no longer get an estimated $300 million in discounts they'd been getting from the wholesalers. Instead, Genentech and the specialty distributors would be able to pocket the money.

Pharmaceutical companies have also been repricing their cancer drugs on a regular basis to boost profits. Prior to 2000, the price of cancer drugs for one year of treatment typically ranged between $5,000 and $10,000. By 2012, the average had risen to $120,000.[37]

Another way of looking at it is the cost per additional year of life made possible by the drugs. In 1995, a group of fifty-eight leading cancer drugs cost on average about $54,100 for each year of life they were estimated to add. By 2013, those drugs cost about $207,000 for each additional year of life.

The rapid increase in costs, coupled with the aging of the U.S. population, led the National Institutes of Health to project in 2011 that medical expenditures for cancer in 2020 will reach at least $158 billion—27 percent more than in 2010—and could go as high as $207 billion. Speaking at the annual meeting of the American Society of Clinical Oncology in Chicago on May 31, 2015, Dr. Leonard Saltz, chief of gastrointestinal oncology at Memorial Sloan Kettering Cancer Center in New York, called the rapid cost of cancer drugs "unsustainable." He said the median monthly price for new cancer drugs in the United States had more than doubled over the past decade—from $4,716 in the period from 2000 through 2004 to $9,900 from 2010 through 2014.[38] That increase, he said, could only be explained by the desire of pharmaceutical companies to boost profits. "Cancer-drug prices are not related to the value of the drug," he said. "Prices are based on what has come before and what the seller believes the market will bear."

At the same time, many patients—including cancer patients—are finding that drug companies are not making adequate amounts of some lifesaving medications because they're not as profitable as they once were. The *Wall Street Journal* reported in May 2015 that BCG, a drug used to treat bladder cancer, is now in short supply because the twenty-five-year-old drug is no longer protected by patent. BCG sells for $145 a vial, a fraction of the $2,700 Genentech charges for a vial of Avastin. As the *Journal* noted, there has been no shortage of Avastin.[39]

If anything, spending will go even higher. In 2014, total prescription drug spending in the United States rose to $374 billion, an increase of 13.1 percent in just one year, according to the IMS Institute for Healthcare Informatics.[40] Driving the big increase were the emergence of Sovaldi and other new expensive specialty drugs and pharmaceutical companies' decision to slap new price tags on their older medications, their older specialty drugs in particular. Indeed, spending on specialty medicines, not just for hepatitis C and cancer but also for other diseases such as multiple sclerosis, jumped an unprecedented 31 percent, according to an analysis by Express Scripts, the pharmacy benefit management firm. The company noted in an earlier report that while specialty drugs accounted for less than 1 percent of all U.S. prescriptions, they accounted for 27.7 percent of the country's total spending on medications in 2013. It projected spending on specialty drugs would increase 63 percent between 2014 and 2016.

Not only are brand-name drugs being priced at unprecedented levels, so are generics, which until recent years had been decreasing in price. A survey conducted by AARP and published in May 2015 showed that one in four generic medicines used widely by older Americans increased in 2013.[41] "This is the beginning of a shift," Leigh Purvis, AARP's director of health services research, told the Associated Press. "What we used to get from generics in the way of savings is going away at the same time that the prices of brand-name drugs are extremely high, and they're going even higher." She called some of the price increases "stratospheric." Among them were two generics used for treating infections whose retail prices increased more than 1,000 percent in 2013.

In his 2015 State of the Union address, President Obama stressed the importance of committing taxpayer dollars to help finance the development of "precision medicine"—personalized therapies to treat a broad range of illnesses. He asked Congress to allocate $215 million to get the initiative under way.

"The possibilities are boundless," he said at a subsequent White House event. "It [precision medicine] gives us one of the greatest opportunities for new medical breakthroughs that we have ever seen." Obama mentioned cystic fibrosis in particular, noting that people with certain mutations in a particular gene are now being treated successfully with a new precision drug called Kalydeco. As the *New York Times* later noted, Obama did not mention that the list price for a one-year supply of the drug is $311,000.[42]

The cost of Kalydeco and other specialty drugs is fueling a huge increase in government spending on the Medicare Part D program. The Obama administration's budget proposal for 2016 had this stunning projection: Part D benefits were expected to increase 30 percent in one year's time—from $63.3 billion in 2015 to $82.5 billion in 2016. Deep inside his $3.99 billion budget request to Congress for 2016, Obama once again proposed giving Medicare the ability to negotiate prices for expensive drugs. But as long as Washington's revolving door keeps spinning, and industries can spend hundreds of millions of dollars to finance the political campaigns of the politicians who are supposed to be regulating them, PhRMA almost certainly will continue to rule Capitol Hill.

CHAPTER 6

Fuel Follies

The United States lacks a clearly defined national energy policy. While Congress has passed laws that purport to create comprehensive goals and accompanying strategies leading to energy independence, each attempt has fallen flat as implementation was resisted by entrenched interests committed to preserving the status quo.

The three energy bills that have passed through Congress in recent years (1992, 2005, and 2007) are known as "Christmas tree" bills, festooned with tax breaks for industries such as solar and wind (in the two most recent bills), conservation incentives like the Energy Star program, and a reiteration of the panoply of allowances for extraction of oil and gas.

But none of them approached the topic from the broader perspective of setting forth guidelines for domestic energy development using legislative carrots, such as tax incentives and federal grants, for research and development while meeting consistent environmental regulation. As a result, our current national energy policy is a hodgepodge of special interest favors granted to companies, and sometimes whole industries, paying homage to lobbying efforts and political contributions as surrogates for sound, decisive policy.

But there are respected voices urging a better approach to a national energy policy. One is James Woolsey, who held a number of positions under Jimmy Carter, Ronald Reagan, and George H. W. Bush before finishing his government career as Director of Central Intelligence under Bill Clinton from 1977 to 1979. Woolsey was known as a neoconservative, a hawk on foreign policy and national defense issues.

After leaving government service he started a conservative think tank called the Foundation for Defense of Democracies in response to the terrorist attacks of September 11, 2001. Since then, he has ascended the bully pulpit to become one of the leading voices elaborating a national security argument for a comprehensive energy policy. Reflecting on the tragedies in New York City, Washington, D.C., and Pennsylvania ten years later, he wrote: "Apart from the heartfelt honoring of those lost—on that day and since—what seemed most striking is our seeming passivity and indifference toward the well from which our enemies draw their political strength and financial power: the strategic importance of oil." He goes on to bemoan the fact that "for 35 years we have engaged in self-delusion."[1]

Woolsey's crusade is echoed by business leaders. The Pew Charitable Trusts gathered a group of experts and executives in 2012 to examine replacing the "patchwork of state policies and cyclical tax incentives, such as the production and investment tax credits" that constitute America's excuse for energy policy with a clear plan that businesses can use to make long-term decisions.[2] Businesses need some degree of certainty and stability to plan for future expansion, without which they tend to be cautious about long-term investment in capital goods and hiring people.

At the Pew meeting was former senator John Warner (R-VA), who had served as secretary of the Navy under Richard Nixon. His summation: "We are hopeful that Congress will formulate a national energy policy that will provide not only economic benefits but strengthen our national security and reduce our dependence on foreign oil."[3]

Woolsey and Warner are talking about oil, which is necessary for the American military's ships, aircraft, and land vehicles. But they are making a more important and less obvious point: Every major energy source in this country—petroleum, natural gas, coal, and renewables—is part of a larger consortium or trade group. Each has a serious and robust statement of national policy promoting the future of that business, but there is no overall melding into a national policy.

To dig more deeply into how special interests are deeply rooted in our moribund energy policy, this chapter will examine how an entrenched industry, coal, has fought tooth and nail to protect its position despite issues clearly affecting the health of our country. As evidence of environmental degradation piled up, the industry turned increasingly to buying influence and political contributions as a way to preserve its declining business.

We'll then shift to the relatively new technology called hydraulic fracturing. When "fracking" began to take the stage, the price of generating electricity using natural gas dropped well below the price of using coal. To protect profits, the new industry did everything within its power to mimic the efforts of Big Coal by frustrating oversight of groundwater contamination and obscuring transparency in identifying toxic chemicals used in the drilling process.

As an example, we will then turn to the state of Pennsylvania, where coal and natural gas coexist in abundant quantities, to show how political contributions have been used to direct energy policy and how the revolving door between government and private industry works to thwart the development of a coherent policy.

Old King Coal

Coal is truly a remarkable substance. Holding a piece of the black, burnished mineral in your hand can be almost mesmerizing. After all, it's the stuff that diamonds are made of. Much of it was formed hundreds of millions of years ago, before the dinosaurs roamed.

Coal has powered the modernization of human civilization, from fueling train engines to electrifying the world. But, as we all know, coal mining and coal burning also have some significant downsides. They contribute to public health problems, global climate change, and the destruction of countless mountains, valleys, and streams. And although the industry is cleaner today than it was fifty or a hundred years ago, that's in part because lawmakers occasionally have been able to overcome industry resistance to pass legislation on behalf of the public interest.

In 1990, for example, President George H. W. Bush signed into law sweeping improvements to the Clean Air Act. He was fulfilling a campaign promise to deal with the problem of acid rain, and the bill mandated dramatic action to reduce the amount of sulfur dioxide spewing into the air from coal-fired power plants. U.S. Environmental Protection Agency studies showed that pollutants generated by Midwestern plants were causing havoc to the Northeast's ecosystems, turning the region's streams, lakes, and forests into spotty wastelands. The legislation had broad bipartisan support, passing the House 401–21 and the Senate 89–11. By 2011 both sulfur dioxide and nitrous oxide emissions had declined to well below the targets established by the new law and, despite howls of protest and dire warnings in the late 1980s and early 1990s from the coal industry, the average price per kilowatt hour of electricity nationwide had not risen one penny for either residential or industrial users.

The 1990 amendments worked because they were based upon sound science and had strong bipartisan support, passing the message to the industry that the nation's elected leadership was committed to solving the problem. Yet, although we can celebrate a reduction in acid rain, two major problems related to coal still needed to be fully addressed: mercury and carbon dioxide emissions.

Coal's Mercury Problem

The EPA estimated that in 1997, about 50 tons of mercury was being released annually by coal-fired utility plants. When combined with organisms that live in oceans, lakes, wetlands, and streams, airborne mercury becomes highly toxic and makes its way into the human food chain, mainly through the consumption of fish.

Several studies have shown a causal relationship between high levels of methylmercury in pregnant women and developmental problems such as diminished language skills and impaired memory function in their offspring. As a result, pregnant women were advised in 2001 by the EPA, the U.S. Food and Drug Administration, and forty-four states to limit their intake of certain fish, particularly higher-level predators such as tuna and swordfish that consume other species, to limit the toxic effects on their unborn children. A later study done for the EPA on methylmercury effects in the United States linked the chemical to diminished IQ and attention deficit disorders in young children.[4]

As bad as it is in the United States, the problem of mercury exposure is much worse in other parts of the world, Asia in particular. Studies done after mercury-laden industrial waste was dumped in two Japanese cities showed children whose prenatal mothers were exposed had severe mental retardation and neurological impairment.

The good news is, as shown on the chart opposite, mercury can be controlled.

So, while the technology exists, the political will has been sidetracked. Scientific and medical studies targeting human health consequences by the National Academy of Sciences, the National Institutes of Health, the FDA, and the EPA have been constantly challenged—by King Coal and utility money shoveled into the political process. Here, in part, is how.

MACT Attack

When President Bill Clinton took office in 1993, it was widely assumed in Washington that dramatic reductions in sulfur dioxide and nitrogen oxide, as a result of the 1990 amendments to the Clean Air Act, were accompanied by diminished amounts of mercury being released into the atmosphere through the installation of scrubbers in coal-fired power plants.

However, according to a study submitted to Congress by the EPA, the nation was being blanketed by about 158 tons of airborne mercury a year from anthropogenic (human-caused) sources, a third of which came from burning coal.[5] In the last month of his presidency, Clinton decided it was time to press for full implementation of the Clean Air Act and regulate mercury emissions from coal-fired power plants. The EPA ruled that power plants would be required to install equipment to meet "maximum achievable control technology"—known as MACT—which, in simple terms, meant that coal-burning electric generating facilities had to meet a standard calculated by averaging the emissions from the best-performing plants across the country.

Bush Retreat

After George W. Bush was elected, aided by $20 million in campaign contributions from King Coal and electric utilities, he took dead aim at the Clinton EPA's MACT rule by appointing a lawyer from the Washington firm of Latham & Watkins, which represented coal-burning utility Cinergy Corporation, to be an assistant administrator at the EPA. His name was Jeffrey Holmstead, and he would be in charge of regulating air and radiation pollution.

Holmstead was well known to the Bush family. As an associate counsel in George H. W. Bush's administration, he had worked on the Clean Air Act amendments of 1990 and become familiar with the concept of cap-and-trade, a system that would allow companies not meeting emission caps to buy pollution credits from companies that were meeting or exceeding emissions goals.

One of Holmstead's principal efforts as Bush's point man on the Clinton MACT standards was to avoid the requirement to set health-protective standards for mercury. He did, by ruling that those emissions would no longer be regulated under Section 112 of the Clean Air Act, but rather under the less stringent Section 111 and by ordering his staff to begin drafting alternatives to MACT.

The process was fraught with problems. The *New York Times* found that Holmstead's office had either altered or deleted information from a National Academy of Sciences report to Congress on mercury and human health, and a large chunk of the alternatives language being drafted—as much as twelve paragraphs—was reported to be lifted directly from Latham & Watkins memos.[6]

After two years, the crowning achievement of Holmstead's brief sojourn at EPA was issued on March 15, 2005: the Clean Air Mercury Rule. Under this alternative proposal, mercury would be regulated in two steps. The first, a nationwide cap of 38 tons (remarkably close to the industry group's recommendation), would be accomplished as a by-product of existing pollution control devices designed to reduce sulfur dioxide and nitrogen. The rule attempted to establish a cap and trade market for polluters to buy credits beginning in 2010 under the assumption that "the ability to bank unused allowances for future use can lead to early reductions of mercury."[7] The second step, to take effect in 2018, had a 15-ton cap "upon full implementation."[8]

Jeff Holmstead resigned from EPA, took a year off, and moving smoothly between government and the private sector, joined the lobbying firm of Bracewell & Giuliani, cofounded by former New York City Mayor Rudy Giuliani. Research by a group called Environment America, based on a review of disclosed lobbying records, showed that by 2011, nine of the twenty-five top mercury-polluting companies in the United States were represented by Jeff Holmstead.[9] We point to his story, specifically, to provide an example of the ease with which the political class in Washington toggles in between representing the narrow desires of special interests and working for the government, where they are employed by us taxpayers to stand for the long-term public interest. Unfortunately, though, for too many in D.C., they see their time in government as just another means of advancing the typically narrow objectives they worked for in the private sector.

Holmstead's successor at the EPA was his personal counsel, Bill Wehrum, again courtesy of the revolving door at Latham & Watkins.

Wehrum did his best to establish a single cap of 34 tons of mercury, but he had to contend with a lawsuit filed by the National Resources Defense Council arguing that Holmstead and the EPA had improperly attempted to regulate mercury under the Clean Air Act's less-demanding Section 111. In December 2009, the U.S. Court of Appeals in Washington agreed with the NRDC and ordered the EPA to create hard and fast rules requiring coal-fired plants to install equipment that would bring emissions down to the MACT standards. The case was one of twenty-six brought by the NRDC against the Bush administration.

Fits and Starts Under Obama

Barack Obama was elected to be an agent of change. It was clear that the nation's courts wanted action on reducing sources of airborne toxins and pollutants despite the continuing pushback from lawmakers representing coal-producing states, and on the campaign trail, Obama had promised to deal with the problem.

Following through during his first year in office, he persuaded congressional representatives Henry Waxman (D-CA) and Ed Markey (D-MA) to introduce legislation to reduce airborne toxins from coal-fired power plants and reduce carbon emissions 80 percent by the year 2050. It was classic market-based cap-and-trade, providing certainty on a nationwide basis as to emissions reduction by allowing flexibility among states and without forcing the controversial issue of a carbon tax.

The bill passed the Democrat-controlled House but languished in the Senate as Republicans joined with coal-state Democrats to slow it down. When Republicans regained control of the U.S. House after the 2010 midterm elections, the new majority introduced a measure to significantly deregulate the coal industry. Their Stop the War on Coal Act picked up support from nineteen Democrats and was eventually passed 233–175 in the House. Part of the reason: Coal state legislators of both parties were lobbied heavily by groups like the Heartland Institute, which got its initial funding from oil and extraction companies. The Institute claimed to have made contact with government officials 291,989 times in 2011. According to the Center for Responsive Politics, in 2011 mining companies spent $16.5 million and electric utilities $74.8 million to affect legislation.[10]

That's, in part, why the Senate never took up Waxman and Markey's bill.

During the 2012 presidential campaign, the industry spent $35 million on ads attacking Obama, alleging that his energy proposals would kill jobs and stifle economic growth. In total, during Obama's first term, the coal industry and its surrogate, the American Coalition for Clean Coal Electricity, more than tripled political contributions, with 90 percent going to Republicans.

By 2014, the Obama White House, having lost both the House and Senate to Republican control, was left only with rulemaking as a path to cleaning up problems created by the coal industry. In July 2015, U.S. Secretary of the Interior Sally Jewell announced new regulations, and a clarification of water quality standards, for mountaintop removal and surface-mining operations called the Stream Protection Rule.

For the first time in thirty years, coal companies would be responsible for monitoring water quality in streams and rivers adjacent to their mines to ensure that drinking water supplies were not affected. Companies would be required to post a financial bond for cleanup as a result of environmental pollution, relieving taxpayers of the financial burden.

The rulemaking was greeted with derision by Big Coal. "This is a rule in search of a problem," said National Mining Association president Hal Quinn. As of the writing of this book, the new regulations were still under mandated review.

The Decline of Coal

The coal industry may have won some key fights in the last decade, but it's down to its last pile of chips and is betting some on carbon capture and sequestration (CCS), a technology that would store carbon dioxide in both natural and constructed underground cavities. A second approach to cleaner coal suffered a major setback in May 2015 when the South Mississippi Electric Power Association pulled its $600 million investment out of the Southern Company's $6.2 billion coal-gasification experiment, forcing a reevaluation of the entire project. According to one source in 2010, the four largest publicly traded coal companies in the United States were worth a total of $21.7 billion, but by 2015 those same four companies had a combined stock market value of only $1.2 billion.[11] Part of the reason for the drop: the price of natural gas, coal's main competitor for electric utility generating plants, had dropped through the floor with the advent of a new technology called hydraulic fracturing. And politics

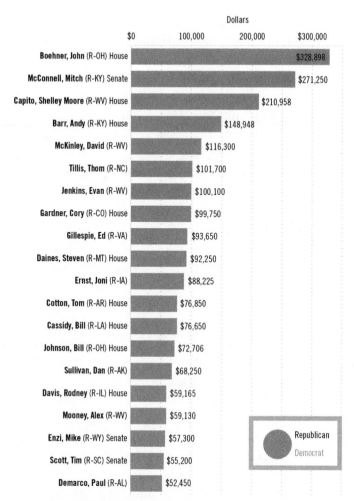

Top 20 Recipients of Coal Mining Contributions 2013–2014
Source: Center for Responsive Politics (opensecrets.org)
Methodology: The numbers above are based on contributions from PACs and individuals giving $200 or more. All donations took place during the 2013–2014 election cycle and were released by the Federal Election Commission on March 09, 2015.

would inevitably play a part as domestic gas drillers flexed their newly acquired muscle, as we shall see now.

Fracking Right

Many of the stories in this book detail shadow relationships, money influencing policy decisions, and crony capitalism at the federal level.

But there is another level of government, and it is as susceptible—in many ways more susceptible—to manipulation by moneyed interests than it is to what goes down in the cloakrooms of the U.S. Capitol and the restaurants of K Street. What follows is the story of one of America's earliest coal-producing states, where the lines become blurred between the revolving doors of public and private interest and where another fossil fuel industry, eager to replace coal, replicated King Coal's playbook with campaign contributions, industry-funded studies, and manipulation of regulations and regulatory bodies to achieve its business objectives.

This story actually began over a century ago, when the state of Pennsylvania provided 80 percent of the coal to fuel the steel mills and railroads that opened up the American West after the Civil War. The state's waterways ended up polluted by the mining of its vast deposits, and cities like Pittsburgh and Philadelphia were enveloped by soot from coal-burning furnaces.

In 1890 the first oil well in the United States was drilled near the town of Titusville in western Pennsylvania, a new find that would lubricate and power smaller engines throughout the world. For the last 150 years, the state has consistently ranked among America's top five producers of hydrocarbons, and by the turn of the twenty-first century it was sitting atop a newer and cleaner source of energy than coal or crude oil: natural gas. Much of it, though, was embedded in rock far below the earth's surface, in some cases almost four miles below. The challenge was how to tap it. The solution was hydraulic fracturing.

The process commonly known as fracking breaks up compressed subsurface rock by high-pressure injection of a combination of water, sand, and chemicals into deep geologic formations to create cracks through which gas and petroleum can flow and accumulate. The hydrocarbons are then captured and brought to the surface. About 50 percent of the chemical soup used in the fracking process is recycled; the other half remains underground, where it sometimes migrates into subsurficial wells and aquifers.

In 2005 a well drilled in Washington County, Pennsylvania, using fracking technology, came in, and came in big—much bigger than expected—setting off a wild boom in six states, all sitting on top of a giant formation called the Marcellus Shale. By 2008, a respected geological survey estimated that the Marcellus held as much as 500 trillion cubic feet of natural gas[12] Pennsylvania's share was estimated to be worth over $500 billion, and getting the gas out of the deep rocks was projected to create 75,000 jobs by 2020.[13]

Big Ed

Ed Rendell is a large, robust man as equally at ease in front of a group of heavy-hitter donors as a television camera. A liberal Democrat in a purple state, he swept into the Pennsylvania governor's office in November 2002 with the support of normally Republican strongholds in suburban Philadelphia, where he had been a well-liked and effective mayor for eight years.

Rendell's years as governor were marked by a number of challenges, and at the end of his first term came one from an unexpected source. Working with his Department of Environmental Protection secretary, Kathleen McGinty, Rendell had been keeping an eye on the developing fracking industry, but it remained a background issue until 2008, when he appointed John Hanger to succeed McGinty. Drilling was picking up, and Rendell told Hanger that the state was woefully unprepared for the boom that had already arrived. Hanger's best bet was to update existing laws like the Oil and Gas Act, but legislation on the books failed to address issues of water contamination and the disposal of the toxic chemical cocktails associated with hydraulic fracturing.

Rendell was on the horns of another dilemma. Although he favored continued growth of the extraction industry with the jobs it brought to his state and the energy independence it promised for the country, he also knew that regulation was critical in order to preserve Pennsylvania's lakes, streams, and drinking water sources; but the banking crisis of 2007–2009 had precipitated a brutal economic recession. Rendell was facing a $4 billion deficit due to lower tax receipts, and he salivated over the stream of potential revenue generated by other states that were successfully levying a tax averaging 5 percent of receipts on gas extraction.

Rendell and Hanger appealed to the legislature for immediate help in both regulating and taxing the burgeoning drilling boom, but the well-paid (fifth-highest in the nation) and well-staffed (first in the nation) Republican-controlled Senate and Democrat-controlled House could not agree on a course of action. With the legislature in paralysis, the state's Department of Environmental Protection, under Hanger's leadership, established a set of enhanced executive regulations to cover both the design and construction of new wells. Rendell pressed the legislature to pass a tax during his last year in office, but the state's lawmakers, many of whom were by then on the receiving end of generous campaign contributions from fracking companies, refused to go along.

Part of the reason was a Pennsylvania State University study released in 2009, funded in part, to the tune of $100,000, by the Marcellus Shale Coalition, the lobbying front for a large group of companies with a direct financial interest. The study's conclusion: energy companies would flee Pennsylvania if a tax was imposed. Hotly debated, the issue became central to the 2010 governor's race pitting Republican Tom Corbett against Democrat Dan Onorato.

Buying the Governor's Office

With the tax on drillers on the campaign's front burner, and Onorato openly favoring it, Pennsylvania's oil and gas industry went all in for Corbett, who opposed any form of levy on oil and gas producers, giving him $1.3 million compared to $130,000 for Onorato. Corbett prevailed by a nine-point margin.

Among Corbett's contributors were a select group of oil and gas executives. The top three were Terry Pegula, founder of East Resources, and his wife ($280,000); Alan C. Walker, former president of Bradford Energy ($112,782); and Ray Walker, senior vice president of Range Resources ($16,800). They joined eleven other campaign donors on Corbett's newly created Marcellus Shale Advisory Commission (MSAC), ten of whom were either lobbyists or executives for oil and gas companies.

MSAC and the gas industry didn't limit 2010 giving to the governor's race, kicking in more than $4.3 million to assorted legislators including Senate president pro tem Joe Scarnati, who got $373,384—nearly 30 percent of the total collected for his upcoming campaign—even though he wasn't on the ballot until 2012.[14]

According to public records, acquired by the Pennsylvania Land Trust, Corbett donor Pegula's company, East Resources, violated environmental regulations 106 times between 2008 and 2010, the third most in the state.[15] Pegula sold part of East Resources to Royal Dutch Shell in May 2010 for $4.7 billion and the balance to American Energy in August, using the proceeds to purchase the NFL's Buffalo Bills and to help Tom Corbett get elected.

Alan Walker, a former board member of the Pennsylvania Coal Association, was rewarded for his support by being named secretary of the

Pennsylvania Department of Community and Economic Development. It was Corbett's first major appointment.

Ray Walker's company, Range Resources, was the largest driller in Pennsylvania. The company had experienced a number of problems, beginning with a wastewater pipe breaking and killing fish in a thousand-yard stretch of stream in a state park. It was also in court with problems in Washington County.

Another of Corbett's first appointments was Michael Krancer, an attorney from the Philadelphia revolving door law firm (as we'll see later) of Blank Rome, to become secretary of DEP. Krancer asserted greater jurisdiction over review of any notices of oil and gas regulatory violations citing companies drilling in the Marcellus Shale. Issuance of a citation would require his, or his deputy's, personal approval.[16] Citations were problematic to begin with, because at the time, the state had only thirty-one inspectors and 125,000 active wells.[17] Federal oversight was lax because the federal Clean Water Act exempted oil and gas drilling operations from many of the mandated precautions to control runoff and wastewater disposal from well sites. With Krancer in place asserting personal jurisdiction over violations, and the EPA's hands tied, the industry breathed a sigh of relief, and Governor Corbett's Marcellus Shale Advisory Commission went to work, holding hearings for the next eighteen months.

By February 2012, Republicans controlled both houses of the Pennsylvania legislature, supported heavily by oil and gas money (see chart next page). The nine members of the Senate Environmental Resources and Energy Committee received $540,894 from extraction companies, or 12 per cent of their total contributions received for the 2012 election.[18] In return, compliant legislators passed Act 13, based partly on recommendations from the MASC, mandating drilling in all zoning areas and giving the State Public Utilities Commission absolute power to override local laws passed to regulate drilling in counties and municipalities.

In the same act, the legislature also proposed an impact fee on drilling that would be adjusted for inflation and market conditions (the price of natural gas). The proceeds would be shared only with municipalities that did not have fracking regulations more stringent than the state's. (Pennsylvania's Supreme Court eventually overrode some of the provisions in Act 13 that limited the ability of local governments to control fracking within their respective jurisdictions, asserting that communities had the right to do so).

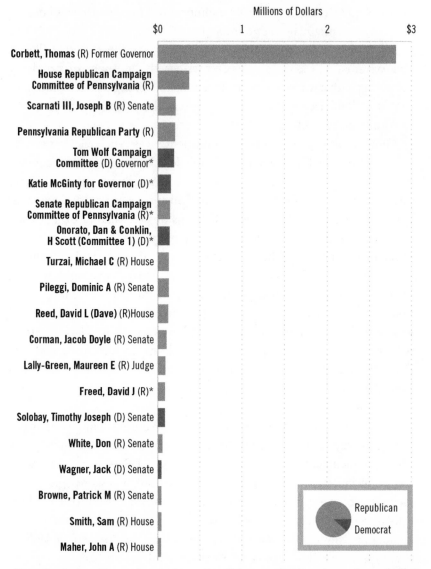

Contributions to Pennsylvania State Candidates and Committees from the Oil and Gas Industry

Source: National Institute on Money in State Politics

Methodology: Contributions made between 2007 and 2014.

Tom Wolf was elected governor in 2014; Katie McGinty was candidate for governor in 2014; Dan Onorato and Scott Conklin were candidates for governor and lieutenant governor in 2010; David Freed was a candidate for attorney general in 2012.

In May 2012, Tim Considine, the author of the 2009 study at Penn State, came out with a second paper from SUNY–Buffalo University claiming that Pennsylvania had achieved a satisfactory level of safety with its new regulatory structure. But that conclusion was questioned when a blogger discovered that the author's department had received nearly $6 million from the oil and gas industry.[19] The blogger's allegation was later corroborated by faculty, who forced cancellation of another Penn State study that was to have been funded by the Marcellus Shale Coalition.[20]

Michael Krancer left DEP in the middle of Corbett's term and was replaced by Christopher Abruzzo, one of the governor's deputy chiefs of staff. Then, in November 2012, two whistleblower employees complained that DEP groundwater test results in Washington County failed to include volatile organic compounds and certain heavy metals including chromium. Later tests showed that seven residents living within one mile of Range's Amwell County drill site and wastewater facility were found to have arsenic, benzene, and toluene—which when inhaled can cause neurological damage—in their systems.[21] The evidence was overwhelming, and the Corbett administration was forced to pursue the matter, finally fining Range Resources, campaign donor Ray Walker's company, $4.15 million for failing to obtain DEP permits to construct six holding ponds that had spilled the fracking fluids. It was the largest fine ever levied on a natural gas driller in Pennsylvania.

Despite the Range Resources settlement, Corbett's coziness with the fracking industry didn't sit well with a lot of Pennsylvania voters. At least partly because of voters' concerns about real and potential environmental hazards, Corbett became a one-term governor. Tom Wolf, a Democrat and wealthy businessman from York, beat him soundly in the 2014 election, despite Corbett's overwhelming advantage in campaign funds raised from energy companies: $1,148,351 to $192,985.[22] Heavy hitter Terry Pegula, former executive of East Resources, contributed $250,000 to the Corbett campaign.

By 2014 Marcellus Shale companies increased their overall political spending in Pennsylvania to over $9 million, as compared to $1.7 million when the boom began in 2007.[23]

One of Wolf's first acts as governor was to ban fracking in Pennsylvania's state parks, and his 2015 budget included a tax on natural gas—making good on a campaign promise. House Speaker Mike Turzai, a Republican from Alleghany County, was in no mood to see the tax implemented. As of the writing of this book, Turzai has refused to allow the tax bill to come

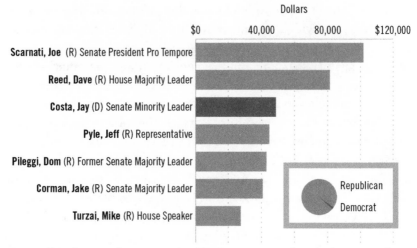

Top Political Contributions to Legislators in Pennsylvania by Natural Gas Interests 2013–2014
Source: Marcellus Money (marcellusmoney.org)
Methodology: Contributions made between 2013 and 2014.

to floor of the House, arguing that it would lead to a loss of jobs. Turzai receved $27,500 from the gas industry in his 2014 bid for reelection.[24]

The Keystone State's Revolving Door

There is no better example of the revolving door between elected officials, appointees to regulatory positions, and the fossil fuel extraction industry than the State of Pennsylvania. Ed Rendell returned, within a week of leaving office, to his Philadelphia law firm, Ballard Spahr, one of the top five energy practice law firms in the United States.[25] In addition to his law practice, Rendell had also been hired as an operating partner of Element Partners for a tidy $30,000 fee. Element Partners, billing itself as providing "Growth Equity for Energy & Industrial Technology,"[26] was financially involved in a number of energy companies including 212 Resources, a company that provided fracking fluid systems to drillers. And to go full circle, another adviser to Element Partners was none other than Rendell's first DEP secretary, Kathleen McGinty. Not an unusual situation in Pennsylvania, as every single secretary of the state's DEP, since its inception, had connections or employment with the natural gas or coal mining industry.

Michael Krancer, the DEP secretary in the Corbett administration, left office in 2012 to return to the law firm Blank Rome, where he was named head of the energy, petrochemical, and natural resources practice representing the industries he was purported to regulate when holding public office. Blank Rome is a member of the Marcellus Shale Coalition. According to Pennsylvania's National Public Radio, the aptly named public relations firm Greentarget put out an email stating that "Michael offers access to regional policymakers that other firms do not have."[27] Pennsylvania state law prohibits former government officials from appearing before the body they worked for, but attorneys are exempted from that section of the ethics code, allowing Krancer full access to state regulatory bodies.

After former Pennsylvania governor Tom Ridge left Washington as George W. Bush's head of Homeland Security, he went into business. He founded Ridge Global, an international consulting and lobbying company specializing in security issues, and joined the board of the nuclear power company Exelon. According to the Public Accountability Initiative, his firms received nearly $900,000 in fees from the Marcellus Shale Coalition.[28]

Today's Postscript is Tomorrow's Promise

We've provided just a few examples of how one state fell into the vacuum created by the lack of a coherent national energy policy. But another state, a thousand miles south of Pennsylvania, is experiencing the same battle. An entrenched and influential industry is using the same techniques of disinformation, industry-funded studies, and lobbying power to defeat a citizens' initiative to bring solar-generated electricity to the Sunshine State.

That is happening because the cost per kilowatt hour (kwH) of solar generation has fallen below ten cents—below electric utility retail prices.[29]

The electric utility industry, however, is doing its best to frustrate the movement to solar by consumers. In Florida, which ranks third in sunshine but thirteenth in solar installations, a compliant legislature has eliminated third-party leasing of solar installations. They have mandated that only utilities can sell electricity to retail customers by banning what are known as power purchase agreements. Florida is only one of four states with a ban on sales by providers other than utilities. Moving the upfront cost to a leasing company would relieve the homeowner or small businessman of the large initial investment, amortization of which would be built into the leasing fee.

According to former state legislators, NextEra, (owner of Florida

Power & Light or FPL) and Duke Energy, the state's two largest electric utilities, have aggressively opposed this option.[30] And the two companies, along with Tampa Electric and Gulf Power, have backed up their opposition with $12 million in campaign contributions to state legislators since 2010.[31]

A group called Floridians for Solar Choice is collecting signatures for a November 2016 ballot initiative to amend the state's constitution to allow citizens to purchase solar-generated electricity from a third party. The group claims that 74 percent of the state's voters support the amendment.[32] Tea party activists have joined Christian conservatives and environmental advocates in support of this measure, claiming it is a matter of free choice. "What's happening now in Florida is really blocking the free market," according to Conservatives for Energy Freedom state director Tory Perfetti.[33] But the Heartland Institute, supported by electric utilities, is cautioning the Florida Tea Party, saying that "tremendously expensive solar power could not compete against more affordable conventional energy alternatives."[34] Heartland is the same organization that lobbied so hard for the Stop the War on Coal Act.

The monopoly utilities in the state have taken a first step in openly opposing the ballot initiative by creating a front group called Consumers for Smart Solar. With a budget in the seven-figure range, the organization is preparing a campaign of disinformation by arguing that solar choice will increase rates to consumers.

The sad tale of Florida's ability to mandate monopoly pricing only happens because of the absence of a comprehensive national policy that would encourage competition to reduce expenses to the consumer as the cost per kwH of solar-generated power continues to decline. The solution appears to be citizen engagement, fueled by outrage at limited available options, pushing back against entrenched interests, sometimes regulated monopolies, willing to spend whatever it takes to preserve the status quo.

Jim Woolsey believes that by freeing the market from the power of foreign cartels, by gradually reducing tax incentives and subsidies, and by having Congress mandate alternative fuels in new cars and trucks, America's competitive spirit will discover new and cost-efficient ways to fuel our needs in the future.

He spoke to the point before the Senate Finance Committee on April 19, 2007: "I would only conclude by noting that I continually find it interesting that there seems to be so much more consensus on what needs to be done in moving decisively to reduce oil dependence than on reasons for doing so. In broad terms the approach suggested above—using a combination of regulatory and market mechanisms to remove barriers to the use of oil alternatives, including electricity, and to promote the development of such renewable technologies—can obtain, I believe, substantial support from a rather wide coalition."

Nine years later, little has been done.

CHAPTER 7

Fat Wallets, Expanding Waistlines

America is one of the fattest countries on earth. More than one third of American adults are obese—roughly defined as thirty pounds above a healthy norm. Another third are overweight.[1] Perhaps most concerning is that 17 percent of children and adolescents are obese.[2] Certain groups are impacted more than others: an astonishing 48 percent of African Americans and 43 percent of Hispanics are afflicted by obesity.

This epidemic has been building for years. Over three decades through the early 2000s, the obesity rate more than doubled for preschoolers and adolescents as it tripled for young children, according to the Institute of Medicine (IOM), a scientific organization the government relies on for advice on health issues.[3]

It is an undisputed fact that corpulence increases the risk of diabetes, heart disease, sleep respiratory disorders, gallbladder disease, and osteoarthritis, as well as some cancers.[4] So the current crop of American kids may be the first to experience a decrease in life expectancy—by as much as five years—unless we undertake "aggressive efforts" to stem the problem, a 2005 study by the National Institutes of Health found.[5] A more recent study says that excessive heftiness can shorten a lifespan by up to eight years.[6]

We already know what "aggressive strategies" are necessary to shrink waistlines. This is not rocket science. Among the main recommendations from the Institute of Medicine to prevent childhood obesity: a varied and nutritious diet, increased physical activity, infant breast-feeding, and reducing the amount of time kids spend staring at screens.[7]

There is reason to believe that increasing numbers of Americans have started following this kind of advice: obesity among low-income preschool children in several states actually decreased by about 1 percent from 2008 to 2011.[8] The Centers for Disease Control and Prevention (CDC) says it's not exactly sure what's behind the improvement, cautioning that cultural factors differ across the country. But it offers some possibilities: publicity leading to greater awareness, state and national initiatives such as First Lady Michelle Obama's Let's Move! campaign (a big push to get kids exercising and eating right), and policy reforms such the 2009 changes made to the federal nutrition program for Women, Infants, and Children, known as WIC, to conform more closely to national dietary guidelines.

Nonetheless, as made clear by a 2013 IOM study, investments in anti-obesity efforts have been sporadic at best. The IOM suggested a solution: the creation of a national "obesity evaluation task force" that would establish common standards to measure our progress on obesity prevention and track goals at national and community levels.[9]

Americans recognize the seriousness of the problem more than ever, according to a 2012 Gallup poll. For the first time, they saw obesity as a more serious societal problem than cigarette smoking. Gallup had been polling on that question since 2003. And 81 percent of Americans said our collective weight was a very serious or extremely serious problem, up more than 20 percentage points from a 2004 poll. More than half think it's very important to have federal programs to address the concern.[10]

But most Americans still eat a shockingly unhealthful diet, with little improvement in consumer choices in recent decades, according to a 2015 Dietary Guidelines Advisory Committee report.[11] We have a school lunch program that is beset by Washington partisan bickering, making it more difficult for kids to get nutritious food at a reasonable price.[12]

We know what "aggressive strategies" need to be implemented. Eight in ten Americans understand we need to take action, and—as is the case with other public health crises—the public believes our government should be playing a role in addressing the crisis. Yet . . .

Enter Big Food

One enormous force distorting the debate on healthy eating is Big Food. The food and beverage industry, along with crop and food producing, processing, and sales companies, spent close to $92 million lobbying Washington in 2014 alone.[13] That figure does not include the U.S. Chamber of Commerce, the lobbying behemoth that often joins Big Food and many other industries in lobbying battles.

On the other side, the most prominent organization lobbying for healthier eating—the Center for Science in the Public Interest (CSPI)—spent $82,000 in 2014. That's less than 1 percent of the lobbying budget for just one company, Coca-Cola, which reported spending $9.3 million lobbying Washington that same year.

Here's another way to look at this David vs. Goliath battle: in 2011, CSPI spent about $70,000 on lobbying. The coalition of companies opposed to new federal guidelines on the marketing of food and beverages—guidelines that would only have been voluntary—spent that much *every thirteen hours* in 2011, according to an analysis by Reuters.

On just one contentious issue we will examine in this chapter—whether the government should establish optional guidelines for how companies can market food to children—the industry and its allies outspent opponents by at least a 17-to-1 margin, according to our own analysis. On this issue, we could find only a dozen groups lobbying on the side of child nutrition, including CSPI, the American Cancer Society, the Environmental Working Group, and associations of dentists, pediatricians, and dietitians. Lobbying against them were more than three dozen food, beverage, and media companies.

Soft Drinks, Too

In recent years, beverage makers have succeeded at another tactic to keep kids and adults alike gulping down their products: spend tens of millions of dollars on misleading public relations campaigns to defeat city and state ballot initiatives to levy a small tax—typically a penny per ounce—on sodas and other sugary beverages.

The trade associations for the beverage makers have one of the biggest PR budgets of any industry. Collectively, they spent $105 million on various PR campaigns between 2008 and 2012. Leading those campaigns has been the American Beverage Association, which along with its state and local affiliates has bankrolled the anti-soda-tax campaigns in cities and states from coast to coast.[14]

It's worth noting that the industry, in reaction to the ballot initiatives and other attacks, has voluntarily taken some steps to keep Americans' waistlines from growing even bigger. The ABA announced in 2010 that as part of a joint initiative with the American Heart Association and the William J. Clinton Foundation, beverage makers had cut 88 percent of the calories from drinks shipped to schools since 2004. (It is ironic that the agency the beverage industry hired to develop and implement its ongoing anti-soda-tax campaign, Goddard Gunster—formerly Goddard Claussen—is the very same firm the health insurance industry hired to create the "Harry and Louise" ad campaign that played a major role in turning the public against the Clinton health care reform proposal in 1993 and 1994.)

Again and again, we have seen sound public health policies backed by expert research fail at the hands of special interests with large sums of money to spend. As Reuters noted in its 2012 report "the food and beverage industries won fight after fight during the last decade. They have never lost a significant political battle in the United States."

Before turning to sugar, both fructose and processed, let's take a hard look at Big Food and how it manipulates dietary guidelines at the federal level.

Big Food and America's "Lunch Ladies"

On the heels of the First Lady's Let's Move! campaign, Congress passed the Healthy, Hunger-Free Kids Act of 2010, a historic law that included a significant increase in federal funding for the school lunch program as well as incentives for schools to provide more nutritious food to an estimated 32 million kids.[15] In exchange for six cents a meal in additional funding for each lunch ($4.5 billion in total federal funding), lunches would have to be more healthful. The specific standards required by the law were unveiled in 2011 by the U.S. Department of Agriculture, which consulted academics, industry representatives, and health care professionals and relied on expert recommendations from the IOM and the Dietary Guidelines for Americans. The USDA would ultimately rule that school meals had to be richer in fruits, vegetables, and whole grains and include less sugar and sodium.

From the moment the bill was introduced in early 2010 by Senator

Blanche Lincoln (D-AR), the food and beverage industry viewed it as a potential threat to profits and began mobilizing to weaken it if necessary. The year before, in response to Congress's exploration of a national soda tax, the food and beverage industry began devoting far more money to influence lawmakers than it had during the Bush years. The industry's spending on lobbying increased 250 percent—from $22 million to $58 million—between 2008 and 2009. Over the next half dozen years, as food and beverage companies perceived a threat to its school district revenues, the industry's lobbying ballooned by more than 140 percent, when you compare lobbying numbers from the first six years under Obama to the first six under Bush.[16]

The increase in lobbying expenditures has been matched by increases in campaign contributions. Food and beverage companies contributed approximately 30 percent more to federal campaigns during the first six Obama years than they did during the last six Bush years.[17]

Although the food and beverage companies had the most to lose—at least in terms of profits—if the rules developed by the USDA forced significant changes in the nutritional value of school lunches, tens of thousands of schools and their lunchroom workers would also be affected. As the legislation was working its way through Congress, the School Nutrition Association (SNA), which represents more than 55,000 workers

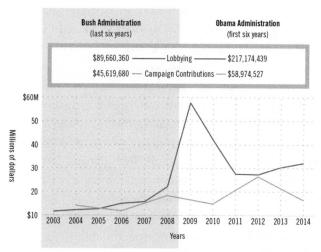

Influence of the Food and Beverage Industry: Lobbying spending and campaign contributions during the Bush and Obama administrations
Source: Center for Responsive Politics (opensecrets.org)

running school cafeterias, initially embraced it. But after the lobbyists for food companies that help fund the SNA came out vehemently against it, and it became clearer how the USDA's rules would change the way the "lunch ladies," as SNA members are often called, ran their school programs, they began to push back. They would soon find themselves allied with Big Food in a pitched battle to keep several of the USDA's school nutrition rules from being implemented.

Once the USDA started unveiling those rules in 2011, both cafeteria food suppliers and the lunch ladies' association had many objections. They didn't like the requirements that sodium levels would have to be halved, fruits and veggies doubled, and fewer calories could come from potatoes.[18]

While the SNA's complaints were making headlines, the food companies were already working behind the scenes in Washington—on Capitol Hill as well as at the Department of Agriculture's offices on Independence Avenue—to keep their bottom lines from taking a hit. The industry's strategy would be to lobby on each part of the lunch tray—from pizza to French fries to pasta—to weaken the rules.

Pizza as a Vegetable

The first big battle between the USDA and industry was over pizza. A loophole in the old rules had made the tomato paste in pizza count as a serving of tomatoes. (During the Reagan years, even ketchup was briefly considered a vegetable.) The USDA's new rules closed the tomato-paste loophole, which meant that pizza could no longer get credit for containing a vegetable. Among the USDA's concerns was the high sodium content—and in some brands, high sugar content—of tomato paste.

The Schwan Food Company, a privately held company with about $3 billion in annual sales and the biggest supplier of frozen pizza to schools, was especially upset with the tomato-paste ruling. In a letter to the USDA, the company, whose brands include Red Baron, Tony's Pizza, and Freschetta, made the case that its products were important because they appeal to kids and keep them buying school lunches.[19] In addition to the letter, Schwan began spending more than it ever had on lobbying. Along with the American Frozen Food Institute, the industry's trade group, it spent about $600,000 on lobbying in 2011, an all-time high.

Another part of Schwan's strategy was to appeal directly to members of Congress from its home state of Minnesota. The company succeeded in getting eight of the ten members of the Minnesota congressional delegation—including its two Democratic senators, Al Franken and Amy Klobuchar—to go to bat for it.[20] Those efforts paid off after Klobuchar pressured Secretary of Agriculture Tom Vilsack to relax the rules. In a June 2011 letter to Vilsack, Senator Klobuchar touted the benefits of tomato paste, criticized the whole-grains mandate as far too tough and called the proposed decrease in sodium unattainable, especially "when serving a dairy based center-of-the-plate item, such as pizza." As Minnesota Public Radio pointed out later, at least one sentence of Klobuchar's letter was identical to the written testimony Schwan would soon provide to a congressional committee that was holding a hearing on the issue.[21]

Neither Schwan nor the American Frozen Food Institute had donated to Klobuchar's campaign before 2009. That was soon to change. By 2013, they had donated thousands of dollars to her reelection campaign.[22] In all, nineteen food and beverage groups gave Klobuchar's campaign $160,000 between 2009 and 2011, double what they'd given her the three prior years. Her office told Reuters there was no connection between the money and her efforts on behalf of the industry.

Once Klobuchar got involved, several other Democrats joined what came to be called the pizza-as-a-veggie campaign, greatly increasing the chances that Schwan and the industry would be able to declare victory.

There was protest from the potato lobby, too, despite a Harvard report that found overconsumption of potatoes contributes to obesity. After pressure from the National Potato Council, Senators Susan Collins (R-ME) and Mark Udall (D-CO) intervened to fight limits on starchy vegetables so that French fries could remain a staple on school lunch menus.[23]

The result of all the lobbying and campaign contributions: House and Senate lawmakers came together in November 2011 to pass a big spending bill that included a rider preventing the implementation of the tomato paste and potato rules.[24]

The Industry's Lunch Ladies Strategy

Part of Big Food's strategy to mobilize against the law, beginning in 2011, appeared to include a push to create a rift within the SNA. It succeeded. In fact, as the *New York Times* reported, food companies like Schwan and ConAgra Foods enlisted dozens of school lunch directors to join an industry-created and -funded group in 2011 called the Coalition for Sustainable School Meals Programs.[25] The new front group was headed by the lobbyist Barry Sackin, a former SNA official. Stanley C. Garnett, the former director of the USDA's Child Nutrition Division who was once an SNA member, was dismayed when several school lunch directors joined the coalition. "They sold their souls to the devil," he told the *New York Times*.[26]

SNA members' willingness to front for the industry should have come as no surprise, however. About half of the organization's budget —$11.2 million in 2013—comes from the industry.[27] The food and beverage companies pay to exhibit their products at the group's annual conference, buy advertising in the group's publications, and provide grants.

In addition, the companies fund the SNA's School Nutrition Foundation. Since 2009 Schwan has provided more than $200,000 in education scholarships for SNA members. The National Dairy Council has provided about $75,000 in grants to the organization since 2008.

The USDA issued more rules in 2012 and 2013, ranging from limits on junky snack foods to a requirement that calories must come from many different food groups. Kids were not happy. In the 2012–2013 school year, participation in the federal school lunch program declined for the first time in more than two decades.

Some of the school lunch directors were not happy, either, and they turned to the industry's friends in Congress to allow them to apply for a waiver from some of the USDA's rules. They found a champion in GOP congressional representative Robert Aderholt of Alabama, who in 2013 became chair of the House Appropriations Committee's Subcommittee on Agriculture. At the time, Alabama ranked eighth-highest in the nation in adult obesity, with 32.4 percent of the adult population carrying too many pounds (up from 11.2 percent in 1990),[28] and led the nation in Type 2 diabetes.[29] A member of the Tea Party caucus, Aderholt said during a meeting of the House Appropriations Committee that, "[The USDA's rules] is where the heavy hand of government is coming down and trying to dictate to local school systems."[30]

Sharing that point of view was Senate Agriculture Committee member John Hoeven (R-ND). Hoeven's state is home to American Crystal Sugar, the nation's largest processor of sugar beets and the industry's largest political contributor.[31] Aderholt, who was first elected in 1996, has received almost $900,000 in campaign contributions from agribusiness during his career, more than from any other sector. Hoeven, who was elected to the Senate in 2010, had received approximately $300,000 from the agribusiness sector by 2014, far more than from any other sector.

Aderholt and Hoeven came through. In late 2014, Congress approved a measure allowing schools to apply for a waiver from the rules requiring the use of whole grains exclusively. It also eased salt restrictions. The SNA issued a press release to thank Aderholt and Hoeven.

Many former SNA presidents were outraged by the changes, however. Nineteen of the former presidents sent a letter to members of Congress reminding them of broad public support for the law, which they called a "strong response to the nation's obesity epidemic," and urging them to oppose efforts to undermine the healthful lunch program. They added: "We must not reverse the progress that was sought by school leaders and is well on its way to success in most schools."[32]

Soon after that letter was made public, the SNA issued a press release saying that while it "supports many of the law's regulatory requirements," its members wanted "greater funding and flexibility to address the financial consequences of overly restrictive regulations."[33] An SNA spokesperson told us in an email that the organization supports calorie limits on school meals, balanced lunches, and caps on saturated and trans fats but wanted more flexible rules on sodium and whole grains. The waiver gave school lunch directors that flexibility, at least temporarily.

Despite the protests over the new rules the USDA reported that more than 90 percent of the nation's schools were able to meet them by 2014. In a fact sheet touting the success of the program, the USDA wrote that "despite concerns raised about the impact of the new standards on participation and costs"—a subtle jab at the SNA—school revenue had actually increased by about $200 million nationwide in the program's first year. The fact sheet cited a Harvard study that concluded that under the new standards, school children were eating 23 percent more fruit and 16 percent more vegetables at lunch.[34]

The relationship between the White House and the SNA had become pretty toxic by 2014. When Sam Kass, a former White House chef, who at the time was the executive director of the Let's Move! campaign, asked to speak at the SNA's annual conference, he was turned down. And while the USDA had a presence at the conference, the event also featured booths, presentations, and speakers from Domino's Pizza, General Mills, ConAgra, Sara Lee, Smuckers, and Sunny Delight, among others. A Cheetos mascot even put in an appearance.

The Big Gulp

As noted earlier, another food fight has been popping up in recent years as states and cities as well as the federal government have sought to reduce obesity-related health care costs. More precisely, it's a drink fight. From Congress to state capitals and city halls, measures have been proposed to tax sugary beverages, which are strongly linked to obesity.

Medical research on the effects of sugar began in the late 1970s with the introduction of high fructose corn syrup into soft drinks. By the year 2000 there was sufficient data (twenty years or more) for scientists to identify the long-term effects of sugar consumption on human health. A 2001 article published in *The Lancet*, a venerable and respected peer-reviewed journal, related sugary drinks to the growing epidemic of childhood obesity.[35] Despite growing evidence, the sugar industry chose to ignore the connection.

But when the World Health Organization (WHO) recommended in 2003 that no more than 10 percent of daily calories should come from sugar, the industry went ballistic. The Sugar Association attacked WHO funding by Congress and even demanded that the secretary of health and human services, Tommy Thompson, force the WHO to withdraw its report. As Kelly Brownell, an internationally renowned expert on obesity and Dean of the Sanford School of Public Policy at Duke University, commented, "This is the WHO that deals with AIDS, malnutrition, infectious disease, bioterrorism, and more, threatened because of its stance on sugar."[36]

The next blow was struck by a U.S.-government-issued report linking sugar-loaded drinks with obesity. The U.S. Department of Health and Human Services and Department of Agriculture, normally tight with the sugar industry, recommended consumption guidelines even lower than WHO's—no more than eight teaspoons per day. The American Heart Association (AHA) followed with a recommendation that women should consume no more than six teaspoons a day and men no more than nine teaspoons, far below the consumption rate of 22 teaspoons per day in 2005. (For comparative purposes, one 16-ounce soft drink contains about 12 teaspoons of sugar.)

A 2009 *New England Journal of Medicine* article suggested that sodas and other sugary beverages "may be the single largest driver of the obesity epidemic."[37] A Yale study concluded that they're "high in calories, deliver little or no nutrition," and increase the "risk for obesity, diabetes, and a number of other serious health problems."[38]

On a second front, medical research began to seek a causal relationship between diabetes and the consumption of added sugars. For years, obesity was believed to be the main cause of type 2 diabetes, but new studies related excess sugar consumption directly to the disease. In March 2013, the open-access scientific journal *PLoS ONE* published a peer-reviewed study from the University of California, San Francisco, isolating the link between high sugar consumption and type 2 diabetes (after adjusting for other factors such as obesity).

Enter the Beverage Lobby

Those and numerous other studies have convinced many health experts and policymakers that efforts need to be made to reduce consumption of drinks that are loaded with sugar, or to reduce the amount of sugar in those drinks, or both. Standing in the way of progress, however, are beverage companies and sugar growers that want nothing to do with initiatives that might have an adverse effect on profits. To supplement their lobbying efforts, they have spent millions of dollars on PR and advertising campaigns to scare voters—and lawmakers—away from any proposal that would make Americans pay even a few pennies more for their products.

A 2015 investigation by the Center for Public Integrity into the world of high-stakes spin found that many trade associations—including the American Beverage Association—frequently have bigger advertising and PR budgets than lobbying budgets. It also found that among trade associations in Washington, few devote more resources to PR and advertising than the ABA, which spent at least $98 million hiring PR firms to influence public opinion and public policy between 2008 and 2012.[39]

It was during those years that the industry was under siege on several fronts. Not only were several states and cities considering a tax on sugar-sweetened beverages, so was Congress. The ABA was so alarmed by proposals for a national soda tax that it increased its Washington lobbying budget of less than $700,000 in 2008 to about $19 million in 2009. To supplement that, Coca-Cola increased its spending from $2.5 million to $9.4 million. Pepsi's lobbying budget went from $1.2 million to $9.4 million. The reason: during the health care reform debate in 2009, some members of Congress proposed an excise tax on sugar-sweetened soft drinks as a means to help pay for reform. But intense lobbying by sugar and soft drink companies stopped the idea dead in its tracks.

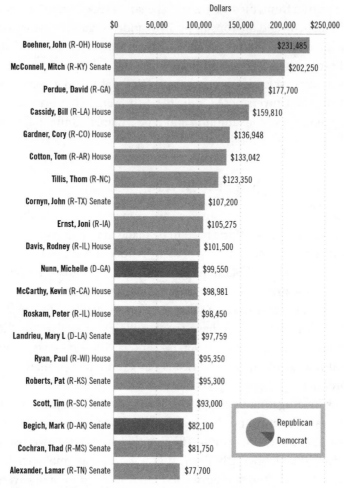

Top 20 Recipients of Food & Beverage Contributions
Source: Center for Responsive Politics (opensecrets.org)
Methodology: The numbers above are based on contributions from PACs and individuals giving $200 or more. All donations took place during the 2013–2014 election cycle and were released by the Federal Election Commission on March 09, 2015.

The idea appeared again when a tax on sugar-loaded soft drinks was proposed by Democrat Rosa DeLauro of Connecticut in 2014. Backed by the Center for Science in the Public Interest and several other advocacy groups, DeLauro's Sugar-Sweetened Beverage Tax (SWEET) Act would impose a one-cent-per-teaspoon tax on sugary drinks and raise $10 billion a year. But after intense lobbying from sugar beet and cane growers and producers, beverage companies and the high fructose corn and sucrose sugar industry, the excise tax effort failed.[40]

Local Governments Step Up to the Plate (but Usually Strike Out)

The ABA and its member companies and local bottlers also poured millions more into lobbying efforts in several states and cities. It has been money well spent. Across the country, soda tax initiatives have failed or been overturned in at least thirty states and cities since the mid-2000s. The ABA's first defeat came during the 2014 elections, when Berkeley, California, became the first city in the United States to approve a soda tax. The one-cent-per-ounce tax on sugar-sweetened beverages, charged to retailers, brought in $116,000 during its first month. The industry had better luck across the bay in San Francisco, where voters rejected a two-cents-per-ounce soda tax measure on the same day that Berkeley residents approved their city's tax. The beverage industry reportedly spent more than $10 million fighting the two measures.

There are factors other than the PR and lobbying campaigns that have contributed to the industry's success: the broad appeal and iconography of Coke and Pepsi, the soda industry's seamless marketing in our everyday lives, and the fact that Americans just don't like being taxed. But it could be argued that the industry's deception-based PR strategy has made the biggest difference.

One of the beverage industry's key tactics has been to hire PR firms to create front groups with misleading names to obscure the industry's involvement, especially its massive funding. The idea is to make voters believe that the front groups are grassroots organizations made up of concerned citizens.

One such group is Americans Against Food Taxes (AAFT), which registered its tax documents at the same address as the American Beverage Association and shared the same president. The group, which also received support from the U.S. Chamber of Commerce, raised about $25 million between 2009 and 2011.[41] One of the ads it ran in Washington—aimed, of course, at members of Congress—featured a young mother saying she couldn't afford the proposed soda tax because "those pennies add up when you're trying to feed a family."[42] The apparent goal was to mislead people into thinking that the tax would apply to all grocery items.

Aiding the beverage industry in its opposition to the national tax were the corn and sugar lobbies, which have big operations in the states of senators that led the tax-writing Senate Finance Committee at the time (Iowa, home to Republican Chuck Grassley, the committee's ranking member, and Montana, home to Democrat Max Baucus, the committee's chairman). The tax "ran into a committee with a lot of farm members," Chuck Marr, director of federal tax policy at the nonpartisan Center on Budget and Policy Priorities, told the Center for Public Integrity.[43]

The AAFT advertised itself as "a coalition of concerned individuals, working families, and large and small businesses" and reported that more than 95,000 individuals had signed its petition. Analysts at the Rudd Center for Food Policy and Obesity at Yale checked that claim and found that 73 percent of the group's member organizations were in the food and beverage industry and just 7 percent were community organizations. Of the community groups where sponsors could be identified, 83 percent were sponsored by Coca-Cola, and 94 percent of them marketed their services to African American or Hispanic populations.[44]

Similar front groups have appeared out of nowhere whenever a city or state has proposed a soda tax. In New York, the beverage industry spent approximately $13 million on lobbying and PR to kill a one-cent-per-ounce tax that then governor David Paterson proposed to offset costs related to diabetes and other obesity-linked diseases. Much of the money went to the firm Goddard Gunster, which set up the front group New Yorkers Against Unfair Taxes.[45,46,47] After the proposal died in the legislature, Paterson compared the soda lobby to a Mack truck. "We got smashed," he said."[48,49]

Goddard Gunster also helped create the California version of Americans Against Food Taxes when El Monte, a Los Angeles suburb, and Richmond in the Bay Area put a one-cent-per-ounce soda tax on their ballots in 2012.[50] The industry's front group in Richmond—the Community Coalition Against Beverage Taxes (CCABT)—even sued the city when the council passed an ordinance requiring special interest groups to disclose their sources of funding on campaign mailers. CCABT claimed the ordinance violated the group's First Amendment rights.[51] According to public disclosure documents made available later, the coalition received 95 percent of its $2.5 million budget from Washington lobbying firms. Just $4,778, or 0.0019 percent, came from local groups. CCABT never mentioned the ABA's support on its website during the campaign.

In all, Big Soda spent more than $4 million opposing the tax proposals in El Monte and Richmond, while advocates spent just $114,000, according to the Berkeley Media Group, which analyzes public health campaigns in the media.[52] Both cities were blitzed. "The conversation here is dominated by the ABA," El Monte mayor Andre Quintero said at the time. "Billboards, cable television ads, events, mailers, canvassing teams, phone banks, legal maneuvers, constant polling ... We are under siege." He added: "It's a domination by corporate interests that's similar to the early 1900s, when the railroad barons rode roughshod on the state." Between the El Monte and Richmond campaigns, it was estimated that the beverage industry spent at least $115 for every vote it got.[53] When all the votes were counted, the tax had been soundly defeated in both cities.

Undoubtedly one of the reasons the industry has spent so much money to defeat the soda tax initiatives is what happened in Mexico after lawmakers there passed a bill that added one peso (about 7 cents) to the price of a liter of sugary beverages. The increase went into effect January 1, 2014. According to Mexico's National Institute of Public Health, purchases of sugary drinks dropped by 10 percent during the first three months of the year compared to the same period in 2013, while consumption of healthier beverages—including water—increased.

A University of California, San Francisco study suggested that a national penny-per-ounce tax in the United States would reduce sugar-sweetened beverage consumption here by 10 to 15 percent. The researchers predicted that would lead to modest weight loss and a significant reduction in diabetes. Over ten years, they estimated there would be 26,000 fewer premature deaths, 95,000 fewer instances of heart disease, and 8,000 fewer strokes.

Guaranteed Profits

There are two kinds of sugar in America's diet, and they are largely undifferentiated and interchangeable: high fructose corn syrup and sucrose. The big difference between the two is how the beet and cane sugar industries (sucrose) approach the marketplace—with a guarantee of profit no matter what the world price.

Sugar (sucrose) is one of our country's oldest crops, highly adapted to the Caribbean and southern United States. It is likely that Columbus brought sugar plants on one of his three voyages to the West Indies. States abutting the Gulf of Mexico provided a hospitable climate and good transportation for the harvest; today, Florida, Louisiana, and Texas are the main cane-producing states. Cane, a perennial crop, can be produced year-round.

Beet (as opposed to cane) sugar can be grown in more temperate climates. It was a staple of the American colonies, particularly those in the Northeast who saw beet sugar as a way of striking an economic blow against the slave-produced cane sugar from southern states and the West Indies. Today it is grown in the northern tier of inland states including Montana, North Dakota, Idaho, Minnesota, and Utah. Beet sugar is an annual crop, harvested before the ground freezes. Together, cane and beet growers form one of Washington's most powerful—and oldest—lobbies.

Protection of the domestic sugar industry goes back to the eighteenth century, when a tariff was established to protect the nascent republic's small sugar farmers. In 1842 a special act of Congress expanded the tariff to protect sugar refineries. The first comprehensive price support program was begun in 1934 under President Franklin Roosevelt. That legislation, the Jones-Costigan Act, remained in place until a 1974 bubble when the world price of sugar went through the roof.[54]

Commodity prices collapsed to more normal levels in 1976, and the sugar industry began hounding Washington to once again protect domestic producers from both the world market and a new product, high fructose corn syrup, which was making inroads into the soft drink industry. Secretary of Agriculture Robert Berglund, a farmer from the beet sugar state of Minnesota, used powers granted him under the Agricultural Act of 1949 to create a complicated interim program that was institutionalized in the Food and Agriculture Act of 1977. The program underwent a major revision with the Farm Bill of 1990 by establishing a quota system to further restrict sugar imports. That act is the basis of the current sugar support policy. It has been modified slightly since then, but the basic structure remains.

In simplified terms, here is how the program works. The secretary of agriculture sets a country-by-country quota system with a two-tiered tariff scheme. Imports up to the quota are allowed; over the limit they are subjected to a punitive tariff. Beet and cane growers in the United States are given crop allotments to try to balance supply and demand. Congress (via farm bills) establishes a minimum price for domestic sugar. Refined and raw sugar are given two separate price floors. For a recent example, in 2013 the price floor for beet sugar was 22.9 cents per pound and for cane sugar 18.75 cents per pound. Based on 2013 prices, domestic beet sugar was pegged at 88 percent and cane sugar at 73 percent above the world market price respectively, and in that year, U.S. consumers paid $1.3 billion more than they otherwise would have for sugar products.

A second element is a complex loan system begun with Berglund's 1977 order. Loans are available to processors who agree to pay the price floor to farmers (provided they meet federal minimum wage requirements for field workers). The lender (the federal government) accepts sugar as collateral, and no interest is charged if the principal is repaid. If market prices are not high enough for farmers to make a profit, as was the case in 1977 and 1978, the loans go into default and the collateral (sugar) becomes the property of the federal Commodity Credit Corporation, which then sells it at a loss, generally for ethanol.

Loans made to processors rather than farmers might lead one to believe that cane and beet growers are disadvantaged. But an examination of the industry belies this conclusion. Cane sugar, as mentioned earlier, is becoming increasingly concentrated and vertically integrated. The biggest producer is the privately owned U.S. Sugar Corporation, founded in 1931 by Charles Stewart Mott, which produces 700,000 tons of cane sugar grown on almost 190,000 acres between Lake Okeechobee and the Everglades in Florida. It even operates its own short line railroad, the South Central Florida Express, which connects its cane-growing and processing operations with larger rail systems to the north and south.

The government's loan program is little more than a pass-through for U.S. Sugar and other big companies, and a guarantee of profit. In 2013, 55 percent of the $1.1 billion in federal loans went to just three companies, according to the *Wall Street Journal*, which obtained documents on the loan program after filing a Freedom of Information Act request. Although the companies—Amalgamated Sugar Co., Michigan Sugar Co., and Western Sugar Cooperative—borrowed more than half of the funds, at interest rates ranging from just 1.125 percent to 1.25 percent, they produce only about 20 percent of the country's sugar. In addition to the cheap loans that year, the USDA announced that it would buy $38 million worth of sugar "in a bid to raise prices," the *Journal* reported.[55]

If this arrangement seems overly complex, it is designed that way. The only people who understand convoluted programs like the U.S. sugar subsidy are the lawyers and lobbyists who wrote the 1990 bill and the sugar barons for whose benefit the bill was written.

Sugar Daddies in Politics

Once the 1990 bill became law, the industry maintained an annual level of around $3 million in direct lobbying expenses. This jumped to $7 million in 2005 when alarm bells went off. The U.S. Commerce Department was studying the loss of confectionery manufacturing jobs. The department reported the next year that for every job created in cultivating and harvesting, three jobs were lost in the United States due to the high price of raw and refined sugar. Sensing increased scrutiny of their guaranteed profit scheme, the beet and cane growers and processors were forking over nearly $8 million to lobbyists by 2008.

The Heritage Foundation found that by 2013, sugar represented 2 percent of the value of domestic crop production but 40 percent of crop industries' lobbying money. The following year, sugar chipped in 35 percent of agribusiness's campaign contributions to candidates.[56] Sugar lobby expenses were at an all-time high of nearly $10 million. It was a big boys' game, with beet producer American Crystal Sugar popping $2.0 million for lobbying and $2.2 million in widely sprinkled campaign contributions, with 55 percent going to Democrats to assure bipartisan support for the subsidy program. Heritage concluded that more than $50 million was spent between 2009 and 2013 to preserve the federally mandated profit margins of the sugar barons.

So why the dramatic increase of sugar money into the politicians' pockets?

Jelly Belly Jobs Go Abroad

Arrayed against sugar's protectionist program are the American Enterprise Institute, the Heritage Foundation, the Koch-brothers-funded Competitive Enterprise Institute, the U.S. Chamber of Commerce, and even the *Wall Street Journal*. But their arguments have little to do with human health and everything to do with the functioning of a free-market economy.

Writing in *American Boondoggle: A Project of the American Enterprise Institute* in a paper entitled "Sweets for the Sweet: The Costly Benefits of the US Sugar Program," Michael Wohlgenant is very blunt: "The only reasonable policy is no policy: the sugar program should be repealed."[57] Wohlgenant, a professor at North Carolina State University, did an exhaustive study of the direct and indirect costs of sugar subsidies, concluding that in 2009, while producers benefited to the tune of $1.43

billion, American consumers paid $2.44 billion more than they should have as a result of higher prices.

Aside from costs to the consumer, the sugar quota, tariff, and subsidy program wrecks another part of the economy. Confirming the Commerce Department's earlier report, U.S. Census Bureau statistics showed that confectionery manufacturing jobs in the United States dropped from around 70,000 to 55,000 between 1998 and 2011. During that same time span, the average price of domestic sugar was twice the world price. To maintain the disparity, sugar's lobbying expenses rocketed from $2.8 million to $7.5 million annually.

Jelly Belly has been a family-owned company for six generations. It sells 20 percent of the jelly beans consumed in the United States, but it is moving operations out of this country while expanding in Thailand, where sugar and labor prices are significantly lower than in the United States. "You can't compete shipping finished U.S. goods," commented CEO Bob Simpson, explaining why Jelly Belly has been forced to raise prices in recent years due to the high cost of domestic sugar.[58]

In another example, "Atkinson Candy Co. has moved 80 percent of its peppermint-candy production to a factory in Guatemala that opened in 2010. That means it can sell bite-sized Mint Twists for 10 percent to 20 percent less. We did it for survival reasons . . . There are 60 jobs down there . . . that could be in the U.S. . . . it's a damn shame," the company's president, Eric Atkinson, told the *Wall Street Journal*.[59]

One of sugar's most organized opponents is the Coalition for Sugar Reform. Its members include an odd assortment of bedfellows: the Club for Growth, Grover Norquist's Americans for Tax Reform, the National Association of Manufacturers, Kraft Foods, the American Beverage Association, and the Everglades Trust. In 2013, Senator Richard Lugar (R-IN) introduced a bill to end the program. The U.S. Chamber of Commerce, in a letter supporting the Sugar Reform Act of 2013, estimated that tens of thousands of jobs were lost in the "sugar-using industry" between 1997 and 2011, a number plucked out of a U.S. Commerce Department report.

Despite carefully documented economic arguments, the bill went down to defeat. In a rare demonstration of bipartisanship, Florida's two senators, Democrat Bill Nelson and Republican Marco Rubio, who is now running for the presidency, voted against reform. As a reward, Nelson received $42,000 from sugar growers. Rubio, who regularly campaigns against government intervention in the economy, was the beneficiary of a New York fundraiser hosted by sugar magnates Pepe and Alfonso Fanjul that raised more than $100,000.

The Competitive Enterprise Institute summed up the defeat: "The sugar lobby's sweet contributions and their day-in-day-out lobbying means broad bipartisan support for continuing the U.S. sugar program in the 2013 Farm Bill . . . Numerous attempts have been made to rein in this egregious program but the sugar industry's intense and consistent lobbying and the huge contributions they make on both sides of the aisle almost guarantee them the program's continuation."[60]

Aside from dollars spent to buy votes in Congress, the clout of the industry is perhaps best illustrated by a moment during Bill Clinton's term in office. The president was in the middle of an *entre nous* with a young White House intern named Monica Lewinsky when the phone rang. According to testimony given to independent counsel Kenneth Starr, Lewinsky recalled that the call came from someone named "Fanuli." In reality, it was Alfonso Fanjul, co-owner of Florida Crystals, the largest cane sugar processing operation in the world. Clinton interrupted the proceedings with his intern and took the call.

Hooking Our Kids

If Jennifer Harris could raise her kids all over again, she says she probably wouldn't have a TV. And she says she definitely wouldn't serve them products that are marketed to kids on TV. Harris says that although Big Food and Big Sugar claim that their marketing leads merely to brand preferences, not necessarily to an increase in consumption, research shows that if you market sugary drinks to kids, they'll consume more of them.

Before going to Yale for a PhD in how companies market food to children, Harris assumed that letting her kids have some sugary cereals wasn't so bad. What she learned as she was getting that degree, however, changed her mind—so much so that she went to work for the University of Connecticut–based Rudd Center for Food Policy, a nonprofit research and public policy organization whose mission is to "improve the world's diet, prevent obesity, and reduce weight stigma." She is now director of the center's food marketing initiative. "As I was learning more about the psychology of [marketing to kids], it just made me realize how really unfair it is to . . . spend all this money to shape kids' minds so it makes them love all these products that are damaging to their health," she told us.

One of the things Harris said she has come to understand is that, with the billions of dollars food companies spend marketing their often-unhealthful products to kids every year, it's a misconception that parents can control what their children eat. "Once they go to elementary school, parents have very little control over what their kids eat, other than at the dinner table," she said.

Big Food spends about $2 billion per year marketing directly to children, and 90 percent of that money promotes foods that are unhealthful, according to Harris. As a consequence, say food marketing experts, kids become "brand-conscious" when they're two years old.[61] By age three, they can start understanding what the brand can say about their personality, and by first grade, they are typically loyal to their favorite soda, cereal, or candy. That loyalty often sticks through adulthood.

Children watch an average of forty thousand ads every year, mostly for toys, cereals, candy, and fast food, according to Dale Kunkel, a University of Southern California professor specializing in the media's effect on children.[62] Kids are also targeted online, particularly through "advergames" that push product while they play, like a "build your own Fruit Loops" game, or a Capri Sun activity that requires access to the computer's webcam but doesn't verify the player's age.[63]

In 2009, in response to rising concern from the health sector and parental advocates, a bipartisan team of senators, Tom Harkin (D-IA) and Sam Brownback (R-KS), asked the government to set some voluntary guidelines for companies marketing to children. In response, a "working group" of officials from the Federal Trade Commission, the Centers for Disease Control and Prevention, the USDA, and the Food and Drug Administration was formed to develop the guidelines, and in 2011, the group submitted its proposals, which were based on well-established research, for public review. Among the group's recommendations was that marketed food should make a meaningful contribution to a healthy diet and should meet specific limits on salt, added sugar, and certain fats.[64]

Of the 29,000 comments the group received, the vast majority were favorable. Many public health organizations also weighed in with praise. "Everyone was pretty much 100 percent behind those guidelines," said Harris.

Industry groups, on the other hand, which submitted about a hundred comments, were not happy. They claimed the proposed standards—

even though they were completely optional—would be unworkable and were not even needed. Food and beverage companies, they said, could be trusted to regulate themselves. The companies then went to work to make sure the proposals would go nowhere. In short order, they teamed up with big media companies, including Viacom and Time Warner, to form the Sensible Food Policy Coalition. The U.S. Chamber of Commerce joined the lobbying effort, too. The companies hired former Obama communications aide turned public messaging expert Anita Dunn to manage the effort.

The main coalition members had already spent nearly $60 million lobbying during the Obama administration through mid-2011, according to the *Washington Post*.[65] The companies would supplement their lobbying budgets with a generous PR and advertising budget to finance the activities of their front group. One of the first orders of business was to commission a study that warned that the guidelines would kill 75,000 jobs and eliminate more than $28 billion in revenue to companies. The coalition also released a list of 88 products it said would be banned under the guidelines, including Cheerios.[66]

On Capitol Hill, the companies focused attention on Senator Dick Durbin, Democrat of Illinois, and Representative Jo Ann Emerson, a Missouri Republican. Both served on committees overseeing FTC funding. Emerson, a former director of state relations and government programs at the National Restaurant Association, which lobbied against the proposal, told Reuters at the time that she feared that even though the guidelines would be voluntary, they would eventually become mandatory. Contributions from food and beverage companies and crop producers poured into Emerson's 2012 campaign. Among the donors was American Crystal Sugar, which was especially worried about the guidelines. Other big contributors to her campaign were cereal maker General Mills and the Dairy Farmers of America.

Dick Durbin had previously received $11,000 from Kraft Foods, based in his home state. The company gave him another $3,000 in 2011. Kraft also lobbied on the marketing guidelines as part of its $2.8 million 2011 lobbying budget.[67]

Tom Harkin, on the other hand, who had once been an industry favorite, became persona non grata after suggesting the guidelines. In the two years prior to his push for them, food and beverage companies had donated more than $75,000 to his campaigns. In 2010 and 2011, they contributed just $3,000.

Industry lobbyists were able to persuade 176 members of the House and almost a third of the Senate, Democrats as well as Republicans, to send letters to the working group opposing the recommendations. The Sunlight Foundation later noticed that Democrats who signed letters critical of the guidelines had received about twice as much campaign money from food lobbying interests as those who didn't.

It was Emerson who would kill the guidelines in the House by inserting a fifty-five-word sentence into a 130-page budget bill in December 2011. Her sentence required the various agencies involved in the guidelines to do a cost-benefit analysis of their recommendations before finalizing them. The effect of Emerson's language was to make it too costly for the agencies to move forward with the guidelines. On the other side of the Capitol, Durbin agreed to go along with Emerson's language. An aide told Reuters that Durbin did so because he believed the industry was moving toward self-regulation. The final recommendations were never released.

Harris said the FTC, one of the working group participants, might have decided to back off from pursuing the guidelines because of a bad case of déjà vu, from when the FTC's authority was neutered by Congress more than twenty-five years earlier after intense pressure from industry lobbyists. The FTC was attempting to ban TV ads aimed at young children, on the basis that the ads were "unfair and deceptive," but broadcasters, ad agencies, and food and toy companies fought back. They tried to stop the agency from holding hearings and lobbied Congress to cut off funding for the agency's initiative. The companies' lobbyists succeeded in getting Congress to pass a law in 1980 preventing the FTC from issuing industry-wide rules on advertising to children.[68,69] "Ever since then, they're still too scared to stick their neck out too far," says Harris.

So we're left with self-regulation. Eighteen big companies, representing most of the food and drink advertising market, have now signed an agreement with the Better Business Bureau pledging either not to directly target its advertising at kids under twelve or to market only what the companies call "better-for-you" foods to them.[70] The companies say progress has been made. Some advocates agree. The Rudd Center found that by 2013, children were watching about 40 percent fewer TV ads for sugary drinks than they did in 2010. But Harris says this self-regulation has many holes. For one thing, the industry classifies children as eleven and younger, and it really covers only TV programming designed for children, not other programs that many children watch.

Why It Matters

When Big Food reaches into its deep pockets, and Big Sugar moves its protectionist-gained taxpayer dollars into lobbying, both can not only halt or move legislation in Washington and state houses across America, but they can also prevent us from acting on the mounting public health problem that is obesity.

Our annual economic productivity loss due to obesity by 2030 is projected to be between $390 billion, according to a study commissioned by the American Public Health Association,[71] and $580 billion, according to the Robert Wood Johnson Foundation, the largest private funder of anti-obesity efforts in the United States.[72]

One out of every five dollars spent on health care goes toward treating obesity-related illnesses, according to research in the *Journal of Health Economics*, and direct medical costs are even greater than those associated with smoking.[73,74,75] Medicare and Medicaid spend nearly $62 billion annually to treat obesity-related diseases.[76] The medical costs for obese people already are $1,429 higher than nonobese people annually, and their prescription drugs are 105 percent more expensive.[77,78]

Costs will only go up if obesity rates rise as they have in the past. According to research by Duke University professor Eric A. Finkelstein and others, 42 percent of the U.S. population could be obese by 2030. If, however, we could keep obesity rates at 2010 levels, we would save about $550 billion in medical spending.

Other nonmedical costs include an estimated $4 billion in increased fuel costs per year attributed to heavy passengers in cars, buses, and planes.[79] Bus manufacturers have to upgrade components of their vehicles to comply with Federal Transit Authority requirements drafted after concerns that additional passenger weight poses a safety threat.[80] New York City is considering upgrading its subway cars with sturdier seats; Blue Bird, maker of the ubiquitous yellow school bus, is widening the front doors on newer models so bigger children can get through them; baseball stadiums, theaters, and airplanes are adding wider seats. Some military leaders have even called this epidemic a national security threat, as one in four young people cannot qualify for service because of their weight and the military spends more than $1 billion a year on obesity-related medical care.[81]

Efforts to tackle this problem, particularly by nonprofits and health care professionals, have had their impact blunted by the food and beverage

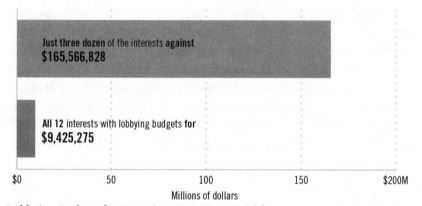

Just three dozen of the interests against
$165,566,828

All 12 interests with lobbying budgets **for**
$9,425,275

$0   50   100   150 $200M

Millions of dollars

Lobbying Budgets for & Against Nutrition Guidelines
Source: Comments received by the FTC in response to issuing nutrition guidelines and federal lobbying disclosures.

industries. It's commendable that the Robert Wood Johnson Foundation has promised to spend more than $1 billion on various anti-obesity efforts by 2025.

But the groups fighting obesity are far outgunned in Washington by industry lobbyists. As we mentioned, the companies and groups against the optional marketing guidelines had a combined annual lobbying budget of about $166 million, compared to $9.6 million for the groups advocating for them.[82] And that discrepancy leaves out PR budgets, all of the undisclosed resources used to support their lobbying efforts, and millions in campaign contributions.

Just as is the case with the other issues we report on in this book—banking, energy, medicine, toxins—it is difficult to imagine how we can make meaningful progress as long as so many of our lawmakers and regulators are in the deep pockets of a few big companies.

The Institute of Medicine released a report in 2012 outlining what it would take to solve America's weight problem.[83] It included some obvious suggestions: encouraging people to get more exercise; getting employers, doctors and nurses, schools, and marketers to encourage healthy living; making nutritious foods accessible to people at all income levels; and "strengthen schools as the heart of health." But lobbying and campaign contributions have halted progress on many of the suggestions.

Of course, government intervention and public programs designed to curb obesity rates will always face some level of disapproval, and they may not always be the best course of action. Any public health campaign must balance outcomes with freedom of choice, recognizing people's individual responsibility for their own health. But in a democracy, we, the citizens, should have the power to enact legislation to tackle a public health crisis—especially one we know so much about solving. It almost seems silly to have to write such a sentence in a nation dedicated to the project of self-government. Yet over and over again, we have seen how special interests with seemingly unlimited funds have been able to shut down our collective ability to act.

CHAPTER 8

Enough to Make You Sick

Soon after installing new flooring in her home, breast cancer survivor Casandra Barrett of Dorr, Michigan, started feeling sick. Her husband, Steve, was having the same symptoms: frequent headaches and a chronic runny nose. The Barretts both suffer from allergies and try to avoid bringing anything into their home that might be toxic. They are especially concerned about Mrs. Barrett, who developed a weakened immune system after undergoing chemotherapy and radiation to treat her breast cancer several years ago. They searched their house to try to identify the source but found nothing obvious.

Then came a blockbuster news segment on CBS's *60 Minutes* in March 2015, reporting that Lumber Liquidators, which manufactured the Barretts' laminate flooring, appeared to be selling a Chinese-made product that was emitting unsafe levels of a known carcinogen, formaldehyde, while labeling it as safe.[1] Formaldehyde helps bind the glues that keep composite wood particles together in laminate flooring. Many Americans turn to this kind of flooring as a cheaper alternative to hardwood.

In the *60 Minutes* segment, one independent lab said the levels of formaldehyde in the Chinese-made flooring tested so high that lab employees thought the instruments were broken. One product registered at thirteen times the limit in California, the only state with a formaldehyde emissions standard for laminate flooring. The Barretts had even checked Lumber Liquidators' website before buying the flooring to make sure it was safe and compliant with California standards.

The Barretts' story is detailed in a class-action lawsuit filed by the law firm Hagens Berman alleging that Lumber Liquidators, which sells more than a hundred million square feet of relatively low-cost laminated flooring every year, defrauded its customers.[2] The company insisted its flooring was safe and sought to prove it by sending free air testing kits to its customers. The lawsuit claimed, however, that the kits were "inherently unreliable" and were actually designed to underreport the formaldehyde levels. With the litigation and negative publicity came a big drop in Lumber Liquidators' stock price. The company eventually pulled the Chinese-made flooring from its shelves.

The bigger picture here is that after years of delays pushed for by the chemical, manufacturing, and furniture industries and their business and political allies, no federal standard for a safe level of formaldehyde exposure for humans exists. That standard would put us all in a safer place, says Tom Neltner, the chemicals policy director at the Environmental Defense Fund. He told us that for starters, state agencies could base enforceable rules on it.

The industry has been so successful that, as of 2015, the Environmental Protection Agency had not finalized its latest scientific assessment, which it began in 1998, of how dangerous formaldehyde is, even after a growing body of research has called it a carcinogen linked to leukemia. The most recent delays, in 2009 and 2011, are significantly due to the power of chemical industry lobbyists and campaign contributors to paralyze our government from taking action.

We also detail the story of how the connections of one deep-pocketed lobbyist can have a big impact on regulations affecting public health. This Washington lobbyist, Charlie Grizzle, gave thousands of dollars in campaign contributions over the years to Senator David Vitter of Louisiana and Representative Mike Simpson of Idaho. The lawmakers led the charge in getting the EPA to delay its assessments, an investigation by the Center for Public Integrity revealed.[3] In Vitter's case, the delay was aimed at formaldehyde. In Simpson's, the scientific assessment of another chemical toxic in high doses—arsenic—was put on hold.

The federal regulation that could have helped prohibit high levels of formaldehyde in flooring was supposed to have been in place by 2013 after Congress passed a law in 2010 mandating formaldehyde emissions standards in that type of flooring. But by 2015, the rule still had not been completed by the EPA. So the agency was left watching from the sidelines when Americans were made aware by *60 Minutes* that dangerously high levels of formaldehyde could be in their homes. On its website, the EPA addressed their concern with this less than comforting statement: "Because national formaldehyde emissions standards will not take effect until after EPA issues its final implementing regulations, EPA is not yet doing any enforcement investigations relating to the formaldehyde emissions standards for composite wood products."[4]

Sowing Seeds of Doubt

Formaldehyde is big business. Nearly 4 billion pounds of it was produced in or imported to the United States in 2011.

It is present in many products—carpets, plywood, nail polish, paper, and pesticides, to name a few—and, as it is a naturally occurring compound, has been thought to be safe at lower levels. A gas that can be condensed into liquid form, formaldehyde is now used primarily in the production of industrial resins. It was a key ingredient in a foam used extensively for home insulation until U.S. Consumer Product Safety Commission banned the foam in 1982. Wood flooring companies sell billions of dollars' worth of products containing formaldehyde every year. In defense of the use of formaldehyde in building materials and many other products, the American Chemistry Council notes that the chemical exists naturally in our bodies.[5] In the past, the council sought to create doubt about the reliability of research linking formaldehyde to leukemia.[6] As Tom Neltner points out, however, "While the industry will tell you that formaldehyde is natural, it's also used to embalm people. They lack a little context."

At higher levels, formaldehyde can cause cancer, according to the National Cancer Institute. An NCI study that followed 25,000 workers for 42 years and was published in 2009 found that workers with the highest exposure to the chemical were 37 percent more likely to die from lymphatic or blood cancer and 78 percent more like to die from myeloid leukemia, a cancer that inhibits the production of normal blood cells.[7]

Less serious but nonetheless troubling, at the levels contained in some of Lumber Liquidators' flooring, formaldehyde can trigger asthma, burning eyes, and nosebleeds as it seeps into the air, the EPA has reported.

Upper respiratory problems were found among the thousands of people who said they suffered from formaldehyde exposure after Hurricane Katrina. All of them had lived at least for a while in trailers the Federal Emergency Management Agency had bought to house displaced residents.

Soon after the families moved into their trailers in late 2005, some started complaining of burning eyes, trouble breathing, and rashes, among other symptoms. Becky Gillette, an Arkansas volunteer with the Sierra Club, became suspicious of materials used in the trailers and bought $39 kits to test for formaldehyde levels. She told us that of the 120 trailers she tested over the years, about nine out of ten exceeded 0.1 parts per million of formaldehyde, the exposure at which the National Cancer Institute says it can have adverse health effects.[8,9] The CDC later confirmed that many occupied trailers had formaldehyde levels above that norm.

Her discoveries helped lead to a class action lawsuit against the manufacturers of the trailers on behalf of 55,000 Gulf Coast residents. In 2012, more than six years after the hurricane, U.S. District Judge Kurt Engelhardt in New Orleans approved a settlement requiring the manufacturers and FEMA contractors who set up and maintained the trailers to pay the plaintiffs $42.6 million. One Mississippi woman, Agnes Mauldin, told Judge Engelhardt that her sixty-six-year-old-mother died of leukemia in 2008 after living in a FEMA trailer.[10] Several other people reported that they or relatives who lived in the trailers were later diagnosed with leukemia.

Gillette doggedly took on bureaucrats in Washington who preferred to deny the problem, and she did not let up. She and Lindsay Huckabee, a Mississippi mother of five whose family fell victim to a toxic trailer, even testified before Congress.[11] Gillette's crusade clearly had an effect on lawmakers. The legislation they passed in 2010 calls for limiting the amount of formaldehyde that can be used in certain wood products, such as the ones used in the trailers. But to Gillette's chagrin, the industry's objections over the specifics of regulations proposed by the EPA continue to delay the law's implementation.

Ubiquitous

At least 2 million Americans are exposed to formaldehyde in the workplace every year, according to the Occupational Safety and Health Administration.[12] It's one of the most common chemicals we encounter. Elizabeth Ward of the American Cancer Society told USA Today in 2009 that it has become "ubiquitous."[13] Two workplaces of particular risk are nail and hair salons. Several hair salon workers have become sick from exposure to a formaldehyde-laced hair straightening product used in so-called Brazilian blowouts. A *New York Times* investigation in 2015 found scores of nail salon employees who complained of nosebleeds and breathing problems.

Many products in our bathroom cabinets contain formaldehyde. And even if it isn't listed as an ingredient, you could still be exposed to the chemical. For example, the ingredient list on a bottle of a popular face wash—one of the commonly used exfoliating scrubs found on pharmacy shelves—doesn't list formaldehyde, but it did contain several other chemicals, including DMDM hydantoin, which the Occupational Safety & Health Administration lists as a chemical that can release formaldehyde.[14] Philip Landrigan, the dean for global health at Mount Sinai Hospital and an expert on toxins, says children, pregnant women, and the elderly are more likely to be sensitive to the chemical's effects, although he added that he doesn't think home testing for formaldehyde is probably necessary unless symptoms develop.

Most Chemicals Go Untested

In addition to formaldehyde, Landrigan says federal limits on exposure to arsenic, which can cause developmental and neurological problems, are past due for an upgrade. An estimated 730 out of 100,000 women get cancer annually as a result of exposure to arsenic—present in water and pesticides—at current maximum exposure levels. High levels of manganese, present in stainless steel utensils and soda cans and also our water supply, has been linked to Parkinson's disease. These are chemicals we *know* can be unsafe. "The great fear is always that there might be other chemicals out there that have never been tested but to which children are exposed," Landrigan said.

Indeed, most of the eighty thousand chemicals in products we use have not been tested. Still, as of 2015, most were not required to be.

And Americans are not exactly happy with that. Three quarters of the people polled in 2012 by Public Opinion Strategies for the Natural Resources Defense Council think the threat posed to people's health by exposure to toxic chemicals is serious. More than two thirds support stricter regulation of chemicals, including a majority of conservatives and Tea Party supporters.[15] In a separate 2012 poll conducted by Lake Research

Partners for the American Sustainable Business Council, three fourths of small business owners support stricter regulation of toxins in everyday products.[16]

Formaldehyde companies have successfully blocked regulation at the federal level for years by presenting studies by industry-funded scientists, by objecting to the EPA's process, and, most important, by persuading members of Congress to write letters and pass legislation that delays the EPA's work. All of this can be hazardous to our health, to say the least. Commenting on the willingness of some members of Congress to go to bat for the chemical companies, the Government Accountability Office noted in 2009 that the EPA assessments that have "been in progress the longest cover key chemicals likely to cause cancer."[17] Advocates say the GAO was referring to the political involvement of Senator Jim Inhofe, Republican of Oklahoma and a member of the Senate Environment and Public Works Committee. In 2004, Inhofe, who now chairs the committee, persuaded the EPA to delay its assessment of formaldehyde until another scientific study was completed. That study was finally published five years later and was unequivocal in calling formaldehyde a carcinogen. The industry also discredited that study, saying it wasn't definitive.

The chemical industry's lobbying effort is well funded. Just ten of the biggest chemical interests that support a new industry-friendly chemical safety bill spent more than $150 million on lobbying in Washington in 2013 and 2014, according to MapLight, a nonpartisan money-in-politics research organization.[18] In contrast, all of the public interest, environmental, and medical associations that lobbied on the bill spent a combined $17.6 million in 2013 and 2014.

The most frequent Washington mouthpiece for the industry is the American Chemistry Council, a trade association with $130 million in assets, and a CEO with a total annual compensation package worth $3.6 million in 2013. The American Chemistry Council is behind another group called the Formaldehyde Panel, a network of more than 150 companies, ranging from small wood manufacturers and the National Funeral Directors Association to big corporate players such as DuPont, 3M, BASF, ExxonMobil, and Chevron.

The American Chemistry Council's toolbox goes beyond lobbying. The group spent $38 million to mount a PR campaign to counter the public's worries about phthalates, a family of chemicals used in plastics that has been linked to development problems in children.[19] The PR firm, Ogilvy, won a coveted industry CLIO award for shifting public opinion against banning the chemicals.

Unlike the chemical industry, environmental and public health groups lack the resources to fund swarms of scientists and consultants to attend every relevant EPA meeting and become intellectual resources for officials, all of which puts them at a disadvantage, Jennifer Sass, senior scientist in the health and environment program at the Natural Resources Defense Council, told us.

The Name of the Game: Delay, Delay, Delay

Charlie Grizzle was an assistant administrator at the EPA during the George H. W. Bush administration. He was appointed to the next Bush president's transition team and then became a "pioneer" for George W. Bush's reelection, a designation for folks bundling in the six figures, the Center for Public Integrity reported.[20,21] He opened his own lobbying firm soon after leaving his post at the EPA and took in well over $1 million in recent years from companies in the chemical and mining industries, among others. From 2004 to 2010, his firm was paid more than $600,000 to work for the Formaldehyde Council, an industry group formed in the face of a regulation threat in 2004.

The Formaldehyde Council members included Georgia-Pacific, a subsidiary of Koch Industries (owned by two of the biggest political donors in recent years, Charles and David Koch), and DuPont, one of the oldest and most successful public companies in the world. It also had furniture and composite wood manufacturers and the National Funeral Directors Association as members. It disbanded in 2010.

More recently, the American Chemistry Council has formed another front group that it named, creatively, the Formaldehyde Panel, and which lists more than 150 companies as members. Most of the companies and organizations comprising the panel are the same ones the Formaldehyde Council claimed. Like the Formaldehyde Council, the Formaldehyde Panel is not required to disclose how much it spends on the effort to resist regulation, and an ACC spokesperson didn't respond when we asked.

In 2009, after the EPA released a draft assessment report concluding that formaldehyde was indeed a known carcinogen, a more dangerous classification than it had previously given the chemical, the Formaldehyde Council issued a statement slamming the study and said the EPA's proposals should be reviewed by the National Academy of Sciences, an independent research organization established by Congress. Such a review could take four years.[22] The Grizzle Company worked to make that happen.

Grizzle's connections helped the formaldehyde makers get the time they wanted. On his website, Grizzle touts his ability to use his "strong Republican credentials" to "bring a client's interests to the immediate attention of the most influential leaders in the White House or Congress." To maintain those strong credentials in Washington, Grizzle has opened his checkbook frequently. He has made more than five hundred individual contributions to candidates and committees since 1989, totaling nearly $400,000, almost all of it to Republicans. (Although he was never elected to public office, he even referred to himself as "the Honorable Charles Grizzle" in at least two disclosures.)

One of the beneficiaries of Grizzle's cash is David Vitter, the senator from Louisiana. Around the time in May 2009 that the National Cancer Institute released its study,[23] Grizzle gave Vitter a $2,400 donation, reports show, part of the $15,000 he and members of his firm have given to Vitter since 2000, most of it since 2008. Campaign contribution reports show that Vitter became a favorite of the chemical industry: he was the second-biggest recipient of campaign money among senators from the chemical manufacturing business in 2010, a reelection year for him, with donations of about $76,000.[24]

In 2009, Vitter used his power in the Senate to block the nomination of an EPA official in an unrelated office until the agency acquiesced to sending the EPA's formaldehyde assessment to the National Academy of Sciences, as the Formaldehyde Council had requested. For lobbyists, kicking a study to the NAS is not a new strategy. "The standard playbook that industry uses first begins with questioning the science, and they can question the science in any one of a number of different forms," Charles Fox, a former EPA administrator, told the Center for Public Integrity. "There is a scientific advisory board at EPA. There's the National Academy of Sciences."

The Natural Resources Defense Council warned that kicking the study to the NAS would mean at least a two-year delay before the EPA could issue a final assessment.[25] That turned out to be wishful thinking. Six years later, the EPA's formaldehyde regulations still had not been made final. "Delay means money," James Huff, associate director for chemical carcinogenesis at the National Institute for Environmental Health

Sciences in the Department of Health and Human Services, told ProPublica in April 2010. "The longer they can delay labeling something a known carcinogen, the more money they can make."

Vitter's rationale for the holdup, his office's spokesman told a reporter at the time, was that "because of the FEMA trailer debacle, we need to get absolutely reliable information to the public about formaldehyde risk as soon as possible." In response to questions we submitted to Vitter's office, his spokesman replied in an email, "During his tenure as Ranking Member of the Environment and Public Works Committee, Senator Vitter had concerns that EPA was failing to utilize strong scientific standards, not using accurate cost benefit analysis, and not adequately regulating. His position on the committee offered him a unique opportunity to provide additional oversight over the standards EPA was employing when making regulations."

The EPA pushed back against Vitter's demands; EPA administrator Lisa Jackson even met personally with Vitter to ask him to stop blocking the nomination of a key official. The EPA said it was "not time for delay."[26]

At least three House Democrats also wrote to Jackson to request a review by the Academy because, they said, it is important for the assessment to be "thorough and accurate." They wrote that since "formaldehyde is found in so many applications from building and construction materials to consumer goods and medications, we are concerned that the public needs the certainty of an NAS review to support broad acceptance" of formaldehyde's "potential health effects." In December 2009, the Society of the Plastics Industry, a trade group representing formaldehyde manufacturers DuPont and BASF, held a fundraiser for Vitter, suggesting donations of $1,000 per person. Later that month, in a letter to the Formaldehyde Council, Jackson acquiesced, writing that she would send the EPA's findings to the National Academy of Sciences for review.

The industry heaped praise on Vitter for his help. "Overcoming the agency's intransigence in engaging NAS on formaldehyde would have been impossible without the timely intervention of U.S. Senator David Vitter," Betsy Natz, the Formaldehyde Council's director, told ProPublica in April 2010. In March 2010, Grizzle cohosted another $1,000-per-plate fundraiser for Vitter, records show, at the exclusive Republicans-only Capitol Hill Club.[27]

In 2011, the National Academy of Sciences completed its review, which criticized the EPA's work on formaldehyde for being disorganized. But its scientists wholeheartedly agreed with the conclusion of the EPA report—

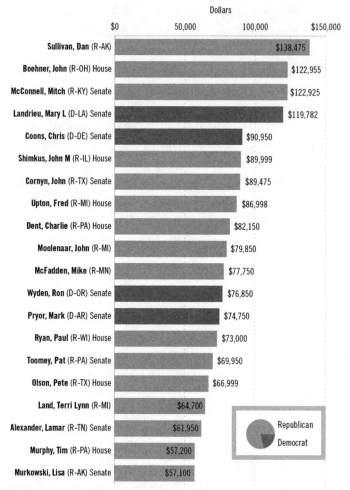

Top 20 Recipients of Chemical Industry Contributions
Source: Center for Responsive Politics (opensecrets.org)
Methodology: The numbers above are based on contributions from PACs and individuals giving $200 or more. All donations took place during the 2013–2014 election cycle and were released by the Federal Election Commission on March 09, 2015.

that formaldehyde can cause cancer. On that point, 51 out of 52 NAS scientists agreed.[28] The NAS also said the issuance of new formaldehyde regulations should not be delayed.[29]

Nevertheless, the chemical lobby continued to have its way in Washington. A few months after the Academy report was issued, an unnamed member of the House Appropriations Committee added a few lines to a 2012 appropriations measure that had the effect of delaying a final assessment not only on formaldehyde, but also on forty-six other chemicals it was in the process of assessing, according to an investigation by the Center for Public Integrity.[30]

Speculation as to the identity of the lawmaker who authored that language has centered on Mike Simpson, the Idaho Republican. Although Simpson, chair of the subcommittee that oversees EPA funding, has not confirmed that he did it, Grizzle admitted lobbying him for it.[31] By that time, Grizzle was working for two pesticide makers whose products contain arsenic, which the EPA was also in the process of evaluating.[32] When the Center for Public Integrity reporter David Heath asked Grizzle if the donations were made to influence the delay, Grizzle replied, "I don't see a connection. I've been a friend and supporter of Congressman Simpson for a long time."

Regardless of which lawmaker wrote the legislation, the result was to almost completely halt the EPA's evaluations of chemicals for three years as the agency was directed to overhaul and improve its scientific process.

The American Chemistry Council has continued to be helpful to Vitter, who decided to run for governor of Louisiana in 2015. The council became the first donor at the over-$100,000 level to a super PAC backing his election.[33] At the time, Vitter was also one of the main point men in Congress in shaping a Chemical Safety Act, which ostensibly would toughen standards for testing and enforcement of the industry. Not surprisingly, it was written in consultation with the council.

Jennifer Sass told us it's hard to blame Jackson for eventually giving in. "When Congress tells you to do something, I'm not sure what you can do," she said.

Floored

Even after the publicity surrounding the FEMA-supplied toxic trailers and the almost $43 million the trailer makers were ordered to pay victims, and even after Congress passed a law to restrict formaldehyde levels in certain wood products, the EPA has yet to issue final regulations. Thanks, of course, to the formidable power and influence of the chemical industry and its friends in business and politics.

In 2015, the *New York Times* reporters Eric Lipton and Rachel Abrams documented the many steps the industry and its allies can take to shape regulations after a law is passed.[34] Those allies in this case include furniture makers and retailers. They joined forces with the chemical companies because the EPA's proposed regulations would affect not only flooring products and cabinetmakers but also lamination facilities that employ a process that adds more formaldehyde to the final product.

The furniture industry, in particular, fumed and used one of the most common tactics of industries under attack: they claimed that new legislation or regulations affecting them would lead to massive layoffs. It's part of a playbook, detailed in *Deadly Spin*,[35] that goes back to efforts by public health officials and consumer advocates to protect people from the harmful effects of cigarette smoke. Formaldehyde producers and users seized on it. The furniture makers said the rule would cost manufacturers up to $200 million per year to implement, considerably more than the tens of millions of dollars estimated by the EPA, the Times reported. The chief lobbyist for the American Home Furnishings Alliance, or AHFA, warned the EPA that if the proposal was not fixed, over a million manufacturing jobs might be impacted.[36]

Executives from La-Z-Boy, Ashley Furniture, and other companies met with House Speaker John Boehner and ten rank-and-file Republicans and Democrats to request that they sign on to a letter pressuring the EPA to fold.[37] They got what they wanted. Members of the House who sent letters included Doris Matsui, a California Democrat, and Alan Nunnelee, a Mississippi Republican. Senate Republicans Roger Wicker of Mississippi, Ron Johnson of Wisconsin, and Roy Blunt of Missouri and Democrats Mark Warner and Tim Kaine of Virginia also sent letters. The furniture executives and lobbyists had reported meeting with all of them except Kaine. All the correspondence echoed the industry's concern that requiring the companies doing the final wood lacquering to test their products would be redundant. They maintain that tests show the lamination process seals in the formaldehyde.

Hundreds of comments were sent to the EPA on the topic from, among others, IKEA, wood products associations, a trade group for mobile home makers, and lobbying powerhouses such as the American Chemistry Council and the U.S. Chamber of Commerce. A few state regulatory agencies, medical associations, and environmental groups sent comments supporting the rule.

All of the influencing and delays has left Becky Gillette demoralized and disgusted with the process. Some members of Congress wanted the rule issued in three years, she told us in the spring of 2015. "It's been five and we've got at least another year to go."

In fairness, Tom Neltner, who negotiated with the industry to help pass the 2010 law, said the EPA's initial proposal may well have been unnecessarily burdensome on hardwood laminators. Another factor, he said, is the EPA's inadequate funding. Still, he added, the chemical industry's well-funded campaign also delayed the process.

The EPA declined to answer many of our questions about those delays. A spokesperson replied only in an email that "since we are looking to revise the standards, all we can say" is "EPA plans to finalize the proposed standards before the end of [2015]."

Is the EPA Its Own Worst Enemy?

The preponderance of resources that the industry can bring to bear and, ironically, the open process that the agency has created to listen to various stakeholders, have further tilted the balance against environmental groups. These factors have also contributed to delays in making rules, the green groups claim.

Advocates such as Richard Denison, a scientist at the Environmental Defense Fund, believes it's a systemic problem. At one of EPA's "stakeholder panels" in 2012, he got up to say so, noting that the average completion time of the assessments is 7.5 years, almost four times the EPA's goal.[38]

On one meeting's agenda, Denison found that as many as six industry representatives from the same consulting firm were scheduled to speak on the same issue. The Center for Public Integrity, analyzing the meetings in recent years, found that 85 percent of the speakers were industry-funded scientists.

This all brings to mind Lee Drutman's book *The Business of America Is Lobbying*. As K Street has drawn the best talent from Congress (with money), Congress has become a kind of "farm system" for lobbying firms, Drutman wrote. "This contributes to a declining government capacity, which means that government policymakers must increasingly rely on lobbyists to help them to develop, pass, and implement policy."[39]

There are other factors pushing the demand up for lobbyists. One is the lobbyists themselves. "More lobbying also makes legislation more complex [in order to accommodate all the lobbying interests]," Drutman wrote.[40] The U.S. Code of Federal Regulations—all requiring specialized knowledge—is now more than 174,000 pages long, he noted, more than doubling since 1975.

That environment, combined with the fact that lobbying itself has become much more competitive and costly, yields a big advantage to trade associations and businesses over public interest groups. They can afford to wield an everything-but-the-kitchen-sink strategy—targeting Congress, the White House, independent agencies—hoping that at least one approach works. As Drutman says, "In an ever-more-complex policy environment, the need for expertise becomes greater, but the gap between public sector and private sector expertise is wider. Again, organizations that can supply the expertise are at an advantage."[41] The nonprofit groups just don't have as much firepower—in terms of scientists, lobbyists, or dollars—to be a source of knowledge for regulators or even to respond to each round of comments submitted to regulators by industry-funded consultants. "A lot of times there are details that I don't have the time to understand," said Tom Neltner of the Environmental Defense Fund. He added: "The public interest community is always outgunned."

Arsenic and Old Science

Arsenic, like formaldehyde, can cause health and developmental problems and at high levels is linked to certain cancers. Columbia University professor Joseph Graziano jokes, darkly, that arsenic makes lead look like a vitamin. That's because, as he told the Center for Public Integrity's David Heath, it "sweeps across the body and impact[s] everything that's going on, every organ system."[42] It's in weed killers marketed to fight your lawn's crabgrass, and, in many places, it's in the water we drink.

A 2008 draft assessment by the EPA estimated that arsenic was seventeen times more potent than previously thought.[43] In assessing the impact of arsenic on women in particular, the agency estimated that if a hundred thousand women were to consume the legal limit of arsenic currently permitted, 730 would get bladder or lung cancer.

After seeing the draft assessment, the producers of arsenic-based pesticides that hired Charlie Grizzle to lobby for them, Drexel Chemical Co. and Luxembourg-Pamol, began to take action, as did mining companies like Rio Tinto, which also would have been affected by the regulation. As the Center for Public Integrity's David Heath reported, a group of lobbyists, including Grizzle, set up a meeting with Representative Mike Simpson, the Republican from Idaho, who by 2015 had received a total of $8,000 in campaign donations from Grizzle, according to data compiled and analyzed by the Sunlight Foundation and the Center for Responsive Politics.

All it took to send the EPA's draft assessment to the National Academy of Sciences for a review was for a congressman to slip one paragraph into in a 221-page spending bill. When Heath asked Simpson about the paragraph, he said he worried about small communities not being able to meet drinking water standards.

Such stealth maneuvers are not uncommon in Congress. A senator, for example, can anonymously put a hold on legislation, completely blocking it. Committee members can insert language written by lobbyists directly into a large spending bill before anyone has adequate time to review it. As Chellie Pingree, a Democrat from Maine, bemoaned to Center for Public Integrity reporter David Heath in June 2014: "It's happening more and more in this Congress that we see less and less of what goes on behind the scenes, that members aren't informed until the last minute. So things like this, major policy changes like this, can happen somewhat in the dark of the night with very little information to the public."

When confronted by a reporter, Simpson said he didn't know that the paragraph inserted into the spending bill kept a weed killer containing arsenic on the market, and he said he had "no idea" that Grizzle had donated to his campaigns.

Delays continued in subsequent years as industry-funded scientists presented their views to the Academy, sometimes without disclosing their financial ties. (The Center for Public Integrity reported that one such scientist suggested that an arsenic dose even higher than the current drinking water standard doesn't cause cancer.) The result: in 2015, seven years after the EPA's draft assessment that arsenic is considerably more dangerous than previously thought, many public health experts said the federal government was continuing to allow too much arsenic in our water and in products like weed killers.

"Nobody's Looking Out for Our Welfare"

"We have a broken Toxic Substance Control Act," says Tom Neltner. That's the big problem that "federal health officials, prominent academics and even many leaders of the chemical industry" agree on, the *Atlantic*'s senior health care editor, Dr. James Hamblin, wrote in 2014.[44]

The obstacles for public health are (1) the vast majority of the eighty thousand industrial chemicals available for use are not regulated or even tested by the government, and (2) companies are not even required to submit most of them for testing.

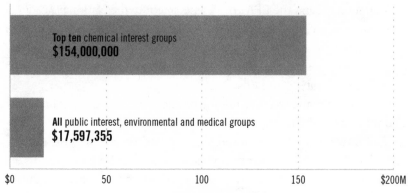

Top ten chemical interest groups
$154,000,000

All public interest, environmental and medical groups
$17,597,355

| $0 | 50 | 100 | 150 | $200M |

Millions of dollars

Sources of Lobbying $$$ on Chemical Safety Reform Legislation
Source: MapLight, authors' analysis (maplight.org)
Methodology: Analysis from organizations disclosing that they lobbied on S. 1009 in 2013 or 2014.

"What most Americans don't realize is nobody's looking out for their welfare," Mount Sinai's Philip Landrigan told us. "The great fear is always that there might be other chemicals out there that have never been tested but to which children are exposed."

In addition, the EPA (like the FDA) has to meet a very high standard before it can ban a toxin. The EPA has banned or limited only five.[45] Weak laws even made it difficult to ban asbestos.

There were signs in 2015 that the chemical safety laws might be strengthened when legislation to update the laws for the first time in thirty-nine years received bipartisan support in the Senate. It would, among other things, require more frequent testing at the federal level and make it easier for the government to pull products off the shelves.

Sponsored by industry favorite David Vitter and New Mexico Democrat Tom Udall, who in the past has supported increased environmental protection, the bill even received kudos of sorts from some environmental advocacy groups, including the Environmental Defense Fund, which view the legislation as an improvement over the broken status quo. Other green groups maintained it was much too weak.[46] Senator Barbara Boxer was pushing a separate, more stringent bill that allowed for testing of more chemicals each year.[47]

Vitter's spokesman wrote that the "legislation provides common-sense reforms that are necessary to update the United States' forty year old chemical regulatory program. Senator Vitter has worked with colleagues across this aisle, stakeholders from all sectors, and the EPA to draft this legislation that will drastically increase EPA's ability to ensure the safety of chemicals being used in the United States." It soon became apparent, however, that the bill was being vetted—and possibly even written, at least in part—by industry lobbyists. Using metadata on a Microsoft Word document circulated by Udall, a reporter for Hearst Newspapers found that the document originated at the American Chemistry Council. Senator Boxer said she felt certain the industry wrote it, citing a Senate information technology staffer who investigated the issue.

Udall, who the *New York Times* suggested had formed an "unlikely alliance" with the chemical industry, maintained that the document originated in his office. One of his aides told Hearst that "it was shared with a number of stakeholders including at least one other senator's office. One of those stakeholders was the ACC."[48] But the council did not deny authoring that draft of the bill. "There's no way for anyone to tell," a council spokesperson said. Others, including Udall's office, said anyone could change some metadata. A spokesperson for Udall said the senator has been engaged with all groups on all sides of the issue.

Regardless of who wrote the bill's language, the end product was more than palatable to the chemical industry. The American Chemistry Council called the bill the "culmination of a multi-year effort" to secure "compromise, common-sense" legislation that it characterized as "a balanced, science-driven solution that reassured the public that our products are safe and that keeps our economy growing."[49]

The ten biggest chemical companies spent $154 million lobbying on the bill over 2013 and 2014, the watchdog group MapLight found. In contrast, public interest, environmental, and medical groups together spent less than $18 million. The environmental groups spent $6.6 million.

Those chemical companies also contributed almost more than $4 million in campaign contributions to several candidates' campaigns in the 2014 election as the sponsors were shepherding the bill through Congress, MapLight found. The ACC also donated $150,000 to a super PAC supporting Vitter's gubernatorial bid in Louisiana.

The ACC also spent $4 million plus on TV and radio advertising in support of the reelection of Udall and the industry's other allies in Congress, the *Times* reported. The ads portrayed Udall as a man who brings "both sides together to get results."[50] According to the *Times*, Udall "emphatically rejects" that he was doing the industry's bidding: "We can't do something that is pie in the sky; we have to deal with reality," he said.

The Price We Pay

In 2007, Lindsay Huckabee of Mississippi, a mother of five whom Becky Gillette called "a real strong mama bear," was invited to testify before Congress. She and her family were among the tens of thousands who had lived in a FEMA trailer after Hurricane Katrina.

Huckabee testified before multiple congressional committees. She told how her son, Michael, was born prematurely, just weeks after she and her family moved into the trailer. She said he had suffered sinus infections and asthmatic bronchitis since he was six days old. Her four-year-old daughter, Leah, had a recurrence of asthma when they moved into the trailer, "more ear infections than I can count," frequent nosebleeds, and several bouts of pneumonia. An ear, nose and throat specialist suggested they move out of the trailer as soon as possible.[51] Lindsay's thirty-year-old husband, a healthy nonsmoker, later developed a mouth tumor that required surgery.[52]

As noted earlier, the prevalence of formaldehyde in a broad range of products and building materials has affected some professions far more than others. Of the 125 nail salon workers interviewed by the *New York Times*, many reported allergies, asthma, and frequent nosebleeds. Others told of worse problems, including miscarriages and children "born special."

Formaldehyde is among a "toxic trio" of ingredients in nail products, including dibutyl phthalate (DBP), which Australia classifies as causing reproductive problems, and toluene, which can lead to developmental problems in fetuses.[53]

There was a bit of good news in 2015. In response to the *Times* article, New York governor Andrew Cuomo signed a bill that would require nail workers to wear gloves and goggles while performing certain tasks and their employers to make respirators available. Still, the health risks for nail and hair salon workers, and consumers of their products, may be even greater than for the rest of us. That's because the U.S. government has even less regulatory power over cosmetics than it has over other consumer products. In fact, except for color additives, the government does not have authority to test what goes into cosmetics before they hit the shelves.[54] The cosmetics industry is self-regulated by an organization that it funds, the Personal Care Products Council, which is also a registered lobbying group.[55] The group insists that the "toxic trio" does not pose a risk to salon workers or their customers.

Researchers have tried to calculate the price we pay for high levels of chemicals. High lead and arsenic exposure has caused neurological problems and are linked to IQ loss. The *Atlantic* reported that "the combined current levels of pesticides, mercury and lead cause IQ losses amounting to around $120 billion annually—or about 3 percent of the annual budget of the U.S. government."[56]

Separately, Philip Landrigan estimated the annual costs of mercury toxicity in children in the United States to be about $5 billion.[57] Researchers writing for *Health Affairs* in 2014 estimated that reducing exposure to BPA, a common chemical in plastics and cans that is linked to childhood obesity and adult heart disease, could save almost $3 billion per year.[58]

There has been progress on some fronts, as Landrigan has noted.[59] The government has made substantial progress in reducing exposure to lead. Every dollar spent to reduce lead hazards produces a benefit between $17 to $220 per person, according to a study by Landrigan and Philippe Grandjean, a Harvard Medical School scientist.[60] Lead-free gasoline alone has generated an economic benefit estimated at $3 trillion since 1980.

Curbing the use of formaldehyde would have measurable health care benefits, according to the Environmental Defense Fund and partner organizations. They maintain that the EPA's proposed rule for wood products would prevent more than twenty-one thousand children from developing asthma each year, resulting in more than $250 million in annual savings.

The cost may also be greater than what current science has shown. Grandjean told the *Atlantic*:

> We don't have the luxury to sit back and wait until science figures out what's really going on, what the mechanisms are, what the doses are, and that sort of thing. We've seen with lead and mercury and other poisons that it takes decades. And during that time we are essentially exposing the next generation to exactly the kind of chemicals that we want to protect them from.

But as long as the vast majority of chemicals that wind up in thousands of consumer products are considered innocent until proven guilty, and as long as the industry and its allies are able to spend whatever it takes to prevent or delay testing and to block legislation and regulation that might affect profits, future generations will be as exposed to poisons as we are today.

PART 3

CHAPTER 9

It's Fixable

You might conclude, at this point in the book, that there's nothing to be done to solve the crisis of money in politics, and that a truly representative republic—a government of, by, and for the people—has become an impossible dream.

You would be wrong.

In fact, the good-government community has spent decades thinking through solutions and creating working models of those solutions at the state and local levels. Such solutions are *technically* easy to implement—establishing a new campaign finance system is a matter of tweaking the tax code and distributing bits of revenue; a new transparency regime is a matter of collecting and sharing data; stronger ethics and lobbying laws are a matter of written words on a page.

Compared to, say, overhauling the ways we produce, distribute, and consume energy in America—which involves hundreds of millions of consumers, thousands of corporations, decades of technological development, trillions of tons of equipment, and a mind-boggling amount of natural resources—campaign finance and ethics laws are remarkably simple to turn into new realities. (And, of course, overhauling our energy infrastructure would be easier if we first reduced the control the energy companies have over politics and policy making.)

Winning back American democracy is not a logistical or technical challenge, it's a matter of political will. That is, our will to make our elected representatives, whose salaries we pay, make it happen.

Remember, we have given ourselves the authority to do it. Look back at the words of the Massachusetts state constitution, which inspired the federal Constitution:

> Government is instituted for the common good; for the protection, safety, prosperity, and happiness of the people; and not for the profit, honor, or private interest of any one man, family, or class of men; therefore, the people alone have an incontestable, unalienable, and indefeasible right to institute government; and to reform, alter, or totally change the same, when their protection, safety, prosperity, and happiness require it.

When we first discussed this quote, in the introduction to this book, we focused on the first part of the sentence—how we've lost government for the common good. But take a look at the last part: *The people alone have an incontestable, unalienable, and indefeasible right to institute government; and to reform, alter, or totally change the same, when their protection, safety, prosperity, and happiness require it.*

Those lines are very reminiscent of the third sentence of the Declaration of Independence:

> That whenever any Form of Government becomes destructive of these ends, it is the Right of the People to alter or to abolish it, and to institute new Government, laying its foundation on such principles and organizing its powers in such form, as to them shall seem most likely to effect their Safety and Happiness.

Democracy requires reinvention and constant vigilance. Like the Founders and the abolitionists, the suffragists and the civil rights activists, when we see a fundamental problem in our system, we fix it. That's the American way. Now we need to fix democracy—before we can fix the other problems we all face.

We also need to define, up front, what winning means. Will we ever "get money out of politics"? No. That phrase is misguiding. Can we limit the amount of coin-operated governing that goes on? Yes. Can we retrain our elected representatives to prioritize our Main Streets over billionaire political donors? Yes. Can we give public-interest legislation a much better shot of winning over the private interests? Yes.

In this respect, maintaining a functioning democracy—which must always include limiting the undue influence of money over politics and policy making—should be seen as a routine function of a civil society. Just as nearly everyone sees schools, libraries, news outlets, green spaces, public health initiatives, hospitals, animal shelters, civic centers, good jobs, secure retirements, public transportation, safe streets, theaters, and art museums as essential components of a thriving community, so should democracy be seen.

Viewing democracy in such a light also helps gauge expectations about what progress means, which then helps reduce the potential for cynicism and resignation. Who among us believes that we can create perfect public health, in which no one is overweight, preventable diseases are eradicated, and everyone is avoiding behaviors that are risky to their health? How about perfect schools, in which all children are achieving their maximum potential? How about a pristine, virginal environment, in which the impacts of human activity are undetectable? How about a 100-percent-efficient and meritocratic economy, in which everyone is justly rewarded for their work and only the best-run businesses flourish?

Goals such as these, of course, are things we would all like to see happen, or most of us would. But we also know that nothing ever reaches a state of perfection. Instead, we keep working on causes and improving systems and pumping money and effort into civic institutions so that they get better over time.

If someone told you they were working on reducing homelessness, would you ever say, "Well, I don't think you'll ever be able to get rid of homelessness, so I don't have time for you." If someone says he or she is the director of an education-reform organization, could you ever imagine saying, "What's the point? There will always be bad students and under-performing teachers, so why bother?" If someone explained to you that they were working on improving air quality, would you ever quip, "It's too late. The air will never be truly clean again because most of the nations on Earth are industrialized." Of course not.

Yet, way too often, when democracy reformers talk about reducing the power of money over politics, many people, especially in Washington, feel perfectly content saying, "Ha! Good luck with that. It'll never happen." It's that very response that has terminally limited the amount of energy and money flowing into the fight for reform. But such a response is appropriate only if the assumption is that the goal is to permanently "get money out of politics." If, instead, the goal, as it is with every other element of a good society, is to keep improving, knowing that a perfect, final destination is unachievable, then we will all be thinking correctly about the challenge ahead.

Which doesn't mean that our task will be easy. This book demonstrates just how powerful Big Money has become. But a movement is building, one that is growing every day, and we'll tell you about it in the next chapter.

One factor that makes our job harder is the current Supreme Court. *Citizens United* was, as we discussed in part 1, a setback. The part of the decision that extended beyond the freedom of the press was naïve and overzealous. Time will show what a mistake it was. The five justices of the majority, without the political experience to understand how the case could warp our democracy, narrowed the ability of legislators to regulate the way money flows to and around the legislative process. But, as you'll learn in the coming pages, those limitations aren't fatal. We can still accomplish 75 percent of what needs to be accomplished to improve the American experiment of self-government.

Also, we should always remind ourselves that the Supreme Court doesn't exist in a vacuum, and like other misguided decisions of yore, like *Plessy v. Ferguson*, which asserted that racial segregation was perfectly constitutional, *Citizens United* will be swept away by the current of time.

Most visible among the efforts to correct the Court's mistake is the movement to overturn *Citizens United* via a constitutional amendment. This strategy has galvanized hundreds of thousands of grassroots activists. A coalition of more than a hundred organizations, called United for the People (united4thepeople.org), is driving the movement, which was sparked more than five years ago by pioneering groups like Free Speech for People. However, amending the Constitution requires approval from two thirds of Congress and then ratification by three quarters of the state legislatures (38 of the 50). Or it requires the calling of a constitutional convention, which means that two thirds of the states (34) would have to agree to do so, and then any amendments that emerge from the convention still need to be ratified by 38 states. So it's a long-term strategy, one that will take many years to accomplish, if indeed it ever succeeds.

More attainable is a three-pronged effort to establish a pro-reform jurisprudence, which groups like the Brennan Center for Justice, the Campaign Legal Center, and Demos are driving.

The first prong of this work is focused on clarifying aspects of the *Citizens United* decision that are demonstrably ill-informed. The most obvious example is one of the central arguments held dear by the five justices: that independent spending is not at all corrupting of candidates and public officials because it is completely unaffiliated with the candidates and their campaigns.

This claim is difficult to square with the current political reality, now that Jeb Bush and Hillary Clinton have super PACs whose "independence" is clearly in name only. All you have to do to prove this lack of independence is search Google for "super PACs and coordination" and you can read hundreds of newspaper articles that document the connections. Jeb raised more than $100 million for his super PAC before he officially filed his candidate paperwork with the government. A nonpartisan group called the Campaign Legal Center has filed complaints against most of the major presidential candidates, on both sides of the aisle, raising the red flag about such coordination.

The second prong of the work is to reassert that Congress has the right—and duty—to make laws preventing corruption or the appearance of corruption. As we mentioned in previous chapters, Fordham University law professor Zephyr Teachout points out in her book, *Corruption in America*, that regulating against systemic corruption is in perfect accord with what the Founders believed, and what served as campaign finance precedent for the hundred years prior to *Citizens United*. The reestablishment of this principle of corruption will require legal scholarship, the shaping of ideas in and around law schools, and the assertion of public opinion—in a 2014 poll, 75 percent of Americans said they believe politicians are "corrupted" by campaign donations and lobbyists.[1]

The third prong of the work is the nominating of judges and Supreme Court justices whose positions on democracy and money in politics are in line with those of the vast majority of the American public. Developing standards for vetting judicial nominees based on their sophistication about the way money and influence manifest themselves in our democracy—the very sophistication that is lacking on the current Court—is necessary to make sure that those on the bench "get it." In the late spring of last year, Vermont Senator Bernie Sanders said, "If elected president, I will have a litmus test in terms of my nominee to be a Supreme Court justice, and that nominee will say that we are all going to overturn this disastrous Supreme Court decision."

Soon after, Hillary Clinton told a group in Iowa: "I will do everything I can to appoint Supreme Court justices who protect the right to vote and do not protect the right of billionaires to buy elections."

As of the writing of this book, no Republican presidential candidates have said they would probe potential justices on their views of money in politics, but there is an increasing amount of discussion among Republicans about taking firmer and clearer stances on the matter. Which is a good sign. If there's a silver lining to *Citizens United*, it's that the decision has ignited an awareness and anxiety about the usurping of our democracy that hasn't existed since Watergate.

So what are the legislative fixes that we can accomplish now, regardless of the Supreme Court?

Broadly speaking, they fall into four categories that embody the principles of a high-functioning democracy: (1) everyone participates, (2) everyone knows, (3) everyone plays by the same commonsense rules, and (4) everyone is held accountable.

Yes, that's four categories. Most people want a single category and ask if there is a silver bullet for this cause—a simple fix that will solve the whole problem. There is not. Most major issues are of such complexity. From public health to education to crime and poverty reduction, it takes all kinds of strategies and policies, applied simultaneously over long periods of time, to make lasting progress. The legislative and judicial fixes we focus on are as varied as the problem. We don't have the space to describe all the efforts to get such fixes enacted and implemented. Instead, we will detail the most promising efforts taking shape across the country.

(1) Everyone Participates

This is the "game changer" category. Unless we create better ways of financing politics in this country, we're never going to be able to rebalance the power dynamic in Washington and the state capitals.

There's no need for us to say anything more about the need to create new ways of financing campaigns than the quote we included in chapter 2 from Representative Jim Himes (D-CT):

> I won't dispute for one second the problems of a system that demands [an] immense amount of fund-raisers by its legislators.

It's appalling, it's disgusting, it's wasteful and it opens the possibility of conflicts of interest and corruption.

This admission is stunning. A sitting member of the United States
Congress telling one of the most respected news outlets in the world that
the way we finance our politics—and therefore, the baseline for our way
of governing—is *appalling, disgusting, wasteful,* and potentially corrupting.

Even when the money isn't given with any transactional intentions—
even if the donor has no expectation of bending legislation or pressuring
a government official for a favor—the process of raising it marinates the
minds of politicians in the concerns of the wealthiest among us. Day after
day after day, four to five hours a day, our elected representatives are
spending their time begging for money primarily from people who can
afford to attend $2,700-a-plate dinners and lunches ($2,700 is the current
limit on what an individual can donate directly to a politician's campaign).
That includes, of course, the lobbyists and political fundraisers who often
"bundle" four-figure checks and then hand over envelopes stuffed with
$100,000 or more in contributions.

The fealty we want politicians to have is to their constituents back
home on Main Street. We want them obsessing about Jane and John Doe,
not David and Charles Koch. We want them spending as little time as
possible dialing for dollars from wealthy people, nearly all of whom live
outside their districts. We want them to have maximum time to study
legislation, attend committee hearings, and reach across the aisle to
engage in the high art of compromise.

The one thing that will most engender such a shift of attention, time,
and loyalty is what some reformers call "citizen funding" of elections. We
prefer the term "citizen funding" rather than "public financing" because
the latter seems generic and somewhat bureaucratic. There are public
restrooms and pools and beaches. There are public works administrations and public programs. Citizens, though, are human beings. In
America, a citizen is an agent of democracy. Such agents—asserting their
agency on the system—are what we need more of today.

Citizen funding programs provide the vast majority of Americans, the
99.7 percent of us who can't afford to write significant checks to politicians, with an incentive to participate. Either by limiting the amount and
type of fundraising a candidate can do or by providing constituents with
funds to contribute as they please, the government is able to redirect a
politician's attention to the rest of us.

There are several types of citizen funding programs, dozens of which are already in place at the state and local levels:

- Clean Elections, in which candidates receive a set amount of money to operate their campaigns. Once they do, they are required to cease raising money from other sources. To qualify for the program they must cross a threshold of viability and popularity by collecting a certain amount of low-dollar private donations and signatures from their districts. Connecticut has the best-functioning of such systems.
- Matching Funds. Candidates opt in to these systems. Once they are in, a government fund matches every dollar raised from citizens, by some multiple, up to a certain amount. In some places the match is as much as six dollars for every dollar raised. New York City's matching-fund system has often been heralded as the best in class, and the politicians who participate in it testify that it has turned their gaze back to their districts.
- Tax Incentives. People get a tax credit or deduction for political contributions, up to a certain amount. In some states, the contribution is eligible to be counted for a credit or deduction only if it's made to a candidate who has agreed to limit his or her campaign spending. Oklahoma and Montana have the most generous incentives, at $100.
- Vouchers. The government provides each citizen with a certificate for $50 or $100, which he or she can then contribute to a candidate or party.
- Hybrids, or some combination of the above approaches.

The criticism of such systems is that they provide "taxpayer-funded welfare for politicians." To which our response is: Your tax dollars will be paying their salaries once they're in office, and they will be allocating trillions of your tax dollars through government spending and contracting. So who would you rather they feel beholden to once they're in office: you, or a bunch of special interests and wealthy benefactors? One of the most important prerequisites of a democracy of, by, and for the people is one funded of, by, and for the people.

Take Connecticut, for example. Its Citizens' Election Program (CEP) is financed through a mix of cash receipts received from unclaimed properties reverted to the state; voluntary contributions from individuals and businesses; donations of surplus funds from dissolved candidate campaigns or political committees; and investment earnings on CEP's resources. In 2014, the program reached an all-time high participation rate with 84 percent of winning candidates using the system, and with striking parity between the two major parties.

A study of CEP by the nonprofit think tank Demos demonstrated just how valued the program is by its participants and how effective citizen funding is at meeting its stated goals: "It is clear," the report stated, "that public financing is a fundamental step towards a more representative legislative process that is more responsive to constituents."[2] According to the think tank, which relied on quantitative data analysis and the reflections of elected officials, CEP brings about a much stronger, more representative legislature in several ways.

First, the program eliminates most of the need to fundraise, allowing candidates to spend more time talking with actual voters. A study by a professor at the University of Maryland found that the average legislator in a typical state spends at least 28 percent of their time fundraising;[3] in a state like Connecticut, with its citizen funding program, that percentage decreased to just 11.[4] Said one member of the state House, "I get all my fundraising done early in the summer and then spend the rest of the time door knocking and talking to constituents, which is where I should be spending my time."[5]

Connecticut's system has also expanded the pool of candidates running for office, because personal wealth and connections are a less necessary component of a successful campaign. Plus, the more candidates run for office, the fewer uncontested or noncompetitive seats there are, expanding choice for voters and allowing fresh voices to compete with incumbents. In a similar vein, CEP has increased the number of donors participating in the process, and incumbents have increasingly shifted away from big-money PACs and toward individual donors.

Because legislators no longer rely on their donations, the influence wielded by lobbyists has waned significantly. Former Connecticut representative Juan Figuero described a system of "shakedowns" where "lobbyists and corporate sponsors had events and you . . . had to go."[6] Now, power dynamics in the statehouse have shifted, and, as a Republican notes, "people concentrate more on the issues . . . the big issues get bipartisan votes."[7] Demos notes, "the actual process of legislating [became] more responsive and substantive." In practice, that means that the policies enacted are more representative of what *all* residents of Connecticut want, not just political donors.

Another Republican legislator explained, "Before public financing, to get donations you had to call people. That would go on. You'd spend half of your time in the election cycle calling up people, raising money instead of going out and knocking on doors. Now, you're getting it from the people and hearing what they want and not from special interests."[8]

In New York City, the effects of the matching funds system have proven to not just remake the way city politics are funded, but also the way politicians think about their constituencies. A data-rich report produced jointly by the Brennan Center for Justice and the Campaign Finance Institute details how politicians who have run on the system said "that by pumping up the value of small contributions, the New York City system gives them an incentive to reach out to their own constituents rather than focusing all their attention on wealthy out-of-district donors, leading them to attract more diverse donors into the political process."[9]

The system has lit up political giving in most of the neighborhoods throughout all of the city's five boroughs. Why? Very simply, because candidates have more incentive to do so than to try to entice wealthy donors to fancy fundraising dinners. Moreover, because the match is six to one, a $100 donor (whose contribution is increased by another $600) all of a sudden starts to look more like a wealthy donor to candidates. As a result, politicians are more inclined to hold large small-dollar fundraisers and rallies back in their districts that regular people can attend, and to reach out more frequently to their constituents with individual fundraising appeals. All of this has a democratizing effect on elected representatives: "The city's public financing system appears to have achieved one of its key goals—strengthening the connections between public officials and their constituents."[10]

Citizen funding programs exemplify the very best of American democracy: public officials fighting hard to earn your support, whether that's in the form of your vote or your donation. And they back up that support by fairly representing you in the halls of government, because their loyalty is to you, the voter.

These programs are proliferating and have earned the support of all sorts of people: in Maryland, Republican governor Larry Hogan became the first gubernatorial candidate in the state to win using public funds. In 2014, Montgomery County, Maryland, enacted its own county-level fair elections program, and Chicagoans passed a resolution in support of such a system by a 58-point margin. Twenty-five states and many more localities have some kind of financing system in place, and activists are pushing for new or strengthened ones in places including Los Angeles, Albuquerque, Santa Fe, and Arizona. By the time this book gets to your hands, this list will likely be longer.

At the federal level, Representative John Sarbanes (D-MD) is currently at work generating support for a bill that would enact citizen funding for members of Congress. We already have public funding for presidential candidates, but for all intents and purposes, it's no longer being utilized; the system failed to keep pace with the astronomical rise in the cost of elections. Sarbanes's bill, H.R. 20, contains three simple provisions: it provides a $25 tax credit to every American to contribute to candidates; it establishes a 6-to-1 matching fund for low-dollar contributions; and it pushes back against outside spending—"dark money" 501(c)(4)s and super PACs—by providing additional resources to qualifying candidates during the sixty-day "home stretch" before an election. By the summer of 2015, the bill had picked up 151 cosponsors in the House.

(2) Everyone Knows

While citizen funding programs are effective at ensuring that candidates remain beholden to the voters who elect them, they don't have any effect on reducing the massive amounts of radicalized "independent expenditures" that outside groups spend to try to elect and defeat candidates. As you have learned in other sections of this book, thanks to the Supreme Court, and to inaction by the Federal Election Commission and the IRS, super PACs and "dark money" 501(c)(4) groups are on the rise.

The one thing we do know is that darkness encourages bad behavior— more extreme messages, which feed the fires of polarization and keep candidates flinching when special-interest groups mention they have a (c)(4) or a super PAC. That's why it's critical that voters know exactly where the money is coming from. And the information should be available online immediately, presented in an intuitive and easy-to-navigate format to give the public the true transparency they need to make informed decisions.

Supreme Court Justice Antonin Scalia isn't on the side of reformers when it comes to most campaign finance issues. But get him talking about disclosure, and he lights up:

> For my part, I do not look forward to a society which, thanks
> to the Supreme Court, campaigns anonymously ... and even
> exercises the direct democracy of initiative and referendum
> hidden from public scrutiny and protected from the account-
> ability of criticism. This does not resemble the Home of the
> Brave.

No matter your pet issue or level of partisanship, if you want to
participate, you should do so in the public square. There is no uncertainty
from the Supreme Court that disclosure is constitutionally sound—
and necessary. It was a fundamental premise of the *Citizens United*
decision, and everyone from New Jersey governor Chris Christie to
American Idol contestant turned politician Clay Aiken agrees. That's
another benefit: this is an area where the left and the right often find
common ground.

A caveat: By themselves, transparency and disclosure will not create
truly representative and responsive systems of governing. Those who
claim otherwise are engaging in wishful thinking. As Harvard professor
Larry Lessig says, recall the BP Deepwater Horizon oil spill of 2010 and
the infamous live video stream that broadcast the torrent of oil as it
billowed into the Gulf of Mexico: "The point is to stop the guck from
pouring into the Gulf, not [just] to see it more clearly."[11]

But sunlight is the baseline for all reform. It's absolutely essential.
Thanks to nonprofit groups like the Center for Responsive Politics,
MapLight, the Sunlight Foundation, and the National Institute on Money
in State Politics, anyone can click around and view much of the political
money that's floating around in the system.

At the state level, transparency laws vary significantly, and few states
deserve praise. The State Integrity Investigation, a project of several
respected good-government groups, is a massive data-driven analysis of
how effective states are at deterring corruption and promoting transparency. Each state government is graded based on 330 specific measures.
The findings are somewhat chilling.

Connecticut ranks best in the nation, mostly due to components of its
clean elections program. Unfortunately, though, it got the only A grade.
Six others received a B- or better. Most of the pack was clustered at the
failing end of the scale. Dead last is Wyoming, where the legislature
exempted itself from open records laws and state officials aren't even
required to disclose their investments (critical information for anyone

attempting to assess conflicts of interest). The state scored an F, along with twenty others earning a D- or worse.

Of the bright spots, California's transparency requirements, managed by the Fair Political Practices Commission (FPPC), demand reporting on just about everything imaginable, from candidates' stock holdings to money flowing in and out of party committees. There's even a rule specifying the font size of the "paid for by" text on mass mailings.

California has also developed ways to tackle the "dark money" problem. They don't distinguish between entities (super PACs, (c)(4)s, (c)(6)s, etc.) or types of spenders (corporate, union, or individual), instead focusing their rules on one question: Is the organization spending money to influence elections? Groups spending more than $50,000 must reveal the names of their donors.

Montana also has a long history of standing up to big money. Their independent streak continued in 2015 with the passage of a state version of the DISCLOSE Act. The bill, introduced by a Republican and passed with bipartisan support, bans dark money outright. As state representative Bryce Bennett (D-MT) said, "If somebody's shooting at you, you deserve to know who's holding the gun."[12] The Montana legislation came into being because a shadowy pro-coal group was illegally coordinating with candidates while spending millions in local elections. But the only reason we know they were breaking the rules is because a box of incriminating documents turned up in Colorado—in a meth house. Voters shouldn't have to depend on the kindness of strangers, meth addicts or otherwise, to learn about political influence.

At the federal level, the landscape lacks adequate sunlight. The Democracy Is Strengthened by Casting Light on Spending in Elections Act of 2010 (DISCLOSE Act) has been floundering on the Hill for five years. It's a pretty straightforward bill that would, among other things, increase transparency around certain kinds of political giving and spending, and discourage political operatives from setting up unaccountable political attack groups.

DISCLOSE came within a single vote of clearing the Senate in 2010, but it has been shelved since then. That's a problem, because right now, only certain types of spenders are subject to disclosure rules, and those rules are not difficult to get around. Some groups have to report to the FEC, others to the SEC. Still others report only to the IRS and often do so months after their spending has taken place.

This independent spending is the guck that's harder to see. Nonprofit 501(c)(4) groups, exempt from donor disclosure rules, are especially easy conduits for "dark" money, which is simply political dollars that can't be traced to their source.

While the Hill falls into an ever-deeper state of dysfunction, though, federal agencies have the opportunity to make progress. The Securities and Exchange Commission could establish a rule mandating that all publicly traded companies disclose their political spending to their share-holders. The idea is a popular one. Since 2011, the SEC has been flooded with positive feedback from state treasurers, institutional and retail investors, former SEC commissioners of both parties, philanthropic foundation leaders, nonprofit advocates, and 1.2 million Americans—the most public comments in the agency's history. A 2014 survey of 1,500 financial analysts found that two thirds support mandatory disclosure of corporate political contributions.[13]

Some businesses already voluntarily disclose this information. The Center for Political Accountability measures the transparency practices of the three hundred largest companies in the S&P 500, and, encouragingly, scores are trending toward more disclosure. Familiar brands such as Capital One, UPS, Aflac, and Microsoft rank strikingly high, and many others have publicly committed to doing even more. But the SEC can, and should, make this reporting mandatory for all.

Another opportunity lies in the hands of the chief executive. With the stroke of his pen, President Obama could sign an executive order mandating that all federal contractors disclose their political activity. These companies receive trillions of taxpayer dollars. We, the taxpayers, have a right to know if and how they are attempting to influence politics and our government. As former Republican senator Larry Pressler (R-SD) wrote in *US News & World Report*, it's a "simple, long-overdue action [that] would go a long way towards restoring a dose of transparency and faith in our democracy."[14]

(3) Everyone Plays by the Same Commonsense Rules

Beyond campaign financing and transparency lies a realm of ideas that is too often overlooked: ethics and lobbying reforms. Many of these involve changing the way lobbyists interact with politicians and government officials.

Americans dislike lobbyists. They dislike them so much that in 2013 the

American League of Lobbyists changed its name to the Association of Government Relations Professionals. As in any industry, there are good lobbyists and bad lobbyists. Some are engaged in the profession because they believe in informing the legislative and regulatory process and in making the best possible arguments for their clients. Others' motives—and means—are less virtuous. They see it as a way to make money, lots of money. And they are willing to pump out endless amounts of false or misleading information to sully and confuse what should ideally be honest policy debates about tough issues.

Earlier in the book, we told you about the political scientist Lee Drutman and his in-depth study of the influence game in his book *The Business of America Is Lobbying*. He found that the balance of lobbying expenditures is vastly tilted toward businesses—80 percent of all reported spending, or $2.6 billion a year—and that the amount of political activity by corporations today is both unprecedented and completely unmatched by environmental, consumer protection, and public interest groups.[15] This inherent imbalance is reflected in the changing culture of Washington. As Demos senior fellow Michael Winship wrote:

> Fifty years ago, people came to Washington drawn by a sense of public service, however they defined it, and they often stayed in the public sector over much of their careers. Now working in government is a brief way station on the road to better things.[16]

Almost all lobbyists claim they get a bad rap. In recent years, though, even the lobbying industry has started to raise red flags about the system within which it is embedded. Jack Quinn, one of D.C.'s most prominent lobbyists and a cofounder of the firm Quinn, Gillespie and Associates, told the website Reddit that political money "has reached the point of being a cancer on our democracy."[17] John Feehery, who, as we noted earlier in the book, was Republican Dennis Hastert's communications director when Hastert was Speaker of the House, wrote in the *Wall Street Journal*, the system is not "just pretty bad. It's really bad." He added:

> If you ask any lobbyist in town about the campaign finance system, they would agree that it is fundamentally broken and needs to be fixed. They would tell you that they don't really want to drain their kid's college fund to give money to political campaigns. They would also tell you that they get hundreds of

requests every month to participate in fundraising efforts, and that they really don't have much of choice but to give in, every once in a while.

So here's our first fix. On behalf of lobbyists' kids' college funds, let's enact at the federal level what many states have in place: bans on campaign contributions from lobbyists. As the former lobbyist Jack Abramoff, who went to jail for crossing the line of influence peddling and is now focusing his energy on fixing the broken system, has said: "If you choose to lobby you need to abstain from campaign contributions. It's your choice either way. But you have to choose one, not both."[18] Twenty-nine states restrict the giving of campaign donations during legislative sessions. South Carolina prohibits lobbyists from making any campaign contributions at any time. The thinking: when an individual has business to do with the government (a registered lobbyist) and then gives money to a politician, it looks like corruption. Let's extend that logic to Washington, D.C., and every state capital in America.

Fix number two: call lobbyists lobbyists. As we reported earlier, 50 percent of politicians and their staff go from Capitol Hill to K Street, often to lobby for the industries they once were regulating, based on their committee assignments. Right now, the "cooling-off" period for former House members and senior Hill staffers is a year; former senators and staff must wait two. Former members of Congress can pass the time during their cooling-off periods by lobbying the executive branch, or state and local officials. And of course they can easily get around the lobbying bans entirely.

So, no more calling these people "policy advisers," or "strategic consultants," or "historians." Any retired congressman or senior staffer who makes contact with the legislative or executive branch for the purpose of influencing official actions is a lobbyist, plain and simple. The Association of Government Relations Professionals agrees. "If you're talking to a lawmaker about an issue or anything, you're lobbying," said AGRP president Dave Wenhold in 2010.[19]

Some members of Congress want to permanently jam the revolving door. In 2014, Senators Michael Bennet (D-CO) and Jon Tester (D-MT) introduced legislation that would institute a lifetime ban on lobbying for former members of Congress. In 2015, Representative Rod Blum (R-IA) introduced similar legislation in the House, observing, "This would be another step in that effort to make Congress more accountable to the people by reducing the incentive for our elected officials to use their position for their own personal gain."[20]

Framing such reform efforts not as campaign-finance-reform initiatives but as ethics and corruption fights can, in some places, help them gain unexpected support. Take Tallahassee, Florida. With the help of the reform group Represent.Us, they started a local campaign to "fight corruption" in their city. What made their strategy so notable, and so successful, was framing the debate around ending conflicts of interest and cronyism. The coalition they formed was a left-right effort including the Tea Party Network, the League of Women Voters, the Florida Alliance of Retired Americans, and Common Cause. And the law they established— with 67 percent of the vote!—requires, as Represent.Us has explained:

> A new, independent cop on the beat policing ethics laws, and ensuring everyone follows them. Lower contribution limits to prevent city candidates from amassing huge war chests from a small handful of special interest donors. And a citizen-funding system that enables anyone with a strong base of supporters to raise significant small contributions from everyday constituents, making city leaders more directly accountable to all voters—not just big donors. That means less cronyism and more efficient use of taxpayer money in the long run.

(4) Everyone Is Held Accountable

All the laws on the books are utterly irrelevant without a strong enforcement mechanism ensuring that everyone is held accountable to the laws.

The most powerful cop on the beat right now, on paper, is the Federal, Election Commission, established, as we explained in part 1, after the Watergate scandals in the early 1970s. Unfortunately it's also the most broken regulatory body in Washington.

We'll let the experts diagnose the problems with the FEC in their own words. Current FEC Democratic chairwoman Ann Ravel calls the agency she heads "worse than dysfunctional."[21] Former Republican chairman Trevor Potter says it's "not healthy for our system."[22] Former Republican commissioner Frank Reiche lamented, "[It's] almost doomed to failure."[23] Former FEC general counsel Larry Noble says politicians are blatantly disregarding campaign finance law because "they are unafraid of enforcement."[24] And the verdict of the watchdog group the Center for Public

Integrity after a months-long investigation: "The FEC is rotting from the inside out."[25]

Potter says the central issues are fundamental philosophical differences and a lack of consensus around what the FEC's job actually is. The Democrats push for strong regulatory oversight, and the Republicans fight for "free speech" above everything else. So, instead, we get complete inaction, which, according to Noble, was the whole point: "It's the perfect agency for Congress—it regulates them and it doesn't do anything."[26]

The FEC's dysfunction has reached Comedy Central levels of self-parody. In 2009, the commissioners failed to come to consensus on whether to accept payment of a fine the candidate in question had already paid. At an event in 2015, they couldn't even agree on whether to serve bagels or donuts. Deadlocks are becoming tradition. With three votes each, the Democrats and Republicans are increasingly unable to pass rulings on either routine or critical election issues. These "no decisions" have increased nearly 20 percent since 2010, and by 2013, 41 percent of the cases before the commission could not garner the necessary four votes to be resolved.

As of the writing of this book, four of the six commissioners are serving on expired terms, and President Obama hasn't nominated anyone to take their places. The agency budget remains flat, while staffing levels (and morale) have fallen to a fifteen-year low. Meanwhile, workloads have exploded—analysts who review compliance issues are facing a quarter-million-page backlog.

Must campaigns disclose funding for online ads? Can foreign nationals donate to a ballot initiative? Just how independent does a super PAC truly need to be? No one knows, because the FEC can't decide. And according to Ellen Weintraub, one of the Democratic commissioners, "people feel free to ignore" the few rules that are left.[27] For example, several candidates for president spent 2015 openly coordinating with, and raising money for, super PACs in complete violation of the law—and in total contradiction of the "independent expenditures" premises of *Citizens United*. Jeb Bush helped his Right to Rise PAC raise almost $100 million as he kissed babies in Iowa and shook hands in New Hampshire, two critical primary states. At one event, Bush said, "I'm running for president in 2016," before quickly adding ". . . if I run."[28]

None of this is meant to depress you, but neither should the magnitude of this enforcement problem be downplayed. The agencies tasked with ensuring that our elections are fair and lawful need to be reformed.

It's a law and order issue—one that anyone who believes in such laws—and order—should get behind.

Larry Noble says that at the end of the day, the effectiveness of enforcement agencies like the FEC comes down to the commissioners who are appointed.[29] Some good-government groups have recommended creating a bipartisan congressional task force to determine the best ways to fix institutional issues in the FEC, including how to replace the ineffectual six-member commission structure. Others have floated the idea adding a seventh commissioner to break deadlocked votes (that seventh, they stipulate, would have to have impeccable nonpartisan credentials).

Of the enforcement agencies at the state level, once again California is a model. We told you about the Fair Political Practices Commission earlier. Kathay Feng of California Common Cause calls it "an extremely effective agency."[30] The FPPC doesn't just review the paperwork—it actively goes after rule breakers. When political contributors hoping to avoid detection funneled over $12 million through out-of-state dark money groups to support two 2012 ballot initiatives in the state, the FPPC investigated and ended up imposing a jaw-dropping $16 million fine. Feng believes it's the largest campaign finance-related fine levied by any state, ever.

There's a lesson to be learned here. When an enforcement agency is given the resources it needs, it can both react quickly to potential infractions and follow through on holding violators accountable. Trevor Potter, in a speech praising the FPPC, helps explain just how important this one-two punch can be:

> The combined effect demonstrated to political players and the citizens of California that the law is enforced in this state. This in turn increases citizens' faith in the institution created to defend their interests.[31]

Our system of self-government relies, in part, on a citizen's belief that someone is enforcing the rules of politics, keeping the game clean. If the FEC were able to replicate California's model, how much of a difference would it make in our elections? Noble is positive that it would help to alleviate cynicism and bring Americans back into the process. "If they had a system that worked, an FEC that was really enforcing the laws," he says, "they might feel more connected to our democracy. They might feel like they have a shot at it."[32]

CHAPTER 10

The Makings of an All-American Movement

I hold it that a little rebellion now and then is a good thing, and as necessary in the political world as storms in the physical ... It is a medicine necessary for the sound health of government.

—THOMAS JEFFERSON

Fellow citizens: it's time for a little rebellion, for a new patriotic force to reclaim our right to self-government.

Many, many times in our past we've had to rise up and transform our democracy. Powerful movements emerged that brought forth heroes like Frederick Douglass, Susan B. Anthony, and Martin Luther King, Jr. Their demands became part of the DNA of our government—the Thirteenth, Fourteenth, and Fifteenth Amendments to the Constitution, ending slavery and extending rights to African Americans; the Nineteenth Amendment, providing women the right to vote; and the Civil Rights Act, putting a legal end to many ingrained practices of discrimination.

We should take a moment to appreciate what remarkable achievements these were, not just for our country but for the course of world history. Just as our revolution had a deep impact on the psyche of Europeans and provided inspiration for the French Revolution and the rejection of monarchy, the American political movements of the nineteenth and twentieth centuries inspired similar action all over the world—and still do.

Our present fight—whether you see it as a fight against cronyism and corruption or a fight for self-government—has the potential to write the next historic chapter.

Sure, you say, but how? How do we build the power necessary to enact the solutions laid out in the previous chapter? How do we move forward?

The beginnings of a movement already exists, comprising liberals and conservatives, Southerners and New Englanders, environmentalists and economic libertarians, business leaders, people of faith, former members of Congress, and everyone in between. From coast to coast, people are agreeing that they might not agree on everything, but they can agree that without a functional democracy, none of us has the power even to be heard, let alone to enact our bright ideas into laws. But the size of the movement right now is more comparable to a battalion than to an army. And it will take an army to win.

We two authors are by no means veterans of social or political movements. We're pretty normal Midwestern and Southern guys who have spent most of our lives in the media, are deeply concerned about the future of the country we love, and are willing to fight to get it back on track. Despite our lack of experience as activists, we do have some suggestions about goals that need to be achieved: (1) change the debate, (2) build a bigger, broader reform movement, (3) win at the state and local levels, (4) win at the federal level, and we can tell you about some groups and leaders who are helping make these things happen.

(1) Change the Debate

As we have shown in previous chapters, the vast majority of Americans are outraged by the current system. However, they don't understand how it connects to their daily lives, and they are skeptical that it can ever be fixed. Too many people have decided that the country might forever work this way, with wealthy people and special interests using their financial power to rig the rules in their favor. The Republican pollster Frank Luntz summed it up nicely in an editorial he penned for the *New York Times* after the 2014 elections:

> The current narrative, that this election was a rejection of President Obama, misses the mark. So does the idea that it was a mandate for an extreme conservative agenda. According to a

survey my firm fielded on election night for the political-advocacy organization Each American Dream, it was more important that a candidate "shake up and change the way Washington operates." I didn't need a poll to tell me that. This year I traveled the country listening to voters, from Miami to Anchorage, 30 states and counting. And from the reddest rural towns to the bluest big cities, the sentiment is the same. People say Washington is broken and on the decline, that government no longer works for them—only for the rich and powerful . . . The results were less about the size of government than about making government efficient, effective and accountable.

We believe this insight is as relevant a mandate for the 2016 elections—perhaps even more relevant than it was in 2014—because 2016 promises to be completely dominated by millionaires and billionaires.

So, step one in changing the debate: Just like the famous journalist Bob Woodward did, let's call it the "governing crisis" that it is. Let's not mince words. Money in politics isn't just something bad that's getting worse—it's paralyzing this country. It's destroying the American experiment. Prominent Republicans and Democrats are increasingly using the term "oligarchy" to describe our current system of governing. Warren Buffett says we're headed toward plutocracy because the political system is so controlled by the wealthy that it's no longer capable of steering the economy back to the middle class. And as you've seen throughout this book, nearly everyone recognizes how hard it is to get anything meaningful done on behalf of the common good these days. We're screwed if we don't fix this problem.

Step two: Recognize the cynicism while simultaneously rejecting it. We understand that this is a tough fight, but it will be a lot less hard as more people join it.

Congressman John Sarbanes, who has long been an advocate of this cause and is the sponsor of the Government by the People Act that we discussed in the previous chapter, speaks candidly about acknowledging the pessimism:

> If I stand in front of an audience of randomly selected Americans, I know that 95 percent of them sitting out there think that Washington is bought and sold by big interests and that their voice is inconsequential. So I can go right to talking about the

minimum wage, job creation, and infrastructure, knowing that
they're saying, "You can't get any of it done, because the system is
rigged."

Or I can start by tapping on the microphone, and saying: "I
know that 95 percent of people in this room think government is
bought and sold by big money special interests. And you're right."
All of a sudden they wake up and say, "Maybe this guy actually
knows how we feel and has something to say to me."

One of the many reasons the two of us prefer to talk about the right
to self-government—as opposed to discussing "money in politics" or
"campaign finance reform"—is because we believe that that's how this
fight should be viewed. It's about patriotism first and foremost, not just
about tweaking a campaign finance law here or there. It's not just about
shining a light on "dark money." It's not simply about enhancing ethics
laws on Capitol Hill and reducing conflicts of interest in the state capitals.
This is about the uprightness of the American way. Self-governing is
about believing in our collective problem-solving abilities. De-rigging the
system allows us to solve more problems. Bare minimum, it allows us to
have fairer fights about fixing problems.

We could repeat here the barrage of voices that we have highlighted
throughout this book that are sounding the alarm. We could list the
striking quotes from commentators ranging from CEOs to dignitaries to
former Supreme Court justices to entertainment moguls to former senators to celebrities to current elected officials to Nobel Prize and Pulitzer
Prize winners to the heads of major nonprofit organizations to leading
philanthropists to presidents and vice presidents. We could print dozens
of pages of public opinion polls that show how Republicans, independents, and Democrats feel the deck is stacked against them. But we don't
need to. This might be one of a dozen or so causes about which Americans
of all stripes agree.

So let's stop saying this is another one of those big problems that seem
hard to fix and realize it's a crisis we *can* fix, *have* to fix, and are willing to
come together to fix. All of the solutions laid out in the previous chapter,
wonky as they are, will hopefully provide inspiration and guidance for
anyone interested in how it can be done.

Step three: Set the problem on the kitchen table. This book is in large
part an effort to do exactly that. We hope we've shown you that we all pay
a price for a political system dominated by those who can afford to play.

We need to make more people aware of the connections between political and policy manipulations and the negative effects in their daily lives— why their neighborhood is still suffering the effects of foreclosure or why their grandma is paying so much for her prescription drugs or why their children are struggling with chronic health issues. Why is this step necessary? Because, although people readily recognize the problem of Big Money, it seems abstract, something that happens far away from home behind closed doors in the halls of power. When they are worried about putting food on the table, getting people motivated around abstractions is almost impossible. However, when they see that the problem is directly linked to pain points in their lives, they become more inspired to fight for reform—especially when they also see that there are many viable solutions at hand. The data to connect the dots is easy enough to find. Just check out the Center for Responsive Politics (CRP), the Sunlight Foundation, MapLight.org, Issue One (run by Nick Penniman), the Center for Public Integrity, ProPublica or the National Institute on Money in State Politics (NIMSP).

Fourth: Let's make this issue a feature of every major political contest. The money raised and spent in 2016 will shatter all records. It'll be a Wild West–style Big Money shootout, right in front of us. The spectacle will offer reformers from all over the country the opportunity to press politicians and to organize pro-reform rallies, affinity groups, house parties, and voting blocs. Call such groups and voting blocs the Patriots for Democracy or something that connects with others at a gut level.

We need to make it crystal clear to politicians that they must take a strong stance on cleaning up Washington (or the state capital, or City Hall) if they want our votes. In the past thirty years, gun rights advocates have successfully made the Second Amendment an issue that can either make or break a political campaign. During that same period of time, "pro-choice" and "pro-life" advocates have accomplished the same thing for their primary issue. Now we have to do likewise for the issue we all have in common: restoring our democracy.

Efforts are already under way in the primary states of New Hampshire (called the New Hampshire Rebellion) and Iowa (called Iowa Pays the Price) to force presidential candidates to take clear, strong stances against the harm that Big Money is doing to the health of our republic. By the time this book is published, we should know whether those efforts have had the desired effect. And the state chapters of liberal organizations such as Common Cause or U.S. PIRG, and conservative organizations such as

Take Back Our Republic, continue to organize around this issue and ensure that politicians are feeling the heat.

Another way to exert pressure on our politicians is to provide feedback to all of the proxies, volunteers, and operatives who work in and around their campaigns. So when some young people knock on your door to talk to you about candidates they're hoofing for, tell them that you want to know what the politician will do to clean up the money-in-politics mess. You know those little handheld electronic devices they carry around while doing their door knocking? The data they collect—including your views on specific issues—is all assessed by the candidates' campaigns as a barometer of what the voters care about. Then lots of that data is dumped into master databases at the national level, where it is commingled with other data from other campaigns all over the country to inform the political parties and presidential candidates about which issues are hot and which are not. Similarly, if you get a fundraising phone call from a campaign, bring the issue up. When a polling firm asks you—those of you who actually still answer your phones—what issues you care about, make sure you mention this as a top priority. If it's not on their standard list of issues—jobs, education, national security, crime, health care, environment—then tell them to add it.

(2) Build a Bigger, Broader Reform Movement

Most of the organizations that work on this cause accomplish a tremendous amount with meager financial support, and there is nothing they would like more than to work themselves out of a job. These groups are full of bright, competent people who could be doing more lucrative work in the for-profit world. Or they could even stay in the nonprofit realm and put their shoulders to the wheels of causes that offer more immediate satisfaction. But, whether for love of country or hatred of corruption, they are spending their weeks—long weeks much of the time—fighting this Goliath. (And don't forget that David won that fight.)

You have doubtless heard of some of them: Common Cause, Public Citizen, Every Voice, People for the American Way. Others, you probably haven't, although the work they do—focused on making campaign finance data easily available to the public—you have probably benefited from. We mentioned them already: the Sunlight Foundation, the Center for Responsive Politics, MapLight.org, the National Institute on Money in State Politics. Others engage in legal battles over campaign finance law:

the Brennan Center for Justice, the Campaign Legal Center, Justice at Stake, Demos.

In recent years, a few organizations have been formed for the primary purpose of amending the United States Constitution, with an emphasis on effectively overturning *Citizens United* by constitutionally granting Congress and the states the authority to regulate and limit campaign fundraising and spending as they see fit. Groups such as Free Speech for People and Move to Amend are leading the charge. They've been remarkably successful in winning symbolic victories. More than six hundred anti–*Citizens United* resolutions have been passed by state and local governments.

A host of organizations that don't normally focus on defending democracy are now pitching in some of their time. In 2013, led by the Sierra Club, Greenpeace, the NAACP, and the Communications Workers of America, an effort called the Democracy Initiative was formed for the purpose of engaging environmental, labor, voting rights, civil rights, and good-government groups into a single coalition. Additional efforts are under way to connect the fight for self-government to #BlackLivesMatter and other vibrant social justice movements, including campaigns for raising the minimum wage and prison reform.

All of this momentum is promising. But don't let it lull you into thinking that that you're not needed. Most of the groups named above have very limited budgets, and most appeal almost exclusively to already activated liberals. As we said, it's a battalion, not an army. And a lot of the troops in it have been fighting this fight for a long time. It's time for new faces and new energy to emerge, especially from unexpected places. As the TV journalist Bill Moyers, who has written and spoken extensively about money in politics over the years, likes to say, our mentality should be: "Is this a private fight or can anyone get in it?"

This is an all-American cause. A democratic republic is the hardware that all of our software runs on. We may not enjoy one another's software choices all of the time, but we can agree that we all need the hardware to work.

Some unexpected organizations have cropped up in recent years, animated by that spirit, with a focus on generating support for reform with new constituencies. These types of groups include Issue One, Take Back Our Republic, and Represent.Us.

Josh Silver, the head of Represent.Us, is the reformer who successfully brought Tea Party activists and progressives together in 2014 to win the "anti-corruption" ballot initiative in Tallahassee, Florida. The experience led him to the conclusion that "This idea that reform is exclusively a pet project of the American left is 100 percent false." Says Silver, "If you ask conservatives where they stand on the policies we need to actually fix this problem, they're overwhelmingly in favor. We need to call out corrupt behavior regardless of party affiliation, and make it clear that we believe it should be illegal for anyone to use money to purchase political influence. Period."

As polling demonstrates, the problem resonates across political boundaries—at least, outside Washington, D.C.

- A comprehensive poll conducted by the *New York Times* and CBS News in the spring of 2015 showed that 84 percent of adults— including 90 percent of Democrats and 80 percent of Republicans— think that money has too much influence in American political campaigns. Even the richest Americans agreed: 85 percent of adults making $100,000 or more believe money has too much influence in the election process.

- In the same poll, another 85 percent said they want to see our campaign finance system either fundamentally changed or completely overhauled. Just a single example of such fundamental change: 80 percent of Democrats, 71 percent of Republicans, and 76 percent of independents favor contribution limits. The *New York Times* reporters Nick Confessore and Megan Thee-Brenan summarized it in their article on the poll: "The findings reveal deep support among Republicans and Democrats alike for new measures to restrict the influence of wealthy givers, including limiting the amount of money that can be spent by 'super PACs' and forcing more public disclosure on organizations now permitted to intervene in elections without disclosing the names of their donors."

- A November 2013 poll by Global Strategy Group showed that Republicans are as likely as any other voters to say that eliminating corruption in politics is very important (86 percent for Republicans, 85 percent for all voters). It also showed that Republicans are about as likely as Democrats to agree that politicians respond primarily to donors (65 percent of Republicans, 70 percent of Democrats) and that they are more likely to represent the moneyed interests than to do what is in the public interest (53 percent of Republicans, 56 percent of Democrats).

- A 2014 poll conducted by Public Citizen found that on a scale of 1 to 10, with 10 being extremely important, Democrats rated reducing the influence of money in politics a 7.7 and Republicans a 7.0.

In our conversations with prominent Republicans, a number of arguments against Big Money came up again and again.

First, there is a rising concern within the party about crony capitalism. We have devoted a lot of space in this book to detailing examples of such cronyism and highlighting the many conservative voices—from Luigi Zingales at the University of Chicago's School of Business to Peter Schweizer at the Hoover Institute—who are sounding the alarm.

Second, the political parties generally spend the same aggregate amount of money in election cycles. Although major Republican donors, such as the Koch brothers are chipping in huge amounts of money to outside groups, it isn't clear that either party has the financial upper hand. Witness the fact (see chart below) that there is nearly always, in aggregate money spent, basic parity between Republicans and Democrats in each election cycle.

Finally, as we have said over and over again, everyone is concerned about the health of the republic. We're all Americans who love this country. And we all—Republican, Democrat, independent—feel as if we have been kicked to the curb. We are losing faith, shutting down, tuning out. Republican

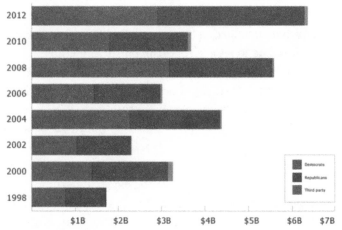

Total Cost of U.S. Elections (by Party) (1998–2012)

senator Lindsey Graham noted this emerging trend in the spring of 2015 when he said: "You're going to have money dumped in this [2016] election cycle that's going to turn off the American people." Graham has said we might need to amend the Constitution to reverse *Citizens United.* Other prominent Republicans who have joined the fight for reform include former senator Alan Simpson (R-WY), one of the leading voices of the need to reduce the national debt. Also in the phalanx is former senator Chuck Hagel (R-NE), who also served as President Obama's Secretary of Defense from 2013–2014. So is former representative Porter Goss (R-FL), who was President George W. Bush's director of the Central Intelligence Agency. Sean Hannity has devoted segments of his show to exposing lobbying and cronyism in D.C., at one point dedicating a whole show to the topic. The one-hour special featured a mini-documentary, produced by journalist Peter Schweizer and Stephen Bannon, then the executive chairman of the conservative site Breitbart News. The way Breitbart.com described the show: "'Boomtown: Washington, The Imperial City' reveals how Washington's power elite leverage their crony connections to vacuum taxpayer wallets, bankrolling their lifestyles of luxury and opulence—all under the guise of what's best for America."

There are more than one hundred such powerful Republican leaders who have gone on the record in support of reform, joining the tens of millions of Republican voters who feel the same.

John Pudner is an example of a reformer who understands the Beltway, but has chosen to work at the grassroots level for most of his career. A Republican political strategist with an uncanny record for winning underdog campaigns, he comes from Richmond, Virginia, and is the oldest of nine children. He cut his teeth in Southern conservative movement circles, where he married his love of grassroots organizing with his love of statistical data to launch surprising insurgent efforts that got him noticed, and got him good consulting contracts.

The biggest electoral feather in Pudner's cap is his work for Republican congressman Dave Brat, who ousted Eric Cantor (R-VA) in the 2014 Republican primary. At the time, Cantor was the Republican majority leader, the second most powerful member of the House, and was believed by all to be immune from serious primary challenges. But Brat and Pudner didn't accept that notion and launched an underfunded, outsider, Tea Party–style campaign that framed Cantor as being out of touch with his constituents and part of a system of cronyism. Brat relished landing lines against Cantor such as "All the investment banks in the New York and D.C.—those guys should have gone to jail. Instead of going to jail, they went on Eric's Rolodex, and they are sending him big checks." It was conservative populism, updated.

Months after Brat's victory, Pudner decided to launch the organization Take Back Our Republic to organize more conservatives to clean up the money-in-politics mess. His view:

> We are simply saying, "Look at the role of money in politics as a part of this—we know it influences the system, but how? Does it lead to increased spending in the interests of those who give money? Does it lead to regulations that benefit certain companies or special interests rather than the general interest? Does it force members of Congress to spend too much time raising money rather than spending time listening to ordinary citizens?" I think the answer is yes.

The organization's board consists of Bush-Cheney Republicans including Mark McKinnon, who was President George W. Bush's communications adviser; Juleanna Glover, who was a senior aide to Vice President Dick Cheney; and Richard Painter, who also served in the George W. Bush White House. Take Back Our Republic is young, but it has accomplished a lot in its short life—setting up chapters throughout the country, shining the light on foreign money affecting U.S. elections, and much more.

Pudner and Brat represent a strong vein of the conservative movement that is as deeply concerned about the dominance of Big Money as are the most progressive Democrats. To them, the Wall Street bailouts are Exhibit A. Hillary Clinton is Exhibit B.

A few weeks after Hillary officially announced her second run for the White House, Mark Meckler, formerly a major figure in the Tea Party Patriots, raked her over the coals in the pages of the *Washington Times*:

> The Clintons only sold nights in the Lincoln Bedroom to just a few hundred of their closest friends, right? And who can forget Clinton scandal figure Johnny Chung's defining quote: "I see the White House as like a subway: You have to put in coins to open the gates."

Other conservative leaders feel as if Big Money makes the party more wedded to the Beltway than to the base. Grassroots Republicans were particularly infuriated by the campaign finance rider we mentioned earlier that was attached to a $1.1 trillion appropriations bill signed by President Obama just before Congress left for Christmas recess in 2014. The provision significantly raised the cap on how much an individual could contribute to national political party committees from $97,200 to $777,600 per year. The conservative talk radio host Mark Levin perhaps best articulated outside-the-Beltway concerns when he called the rider "an outrage among many outrages" and an attempt by Mitch McConnell "to destroy any conservative—any group—that seeks to challenge an incumbent, to destroy the entire primary process."

Concerns of how money in politics leads to an increasingly rigged economic game are starting to mobilize business leaders as well. We've discussed in previous chapters some of the voices of business and finance speaking out against Big Money. Voices like theirs are backed up by pro-business groups like the Committee for Economic Development (CED). A 2011 report issued by the group, titled "Hidden Money," stated: "The influence of money [in Washington] can sustain inefficient or outmoded businesses, thereby subverting and frustrating the creative innovation that encourages new investment, spurs business development, and keeps jobs and investment at home."

In 2013, the CED conducted a survey of three hundred business executives—not just people who work in the corporate world, but folks who inhabit corner offices—about the influence of money in politics. The results were so stunning, and so thoroughly defied the conventional wisdom in Washington that "campaign finance reform" is somehow anti-business, that it's worth printing here one of the PowerPoint slides from the survey.

It's probably no surprise that a similar study conducted a year later by a group called Small Business Majority produced similarly resounding results: 72 percent of small business owners said major changes were needed to the campaign finance system; only 4 percent said the current system is fine.

As you can imagine, there are forces within the business community that want to keep the current system in place, perhaps because they benefit from it. The U.S. Chamber of Commerce, which spent $32 million in the 2014 midterm elections, has been customarily hostile to most campaign finance reform efforts, even the most modest efforts to increase transparency, claiming that such reforms would defang businesses. At an event hosted by the Chamber late in 2014, the group's head, Tom Donahue,

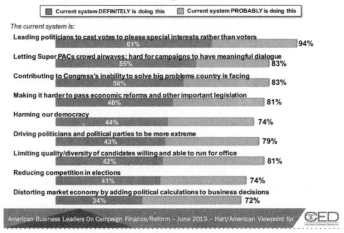

What Business Leaders Think of the Political System
Source: Committee for Economic Development's presentation, *American Business Leaders On Campaign Finance And Reform.*

hyperbolically stated: "They say it's about transparency, that's a laugh . . . the ultimate goal is to ban all corporate political speech and lobbying spending." As far as we know, not a single piece of legislation has ever been proposed that would do either of those things. No one in the reform community is talking about ending lobbying; they are talking about reforming it and delinking lobbying and money. Similarly, no one is talking about ending "corporate political speech." If corporate interests want to run campaigns to weigh in on legislation they either like or don't like, they should do so, just as nonprofit corporations like environmental and consumer watchdog groups should.

But, beyond the hyperbole, the Chamber wields an enormous megaphone in Washington and wants to convince business leaders that reducing the role of money in politics is somehow anti-corporate, as opposed to pro-America and anti-cronyism. Encouraging more business voices to emerge—like the vast majorities that are represented in the CED poll we just highlighted—is essential.

Just as we need more business leaders to stand up and speak out, we also need more representatives of mainstream groups to do so. We're thinking of groups, some of which are referred to throughout this book, that work to improve air quality, reduce obesity, get fewer kids to smoke, protect people from toxins in their food, improve product safety, engage young people in public service, alleviate poverty, improve education—all should see themselves as active players in improving the functioning of our government and the political system on which it rests.

Take Alan Khazei as an example of someone who has realized such connections. In 1988, after attending Harvard College, he and his room-mate, Michael Brown, cofounded City Year—at the time, a first-of-its kind program to engage other college-aged kids from all backgrounds in a year of community service. The idea took off quickly, and in 1991 it caught the eye of then Arkansas governor Bill Clinton, who wanted to see up close how the program worked. As Clinton has said of his subsequent trip to Boston: "The lights came on in my mind and I said 'this is what I want to do.'"

Two years later, President Clinton, Eli Segal, Alan Khazei, Michael Brown, and others worked together to replicate City Year at the national level—the program was called AmeriCorps. To date, more than 900,000 people have served in AmeriCorps and have dedicated more than 1 billion hours of community service to our country.

Khazei now heads a group called Be the Change, which is committed to building coalitions on behalf of complicated issues such as national service, combating poverty, and empowering veterans. He feels that remaking the relationship between money and politics is necessary for anyone—or any organization—working to improve the public good. He told us,

> I've long believed we need two major reforms to make our democracy work and truly citizen-led: universal national service, in which there is an opportunity and expectation that all young people will spend a year in service to our communities and country; and reform of our currently corrosive money-in-politics system. If we don't enact sweeping campaign finance reform we will never see progress on the major challenges facing our country—in education, the environment, fighting poverty, income inequality, health care and more because the special inter-ests and powerful lobbies will continue to get their way, crowding out the desires, hopes and dreams of the American people.

Good-government groups have been at this fight for a long, long time. Reinforcements from conservatives, business leaders, and mainstream nonprofit groups are needed to amplify the dire need for reform and make those calls reverberate across all sectors. When elected officials get phone calls from business leaders and public health leaders and

Republican leaders in their districts, that's when a new political reality will start to set in: Deal with this problem, or we'll all work together to find someone who will.

(3) Win at the State and Local Levels

Money's dominance of politics in the last forty years has been more defined by losses—many of them delivered by the Supreme Court—than by wins. That's why we're in the dismal shape we're in. We've let it go too long.

Obviously, we have to reverse the trend. Given how dysfunctional Washington currently is, cities and states provide the best near-term opportunities to pass transformational legislation or win major ballot initiatives. They are, as Justice Louis Brandeis once said, the laboratories of democracy. Such wins will demonstrate that there is a growing political will for reform.

This theory of change—from the states up to the federal level—has been embraced by many other movements throughout history. Regardless of where you stand on the issue of same-sex marriage, it has been one of the most successful social justice movements of our time. In 2003, not a single state allowed same-sex couples to marry, and less than 40 percent of Americans believed gays should have the right to do so. In the 2004 elections, the Republican strategist Karl Rove successfully deployed it as a key "wedge" issue to increase evangelical turnout for George W. Bush's reelection. A mere decade later, thirty-seven states allow same-sex couples to wed, the Supreme Court has validated the right to marriage for all, and public support for marriage equality is at an all-time high—more than 60 percent.

The recent wave of big victories for gay rights came after years of small ones. Bill Smith, who now runs a Washington strategy firm called Civitas Public Affairs, has spent nearly two decades immersed in political and grassroots organizing on behalf of the cause. Some of his time is now spent working on reducing the role of money in politics. About the need to start putting state and local points on the board, he told us:

> There's nothing that creates a winning culture better than winning. LGBT movement strategists knew that we couldn't go from an audacious idea to a national victory overnight. So while we created a steady drumbeat in the national conversation, we focused most of our energy on winning in the states, through legislatures, courts, and eventually at the ballot box. Recognition

of domestic partnerships, even at the municipal level, was a win. Civil unions in state legislatures were wins, and of course full marriage rights in a state were wins. Every win created momentum, and even in our losses we learned lessons along the way to get better at the game.

We need to amplify and broadcast wins when we get them, particularly to combat the forces of resignation and cynicism. As we covered in the last chapter, solutions are being implemented all over the country, but the movement is doing a poor job of making sure citizens are informed about them.

In the previous chapter we highlighted many effective laws that are already in place in states and cities. Reform advocates have set their sights on winning major reform measures in more than a dozen states by the end of 2016. They are also aiming at counties and cities, including Denver, San Diego, Buffalo, Chicago, and D.C. Such efforts are inherently fluid, so by the time this book is published, some of the goals might have shifted. But the agenda is ambitious, and it needs all the financial and grassroots support that can be mustered. Strong victories in November of 2015 in Seattle, Maine, and San Francisco—in which reformers passed new ethics, lobbying, disclosure, and campaign finance laws—should encourage more action and investment.

(4) Win at the Federal Level

Although we believe the best chance for major legislative progress in the near term is at the state level, we are by no means writing Washington off. Winning incremental victories in D.C. in the coming year is extremely important for building the kind of momentum inside the Beltway that will be needed to pass new and powerful laws down the road.

Remember, from the previous chapter, that President Obama has until January of 2017 to use his authority over the executive branch to increase transparency with federal contractors. "President Obama could bring the dark money into the sunlight in time for the 2016 election," noted Michael Waldman of the Brennan Center for Justice at the New York University School of Law. "It's the single most tangible thing anyone could do to expose the dark money that is now polluting politics."[1]

Also remember that the head of the Securities and Exchange Commission has a similar opportunity to take meaningful action by making a rule that would force corporations to disclose their political activity to their share-holders. Three former SEC chiefs, including Republican chairman William Donaldson, have pressed the SEC to approve the measure and more than a million comments have been submitted to the SEC in favor of it.

All of these are small steps that will help build momentum for an eventual major push for federal legislation that overhauls the way we finance politics in America. We firmly believe that the mightiest reform of all is some kind of citizen-funded system—one that positions regular people, who reside in the districts that our elected officials serve, at the center of political funding, and therefore political power.

We by no means mean to diminish the importance of transparency, stronger ethics and lobbying laws, and functional enforcement agencies. As we have said, there is no single silver bullet. But unless the funding of politics is placed in the hands of the many instead of being dominated by the few, we will never achieve, as Lincoln envisioned, a government of the people, by the people, for the people.

How will we know when we have developed the power to get such legislation passed? We'll know when politicians are winning elections in part because of their stance on the issue. We'll know when ending the reign of Big Money is regularly ranking in the top five concerns Americans are expressing in national polls. We'll know when legislative victories at the local and state level suddenly seem to be occurring everywhere. We'll know when the problem is seen as an all-American cause to preserve the right of self-government, with liberals, centrists, and conservatives putting their other differences aside to fight side by side on behalf of that right.

David Donnelly, who runs the group Every Voice, is a veteran of the reform movement. He's been working at it for twenty years and has helped establish some of the strongest citizen-funded systems in the country. In reflecting on the nature of the battle ahead, he told us:

> We need to build a broad-based, diverse movement of millions of Americans from all walks of life. And to do that, we must show that winning is possible and it starts in city councils, state legislatures, and through citizen-initiated petitions at the ballot box. When we pass real reform—including small donor policies—at the local and statewide level, we inspire hope that everyday people can get more involved in politics and have their voices heard. But winning isn't just about showing we can win; it's about building the apparatus and momentum to move Congress and the White

House. What we're doing now are the first flames of a prairie fire
that will sweep across the country and reach Washington, D.C.

Remember, this is what we Americans do.

> *The gap between rich and poor has never been wider . . . legislative
> stalemate paralyzes the country . . . corporations resist federal regu-
> lations . . . spectacular mergers produce giant companies . . . the
> influence of money in politics deepens.*

The above snippets sound as if they were torn from recent news reports.
Actually, they're from Doris Kearns Goodwin's book *The Bully Pulpit*,
about Teddy Roosevelt, William Howard Taft, and the early-twentieth-
century era of investigative journalism. While reading the book, and
others about that time period, we were continually struck by the remarkable similarities between then and now. We described some of them in
part 1, but want to reiterate the point here.

America's last Gilded Age gave rise to rebellious fires, the flames of
which eventually spread to Teddy, a well-to-do Republican and progressive who was the single greatest champion of campaign finance reform
this country has ever seen. He didn't believe in reform as an end in itself.
He saw it as a means to reclaim the right to self-government, and the right
for every person to have an equal opportunity to get ahead in life—what
he termed a "square deal." In his words:

> Now, this means that our government, national and State, must
> be freed from the sinister influence or control of special interests.
> Exactly as the special interests of cotton and slavery threatened
> our political integrity before the Civil War, so now the great
> special business interests too often control and corrupt the men
> and methods of government for their own profit. We must drive
> the special interests out of politics . . . For every special interest is
> entitled to justice, but not one is entitled to a vote in Congress, to
> a voice on the bench, or to representation in any public office.

We're not sure where the next Teddy Roosevelt might come from, but we
do know that the fires have been lit. Throughout this book, we've cast a
spotlight on some of the colossal collateral damage that results from
coin-operated governing: money over merit; influence over evidence;

creeping cronyism; demoralized and distracted elected officials; and a pervasive sense throughout the country that things might never get better because we, the people, no longer have the power to make things better.

No one wants to stay stuck here. This is not the American mindset that has made us the envy of the world. We're the ones who overthrew a monarch and flew to the moon. We often let our differences divide us, we sometimes overreach, and we don't always fix things correctly. But then we try again, knowing that we might never arrive at a perfect union but that we always want to keep moving in that direction.

It's time to put aside our differences and move confidently together in that direction once again.

We started the book by quoting the Massachusetts constitution, which John Adams helped write. We want to remind you of that quote again:

> Government is instituted for the common good; for the protection, safety, prosperity, and happiness of the people; and not for the profit, honor, or private interest of any one man, family, or class of men; therefore, the people alone have an incontestable, unalienable, and indefeasible right to institute government; and to reform, alter, or totally change the same, when their protection, safety, prosperity, and happiness require it.

As we noted, these words were inspired by the Declaration of Independence and then provided inspiration for the crafting of the federal Constitution, seven years later. For us, these beautiful words best articulate our country's vision of a vibrant society. They also inspire all of us to constantly realize that we have an unalienable right to "reform, alter or totally change" our government when it has betrayed the common good. That's a weighty task, no doubt. But we should be comforted by the ease with which it is stated in so many of the founding documents and Founders' letters. The message to us citizens is: if it breaks, fix it, or get rid of it!

We hope you'll find it in your heart to join the very American struggle to fix our broken government.

Acknowledgments

This book was not just collaboration between the two of us. Many people chipped in, and to them we are immensely grateful. So, at the risk of sounding like two actors who just won Oscars and are trying to not get cut off by the music, here we go.

Thanks to: Anton Mueller, our editor at Bloomsbury, for his deep and thoughtful feedback and his patience; George Gibson, the publishing director of Bloomsbury USA, for his enthusiasm about this book and this topic; Gabrielle Sellei, our lawyer, who acted as so much more than that throughout this whole process; Nick Penniman IV, Nick's dad, for his contributions and thoughts about energy policy and corporate subsidies; Keenan Steiner for his copious research, reporting and insights and his lithe style; Laurie Roberts for helping us lay out the wonkery; Leigh Beasley for her "shock and awe" help early on; Erik Lampmann for his ruminations on cronyism; Jack Noland for his historical research and willingness to chip in whenever and wherever; Kyle Enochs for the same; Caitlyn Weber for the terrific info graphics and charts you see throughout the book; and Gleni Bartels for her expert eye and firm yet friendly nudging as the book trekked through production. Nick offers a special thanks to the staff and board of his organization, Issue One, for allowing him to write this book while also managing the expansion of a very busy startup nonprofit group.

We, of course, owe a huge debt of gratitude to our dear families, who cheered us on and gave us the time and space we needed to get this book into the end zone. Sarah, Nicky, Mac, Winnie, Linda, Da, Lou, Alex, and Morgan. Boundless love and thanks.

Notes

Introduction

1 https://www.opensecrets.org/overview/blio.php.

1. How We Got Here

1 "To George Logan," in *The Works of Thomas Jefferson: Volume* XII, Thomas Jefferson, edited by Paul Leicester Ford (G. P. Putnam's Sons, 1905), 44.

2 "George Washington Plied Voters with Booze," Paul Bedard, *US News & World Report*, November 8, 2011, http://www.usnews.com/news/blogs/washington-whispers/2011/11/08/george-washington-plied-voters-with-booze.

3 Robert E. Mutch, *Buying the Vote: A History of Campaign Finance Reform* (Oxford University Press, 2014), 46.

4 Zephyr Teachout, "The Anti-Corruption Principle," *Cornell Law Review* 94:341, accessed July 14, 2015, 374, http://www.lawschool.cornell.edu/research/cornell-law-review/upload/Teachout-Final.pdf?q=anti-corruption percent7Bporsyar_end percent7D.

5 Doris Kearns Goodwin, *The Bully Pulpit: Theodore Roosevelt, William Howard Taft, and the Golden Age of Journalism* (Simon and Schuster, 2013), 299.

6 Rebecca Edwards and Sarah DeFeo, "Trusts & Monopolies," *1896: The Presidential Campaign: Cartoons & Commentary*, 2000, http://projects.vassar.edu/1896/trusts.html.

7 Matthew O'Brien, "The Most Expensive Election Ever . . . 1896," *Atlantic*, November 6, 2012, http://www.theatlantic.com/business/archive/2012/11/the-most-expensive-election-ever-1896/264649/.

8 Mutch, *Buying the Vote*, 1.

9 Kenneth P. Vogel, *Big Money: 2.5 Billion Dollars, One Suspicious Vehicle, and a Pimp–On the Trail of the Ultra-Rich Hijacking American Politics*, PublicAffairs, 2014, 39.

10 John Milton Cooper Jr., "Theodore Roosevelt," *Encyclopaedia Britannica Online*, August 25, 2014, http://www.britannica.com/EBchecked/topic/509347/Theodore-Roosevelt/8429/The-Square-Deal#ref673089.

11 "The Northern Securities Case," Theodore Roosevelt Center, http://www.theodorerooseveltcenter.org/Learn-About-TR/TR-Encyclopedia/Capitalism-and-Labor/The-Northern-Securities-Case.aspx.

12 *A Compilation of the Messages and Speeches of Theodore Roosevelt,* vol. 1, edited by Alfred Henry Lewis, Bureau of National Literature and Art, 1906, 500.

13 "United States Presidential Election of 1904," *Encyclopaedia Britannica Online*, http://www.britannica.com/event/United-States-presidential-election-of-1904.

14 Mutch, *Buying the Vote*, 43.

15 "The Root of All Evil," *New York Times*, August 13, 1875.

16 "Fifth Annual Message," Theodore Roosevelt, UCSB American Presidency Project, December 5, 1905, http://www.presidency.ucsb.edu/ws/?pid=29546.

17 "Sixth Annual Message," Theodore Roosevelt, UCSB American Presidency Project, December 3, 1906, http://www.presidency.ucsb.edu/ws/?pid=29547.

18 Mutch, *Buying the Vote*, 74–76.

19 Ibid., 93.

20 "Message to Congress on the Hatch Act," Franklin D. Roosevelt, UCSB American Presidency Project, http://www.presidency.ucsb.edu/ws/?pid=15781.

21 Mutch, *Buying the Vote*, 106–107.

22 Ibid., 109.

23 Harry S. Truman, "On the Veto of the Taft-Hartley Bill," U.Va. Miller Center, June 20, 1947, http://millercenter.org/president/truman/speeches/speech-3344.

24 U.S. Government Brief in *United States v. Congress of Industrial Organizations*, quoted in Mutch, *Buying the Vote*, 109.

25 Mutch, *Buying the Vote*, 50.

26 "Appendix 4: Brief History," Federal Election Commission, http://www.fec.gov/info/appfour.htm.

27 "How Presidential Public Financing Works," *Public Citizen*, July 2012, https://www.citizen.org/documents/presidential-election-public-financing-how-it-works.pdf.

28 Comptroller General of the United States, "Report of the Office of Federal Elections of the General Accounting Office in Administering the Federal Election Campaign Act of 1971," U.S. Government Accountability Office, 1975, 23–24.

29 "Appendix 4," Federal Election Commission.

30 "About the FEC," Federal Election Commission, http://www.fec.gov/about
.shtml.

31 Mutch, *Buying the Vote*, 9.

32 James Taranto, "Nine Decades at the Barricades," *Wall Street Journal*,
August 1, 2014, http://www.wsj.com/articles/the-weekend-interview-nine-
decades-at-the-barricades-1406931516.

33 *Nixon v. Shrink Missouri Government PAC*, 528 U.S. 377 (2000) (J. P. Stevens,
concurring).

34 "Lincoln Bedroom Guests Gave $5.4 Million," *CNN AllPolitics*, February 26,
1997, http://www.cnn.com/ALLPOLITICS/1997/02/26/clinton.lincoln/.

35 Doug Weber, "Unlimited Presidential Spending: The Curse of Steve
Forbes," Center for Responsive Politics, December 27, 2011, http://www
.opensecrets.org/news/2011/12/unlimited-presidential-fundraising/.

36 Mutch, *Buying the Vote*, 10.

37 R. Sam Garrett, "The State of Campaign Finance Policy: Recent
Developments and Issues for Congress," Congressional Research Service,
April 30, 2015.

38 Robert Kelner and Raymond La Raja, "McCain-Feingold's Devastating
Legacy," *Washington Post*, April 11, 2014, http://www.washingtonpost.com
/opinions/mccain-feingolds-devastating-legacy/2014/04/11/14a528e2-c18f-11e3-
bcec-b71ee10e9bc3_story.html.

39 "Happy Corporations," *New York Times*, June 17, 1906.

40 Mutch, *Buying the Vote*, 173–74.

41 James Bennet, "The New Price of American Politics," *Atlantic*, October
2012, http://www.theatlantic.com/magazine/archive/2012/10/the/309086/.

42 *Citizens United v. Federal Election Commission*, 558 U.S. 310 (2010).

43 Ibid.

44 Michael McConnell, "Reconsidering *Citizens United* as a Press Clause
Case," *Yale Law Journal*, vol. 123, no. 2, November 2013.

45 Ibid.

46 *Citizens United v. Federal Election Commission*, 558 U.S. 310 (2010) (J. P.
Stevens, concurring in part, dissenting in part).

47 Ibid.

48 "Democracy Corps Supreme Court Project: Frequency Questionnaire,"
Greenberg Quinlan Rosner Research, May 7, 2014, http://www.democracycorps
.com/attachments/article/979/042214percent20DCORPSpercent20SCOTUS
percent20FQ.pdf.

49 Norman Ornstein, "Citizens United: Corrupting Campaign Clarity," *Roll Call*, June 15, 2011, http://www.rollcall.com/issues/56_139/citizens_united_corrupting_campaign_clarity-206476-1.html.

50 Zephyr Teachout, *Corruption in America* (Cambridge, MA: Harvard University Press, 2014).

51 Jeffrey Rosen, "Ruth Bader Ginsburg Is an American Hero," interview with Ruth Bader Ginsburg, *New Republic*, http://www.newrepublic.com/article/119578/ruth-bader-ginsburg-interview-retirement-feminists-jazzercise.

52 Dave Helling, "Jack Danforth says the Citizens United campaign spending decision 'should not stand,'" *Kansas City Star*, June 17, 2015, http://www.kansascity.com/news/local/news-columns-blogs/the-buzz/article24793228.html#storylink=cpy.

53 "More Voters Think They're on the Same Page with Congress," *Rasmussen Reports*, March 31, 2015, http://www.rasmussenreports.com/public_content/archive/mood_of_america_archive/congressional_performance/more_voters_think_they_re_on_the_same_page_with_congress.

54 Stan Greenberg, James Carville, David Donnelly, and Ben Winston, "Voters Ready to Act against Big Money in Politics: Lessons from the 2014 Midterm Election," Democracy Corps, GQRR, Every Voice, November 10, 2014, http://everyvoice.org/wp-content/uploads/2014/11/EveryVoicePostElectMemo.pdf.

2. Rigged

1 Inflation Calculator, U.S. Bureau of Labor Statistics, accessed March 19, 2015.

2 "Pressure Groups Spent $3.85 Million on Lobbying in 1960," *CQ Almanac 1961*, 17th ed. (Washington, DC: *Congressional Quarterly*, 1961), 958, http://library.cqpress.com/cqalmanac/cqal61-879-29202-1371585.

3 "Lobbying Database," Center for Responsive Politics, accessed March 19, 2015.

4 "Annual Lobbying by US Chamber of Commerce," Center for Responsive Politics, accessed March 19, 2015.

5 Peter Schweizer, *Extortion: How Politicians Extract Your Money, Buy Votes, and Line Their Own Pockets* (Houghton Mifflin Harcourt, 2013).

6 "461: Take the Money and Run for Office," *This American Life*, March 30, 2012, http://www.thisamericanlife.org/radio-archives/episode/461/take-the-money-and-run-for-office.

7 Ryan Grimm and Sabrina Siddiqui, "Call Time for Congress Shows How Fundraising Dominates Bleak Work Life," *Huffington Post*, January 9, 2013, http://www.huffingtonpost.com/2013/01/08/call-time-congressional-fundraising_n_2427291.html.

8 http://www.huffingtonpost.com/dan-glickman/congressional-campaign-funding_b_1830462.html.

9 Stephen Koff, "Senator George Voinovich talks about his decision to retire" (video), Cleveland.com, January 12, 2009, http://blog.cleveland.com/openers /2009/01/voinovich_talks_about_his_deci.html.

10 Lawrence Lessig, "Democracy After Citizens United," *Boston Review*, September/October 2012, http://new.bostonreview.net/BR35.5/lessig.php.

11 Rebecca Kaplan, "Watchdog groups: Jeb Bush, others violating campaign finance laws," *CBS News*, March 31, 2015, http://www.cbsnews.com/news /watchdog-groups-jeb-bush-others-violating-campaign-finance-laws/.

12 Thomas Beaumont, "Jeb Bush prepares to give traditional campaign a makeover," Associated Press, April 21, 2015, http://bigstory.ap.org/article/4098 37aa09ee405493ad64a94b8c2c3d/bush-preparing-delegate-many-campaign-tasks-super-pac.

13 Richard L. Hasen, "Jeb the Destroyer: Jeb Bush is tearing down what little campaign finance law we have left," *Slate*, April 22, 2015, http://www.slate.com /articles/news_and_politics/politics/2015/04/jeb_bush_destroying_campaign_ finance_rules_his_tactics_will_be_the_future.single.html.

14 "Republicans Thwart New Campaign Finance Disclosure Rules As DISCLOSE Act Fails Procedural Vote in Senate," Michael Beckel, OpenSecrets .org, July 27, 2010, http://www.opensecrets.org/news/2010/07/republicans-thwart-new-campaign-fin/.

15 http://www.kentucky.com/2010/08/01/1372068/mcconnells-hypocrisy-on-campaign.html.

16 http://www.bloomberg.com/politics/articles/2014-10-14/the-darth-vader-moment-that-made-mitch-mcconnell.

17 https://www.youtube.com/watch?v=0_gPNGV79k0.

18 "Common Cause, Allies Urge Obama to Order Federal Contractors to Disclose Political Spending," *Common Cause*, March 2, 2015, http://www .commoncause.org/press/press-releases/common-cause-allies-urge-president-disclose-political-spending.html?.

19 Keenan Steiner, "New appointees are long overdue but is the FEC broken?" Sunlight Foundation, April 30, 2013, http://sunlightfoundation.com /blog/2013/04/30/new-appointees-are-long-overdue-but-is-the-fec-broken/.

20 Eric Lichtblau, "F.E.C. Can't Curb 2016 Election Abuse, Commission Chief Says," *New York Times*, May 2, 2015, http://www.nytimes.com/2015/05/03/us /politics/fec-cant-curb-2016-election-abuse-commission-chief-says.html?_ r=0.

21 Ben Weider, Kytja Weir, Reity O'Brien, and Rachel Baye, "National donors pick winners in state elections," Center for Public Integrity, January 28, 2015, http://www.publicintegrity.org/2015/01/28/16661/national-donors-pick-winners-state-elections.

22 Zach Holden, "Overview of Campaign Finances, 2011-2012 Elections," National Institute on Money in State Politics, May 13, 2014, http://www .followthemoney.org/research/institute-reports/overview-of-campaign-finances-20112012-elections.

23 Edwin Bender, "Evidencing a Republican Form of Government: The Influence of Campaign Money on State-Level Elections," *Montana Law Review*, Winter 2013, http://scholarship.law.umt.edu/cgi/viewcontent.cgi?artic le=1007&context=mlr.

24 Zach Holden, "Overview of Campaign Finances, 2011-2012 Elections," National Institute on Money in State Politics, May 13, 2015, http://www .followthemoney.org/research/institute-reports/overview-of-campaign-finances-20112012-elections/.

25 Liz Essley Whyte, "Big business crushed ballot measures in 2014," Center for Public Integrity, February 5, 2015, http://www.publicintegrity .org/2015/02/05/16693/big-business-crushed-ballot-measures-2014.

26 Fredreka Schouten, "Federal super PACs spend big on local elections," *USA Today*, February 25, 2014, http://www.usatoday.com/story/news/politics /2014/02/25/super-pacs-spending-local-races/5617121/.

27 Ibid.

28 Theodore Schleifer, "Super PACs coming to a city near you," CNN, May 19, 2015,http://www.cnn.com/2015/05/19/politics/super-pac-local-elections-2015/.

29 Bert Brandenburg, "Justice for Sale: How elected judges became a threat to American democracy," *Politico*, September 1, 2014, http://www.politico.com /magazine/story/2014/09/elected-judges-110397.html#.VWjJPVxVhBd.

30 Adam Liptak, "U.S. Supreme Court Is Asked to Fix Troubled West Virginia System," *New York Times*, October 11, 2008, http://www.nytimes .com/2008/10/12/washington/12scotus.html.

31 "Money & Elections," *Justice at Stake*, http://www.justiceatstake.org/issues /state_court_issues/money-and-elections/.

3. Oligarchy, Gridlock, Cronyism

1 http://www.tulsaworld.com/test/okpreps/volleyball/lee-h-hamilton-money-and-politics-we-need-change-now/article_8db057f6-5c89-5131-adb4-b9520e94827f.html.

2 http://www.politico.com/story/2014/12/top-political-donors-113833. html#ixzz3fbgYpPBH.

3 Philip Rucker, "Governors Christie, Walker and Kasich woo billionaire Sheldon Adelson at Vegas event," *Washington Post*, March 29, 2014, http://

www.washingtonpost.com/politics/governors-christie-walker-and-kasich-woo-adelson-at-vegas-event/2014/03/29/aa385f34-b779-11e3-b84e-897d3d 12b816_story.html.

4 Matea Gold and Philip Rucker, "Billionaire mogul Sheldon Adelson looks for mainstream Republican who can win in 2016," *Washington Post*, March 25, 2014, http://www.washingtonpost.com/politics/billionaire-mogul-sheldon-adelson-looks-for-mainstream-republican-who-can-win-in-2016/2014/03/25/e2f47bb0-b3c2-11e3-8cb6-284052554d74_story.html.

5 "The World's Billionaires," *Forbes*, http://www.forbes.com/billionaires/.

6 Nathan Vardi, "Sheldon Adelson Says He Is 'Willing to Spend Whatever It Takes' to Stop Online Gambling," *Forbes*, November 22, 2013, http://www.forbes.com/sites/nathanvardi/2013/11/22/sheldon-adelson-says-he-is-willing-to-spend-whatever-it-takes-to-stop-online-gambling/.

7 Tim Dickinson, "Inside the Koch Brothers' Toxic Empire," *Rolling Stone*, September 24, 2014, http://www.rollingstone.com/politics/news/inside-the-koch-brothers-toxic-empire-20140924?page=2.

8 Kenneth P. Vogel and Simmi Aujla, "Koch conference under scrutiny," *Politico*, January 27, 2011, http://dyn.politico.com/printstory.cfm?uuid=2EDE2 F1B-BE40-42F0-AF83-BAB96054F413.

9 Nicholas Confessore, "Koch Brothers' Budget of $889 Million for 2016 Is on Par with Both Parties' Spending," *New York Times*, January 26, 2015, http://www.nytimes.com/2015/01/27/us/politics/kochs-plan-to-spend-900-million-on-2016-campaign.html?_r=0.

10 Andrew Restuccia and Elana Schor, "Tom Steyer backs Hillary Clinton despite Keystone caution," *Politico*, May 6, 2015, http://www.politico.com/story/2015/05/tom-steyer-hillary-clinton-keystone-117707.html#ixzz3bHD9ke1A.

11 Timothy Cama, "Billionaire environmentalist to host Clinton fundraiser," *The Hill*, April 29, 2015, http://thehill.com/policy/energy-environment/240460-billionaire-environmentalist-to-host-clinton-fundraiser.

12 Ed Rogers, "The Insiders: I'm embarrassed by our campaign finance system," *Washington Post*, April 21, 2015, http://www.washingtonpost.com/blogs/post-partisan/wp/2015/04/21/the-insiders-im-embarrassed-by-our-campaign-finance-system/.

13 Jesse H. Rhodes and Brian F. Schaffner, "Economic Inequality and Representation in the U.S. House: A New Approach Using Population Level Data," April 7, 2013, http://people.umass.edu/schaffne/Schaffner.Rhodes.MPSA.2013.pdf.

14 Paul Wiseman, "Unemployment rate for recent college grads rose in 2014," *Columbus Dispatch*, April 16, 2015, http://www.dispatch.com/content/stories/business/2015/04/16/0416-college-unemployment.html.

15 Lynn Sweet, "Inside the Fall of Aaron Schock," *Chicago Sun-Times*, Agust 23, 2015, http://chicago.suntimes.com/politics/7/71/900454/inside-fall-of-aaron-schock-investigation-ben-cole.

16 "Press Conference by the President," *The White House*, October 8, 2013, https://www.whitehouse.gov/the-press-office/2013/10/08/press-conference-president.

17 Ed O'Keefe, "Tom Harkin: It's somebody else's turn," *Washington Post*, January 26, 2013, http://www.washingtonpost.com/blogs/post-politics/wp/2013/01/26/tom-harkin-its-somebody-elses-turn.

18 Joseph Stiglitz, "Rewriting the Rules of the American Economy: An Agenda for Growth and Shared Prosperity," working paper, p. 15, accessed May 25, 2015, http://www.rewritetherules.org/report.

19 Bill Moyers, "David Stockman on Crony Capitalism," *Moyers & Company*, March 9, 2012, http://billmoyers.com/segment/david-stockman-on-crony-capitalism.

20 Luigi Zingales, *A Capitalism for the People: Recapturing the Lost Genius of American Prosperity* (New York: Basic Books, 2012), 2.

21 Desmond Lachman, "America's crony capitalism challenge," American Enterprise Institute, October 27, 2014.

22 Zingales, *Capitalism for the People*, 138.

23 Catherine Rampell, "Tax Breaks: A Primer," *New York Times*, February 22, 2012, http://economix.blogs.nytimes.com/2012/02/22/tax-breaks-a-primer/.

24 Timothy P. Carney, "The Case Against Cronies: Libertarians Must Stand Up to Corporate Greed," *Atlantic*, April 30, 2013, http://www.theatlantic.com/business/archive/2013/04/the-case-against-cronies-libertarians-must-stand-up-to-corporate-greed/275404/.

25 Timothy P. Carney, *The Big Ripoff: How Big Business and Big Government Steal Your Money* (Wiley, 2006).

4. Too Big to Beat

1 Jon Prior, "Fannie and Freddie to pay back taxpayers," *POLITICO*, February 21, 2014, http://www.politico.com/story/2014/02/fannie-mae-freddie-mac-bailouts-103768.html.

2 William D. Cohan, "The Final Days of Merrill Lynch," *Atlantic*, September 2009, http://www.theatlantic.com/magazine/archive/2009/09/the-final-days-of-merrill-lynch/307621/.

3 Matthew Karnitschnig et al., "U.S. to Take Over AIG in $85 Billion Bailout; Central Banks Inject Cash as Credit Dries Up," *Wall Street Journal*, September 16, 2008, http://www.wsj.com/articles/SB122156561931242905.

4 Chris Isidore, "Poll: 60% say depression 'likely,'" *CNN Money*, October 6, 2008, http://money.cnn.com/2008/10/06/news/economy/depression_poll/.

5 Tami Lubhy, "Foreclosures soar 76 percent to record 1.35 million," *CNN Money*, December 5, 2008, http://money.cnn.com/2008/12/05/news/economy /mortgage_delinquencies/.

6 Robin Sidel and Saabrina Chaudhuri, "U.S. Bank Profits Near Record Levels," *Wall Street Journal*, August 11, 2014, http://www.wsj.com/articles /u-s-banking-industry-profits-racing-to-near-record-levels-1407773976.

7 "Dow Jones Industrial Average," *Barron's* Market Data Center, http://online .barrons.com/mdc/public/npage/9_3050.html?symb=DJIA.

8 Floyd Norris, "Corporate Profits Grow and Wages Slide," *New York Times*, April 4, 2014, http://www.nytimes.com/2014/04/05/business/economy /corporate-profits-grow-ever-larger-as-slice-of-economy-as-wages-slide.html.

9 Elise Gould, "Average Real Wage Growth in 2014 Was No Better Than 2013," Economic Policy Institute, January 15, 2015, http://www.epi.org/blog/average-real-hourly-wage-growth-in-2014-was-no-better-than-2013/.

10 "Most Say Government Policies Since Recession Have Done Little to Help Middle Class, Poor," Pew Research Center, March 4, 2015, http://www.people-press.org/2015/03/04/most-say-government-policies-since-recession-have-done-little-to-help-middle-class-poor/.

11 Leslie Wayne, "Lobbyists for Financial Institutions Swarming All Over the Bailout Bill," *New York Times*, September 27, 2008, http://www.nytimes .com/2008/09/27/business/27lobbyists.html.

12 "American Bankers Assn," OpenSecrets.org, http://www.opensecrets.org /lobby/clientlbs.php?id=D000000087&year=2008.

13 "US Chamber of Commerce," OpenSecrets.org, https://www.opensecrets .org/lobby/clientsum.php?id=D000019798.

14 "Ranked Sectors: 2008," OpenSecrets.org, http://www.opensecrets.org /lobby/top.php?showYear=2008&indexType=c.

15 "Top Spenders: 2008," OpenSecrets.org, http://www.opensecrets.org /lobby/top.php?showYear=2008&indexType=s.

16 Harry Bradford, "10 Worst Single-Day Drops In Dow Jones History," *Huffington Post*, August 5, 2011, http://www.huffingtonpost.com/2011/08/05 /dow-jones-biggest-drops-falls_n_919216.html.

17 Paul Blumenthal, "Plunge in Wall Street Money Bolsters Populist Shift Among Democrats," *Huffington Post*, January 10, 2015, http://www.huffington post.com/2015/01/10/democrats-wall-street_n_6445276.html?ncid=tweetlnku shpmg00000016.

18 Ibid. "Top Organization Contributors," OpenSecrets.org, http://www .opensecrets.org/orgs/list.php.

19 Russell J. Funk and Daniel Hirschman, "Derivatives and Deregulation: Financial Innovation and the Demise of Glass-Steagall," *Administrative Science Quarterly*.

20 Jerry Markham, "The Subprime Crisis—A Test Match for the Bankers: Glass-Steagall vs. Gramm-Leach-Bliley," 2009, http://scholarship.law.upenn .edu/cgi/viewcontent.cgi?article=1365&context=jbl.

21 Robert Dreyfuss, "How the DLC Does It," *American Prospect*, December 19, 2001, http://prospect.org/article/how-dlc-does-it.

22 James Shoch, *Trading Blows: Party Competition and U.S. Trade Policy in a Globalizing Era* (Chapel Hill: University of North Carolina Press, 2001).

23 "Finance/Insurance/Real Estate," OpenSecrets.org, http://www.opensecrets .org/industries/totals.php?cycle=2014&ind=F.

24 Jacob S. Hacker and Paul Pierson, *Winner-Take-All-Politics: How Washington Made the Rich Richer—and Turned Its Back on the Middle Class* (New York: Simon and Schuster, 2011).

25 John J. Pitney Jr., "Democrats Bring Back Their Hit Man: Tony Coelho, who rapped GOP ethics but took tainted S&L perks, returns to guide party," *Los Angeles Times*, August 16, 1994, http://articles.latimes.com/1994-08-16 /local/me-27581_1_tony-coelho.

26 Ibid.

27 Hacker and Pierson, *Winner-Take-All-Politics*, 177.

28 Bill Sing, "Coelho Joins Investment Firm," *Los Angeles Times*, October 3, 1989, http://articles.latimes.com/1989-10-03/business/fi-650_1_investment-banking-experience.

29 Ibid.

30 Ibid.; "National Republican Senatorial Cmte," Center for Responsive Politics, http://www.opensecrets.org/parties/indus.php?cmte–RSC&cycle=2008

31 Authors' analysis of House Financial Services Committee membership: Ryan Grim and Arthur Delaney, "The Cash Committee: How Wall Street Wins on the Hill," *Huffington Post*, March 18, 2010, http://www.huffingtonpost .com/2009/12/29/the-cash-committee-how-wa_n_402373.html.

32 Ibid.

33 Ibid.

34 Ibid.

35 Ibid.

36 Phil Angelides and Bill Thomas, "Financial Crisis Inquiry Report," Financial Crisis Inquiry Commission, Washington, D.C., January 2011, http:// www.gpo.gov/fdsys/pkg/GPO-FCIC/pdf/GPO-FCIC.pdf. Ibid.

37 "Byron Dorgan's Prophetic Words," Lauren Feeney, Moyers and Company, January 27, 2012, http://billmoyers.com/content/a-senators-prophetic-words-then-and-now/.

38 Stephen Labaton, "Congress Passes Wide-Ranging Bill Easing Bank Laws," *New York Times*, November 5, 1999, http://www.nytimes.com/1999/11/05/business/congress-passes-wide-ranging-bill-easing-bank-laws.html.

39 "The Long Demise of Glass-Steagall," PBS *Frontline*, http://www.pbs.org/wgbh/pages/frontline/shows/wallstreet/weill/demise.html.

40 Eric Lipton and Stephan Labaton, "Deregulator Looks Back, Unswayed," *New York Times*, November 16, 2008, http://www.nytimes.com/2008/11/17/business/economy/17gramm.html?pagewanted=all.

41 "Citigroup Inc," OpenSecrets.org, http://www.opensecrets.org/orgs/totals.php?id=D000000071&cycle=2014.

42 Ibid.

43 "Commerical Banks," OpenSecrets.org, http://www.opensecrets.org/lobby/indusclient.php?id=F03&year=2008.

44 Stephen Labaton, "Agreement Reached on Overhaul of U.S. Financial System," *New York Times*, October 23, 1999, http://partners.nytimes.com/library/financial/102399banks-congress.html.

45 Ellen Schloemer et al., "Losing Ground: Foreclosures in the Subprime Market and Their Cost to Homeowners," Center for Responsible Lending, December 2006, http://www.responsiblelending.org/mortgage-lending/research-analysis/foreclosure-paper-report-2-17.pdf.

46 Ibid.; Glenn R. Simpson, "Lender Lobbying Blitz Abetted Mortgage Mess," *Wall Street Journal*, December 31, 2007, http://www.wsj.com/articles/SB119906606162358773.

47 "Countrywide Financial," OpenSecrets.org, https://www.opensecrets.org/lobby/clientsum.php?id=D000021941&year=2006.

48 Simpson, "Lender Lobbying Blitz."

49 Ibid.

50 Joe Nocera and Bethany McLean, "All the Devils Are Here: The Hidden History of the Financial Crisis," *Portfolio*, 2011.

51 Board of Governors of the Federal Reserve System, Press Release, December 18, 2007, http://www.federalreserve.gov/newsevents/press/bcreg/20071218a.htm.

52 "Gretchen Morgenson on Corporate Clout in Washington," *Moyers and Company*, March 9, 2012, http://billmoyers.com/segment/gretchen-morgenson-on-industry-influence/.

53 Ibid.

54 Ibid.; "How Wall Street Defanged Dodd-Frank," Gary Rivlin, *The Nation*, April 30, 2013, http://www.thenation.com/article/174113/how-wall-street-defanged-dodd-frank.

55 Ibid.

56 "US Chamber of Commerce," Center for Responsive Politics, https://www.opensecrets.org/lobby/clientsum.php?id=D000019798&year=2015.

57 "American Fedn of State, County & Municipal Employees," Center for Responsive Politics, https://www.opensecrets.org/orgs/lobby.php?id=D000000061.

58 Kevin Conner, "Big Bank Takeover," Institute for America's Future, http://ourfuture.org/files/documents/big-bank-takeover-final.pdf.

59 "Citigroup Inc," Center for Responsive Politics, https://www.opensecrets.org/orgs/summary.php?id=D000000071.

60 Les Christie, "Foreclosures up a record 81 percent in 2008," CNN, January 15, 2009, http://money.cnn.com/2009/01/15/real_estate/millions_in_foreclosure/.

61 Paul Kiel and Olga Pierce, "Dems: Obama Broke Pledge to Force Banks to Help Homeowners," *ProPublica*, February 4, 2011, http://www.propublica.org/article/dems-obama-broke-pledge-to-force-banks-to-help-homeowners.

62 "Senator Obama Speaks in Golden, Col. on the Economy," CQ Transcriptwire, *Washington Post*, September 16, 2008, http://www.washingtonpost.com/wp-dyn/content/article/2008/09/16/AR2008091601767.html.

63 Adam J. Levitin, "Resolving the Foreclosure Crisis: Modification of Mortgages in Bankruptcy," *Wisconsin Law Review*, 2009:3, http://wisconsinlawreview.org/wp-content/files/1-Levitin.pdf.

64 Kiel and Pierce, "Dems: Obama Broke Pledge."

65 Brady Dennis and Renae Merle, "House Democrats push bill to use TARP funds for homeowner mortgage relief," *Washington Post*, December 8, 2009, http://www.washingtonpost.com/wp-dyn/content/article/2009/12/07/AR2009120703903.html.

66 Shaila Dewan, "Lew Unveils Small Steps to Augment Loan Modification Program," *New York Times*, June 26, 2014, http://www.nytimes.com/2014/06/27/business/treasury-secretary-unveils-small-steps-to-augment-loan-modification-program.html?_r=0.

67 Arthur Delaney, "HAMP: Obama Administration Lets Bank Out of Doghouse for Bad Mortgage Servicing," *Huffington Post*, March 2, 2012, http://www.huffingtonpost.com/2012/03/02/hamp-mortgage-barack-obama_n_1316873.html.

68 Olga Pierce and Paul Kiel, "By the Numbers: A Revealing Look at the Mortgage Mod Meltdown," *Pro Publica*, March 8, 2011, http://www.propublica

.org/article/by-the-numbers-a-revealing-look-at-the-mortgage-mod-meltdown.

5. Drugged

1 FastStats, Centers for Disease Control and Prevention, last updated April 29, 2015.

2 http://www.oecd.org/unitedstates/Briefing-Note-UNITED-STATES-2014.pdf.

3 The $3,484 figure is for 2012, the most recent year for which this OEDC information was available as this book was going to print.

4 Sheryl Gay Stolberg, "A Delicate Dance for 2 Health Lobbyists," *New York Times*, October 27, 2009.

5 https://www.opensecrets.org/politicians/summary.php?cid–00005372&cycle=2004.

6 Paul Blumenthal, "The Legacy of Billy Tauzin: The White House-PhRMA Deal," Sunlight Foundation, February 12, 2010.

7 http://www.opensecrets.org/lobby/indusclient.php?id=H04&year=2009.

8 https://www.opensecrets.org/lobby/top.php?showYear=a&indexType=s.

9 Megan R. Wilson, "PhRMA comes out on top in trade group rankings," *The Hill*, July 24, 2013.

10 Bruce Bartlett, "Medicare Part D: Republican Budget-Busting," *New York Times*, November 19, 2013.

11 "Former Medicare administrator takes health care job at law firm," Baltimore *Sun*, December 19, 2003.

12 Richard S. Foster, "Actuary in the Hot Seat," *Contingencies*, November/December 2004.

13 Noah Glyn, "Drug Deals," *National Review*, January 30, 2013.

14 Ibid.

15 Robert Pear, "Insurers and Drug Makers See Gain in Bush Victory," *New York Times*, November 5, 2004.

16 "Under the Influence," *60 Minutes*, season 30, episode 25, April 1, 2007.

17 *Congressional Record*, Senate, April 18, 2007.

18 Peter Baker, "Obama Was Pushed by Drug Industry, Emails Suggest," *New York Times*, June 8, 2012.

19 Ibid.

20 Paul Blumenthal, "The Legacy of Billy Tauzin: The White House–PhRMA Deal," Sunlight Foundation, February 12, 2010.

21 Dean Baker, "Reducing Waste with an Efficient Medicare Prescription Drug Benefit," Center for Economic and Policy Research, January 2013.

22 "Billy and the Beanstalk: Big Pharma's lobbyist has sold his CEOs on a political fantasy," *Wall Street Journal*, August 13, 2009.

23 Richard Anderson, "Pharmaceutical industry gets high on fat profits," BBC News, November 6, 2014.

24 Keith Speights, "10 Most Profitable Companies in Healthcare," *Motley Fool*, May 7, 2015.

25 Source: Yahoo! Finance, accessed July 15, 2015.

26 Marcia Angell, *The Truth About Drug Companies* (New York: Random House, 2004).

27 "Treating HCV—Is the Price Right?" Michael Smith, *MedPage Today*, February 18, 2014.

28 http://www.who.int/mediacentre/factsheets/fs164/en/.

29 Merrill Goozner, "Why Sovaldi shouldn't cost $84,000," *Modern Healthcare*, May 3, 2014.

30 Emory News Center, http://news.emory.edu/stories/2012/03/tech_transfer_highlights/campus.html.

31 Goozner, "Why Sovaldi shouldn't cost $84,000."

32 http://www.ncbi.nlm.nih.gov/pubmed/25646109.

33 Charles Ornstein, "New hepatitis C drugs are costing Medicare billions," *Washington Post*, March 29, 2015.

34 Andrew Ward, "Drug Pricing: Bitter Pill," *Financial Times*, July 31, 2014.

35 Dr. Val Jones, "When Chemo Saves Your Life: An Interview with Billy Tauzin," *Better Health*, January 29, 2009.

36 Bob Herman, "Genentech's distribution change for cancer drugs upsets hospitals," *Modern Healthcare*, September 30, 2014.

37 Jim Landers, "Your money or your life: Patients face painful choice," *Dallas Morning News*, April 3, 2015.

38 "High Price of Cancer Treatment Drugs Is 'Unsustainable,' Doctor Says," NPR, June 1, 2015.

39 Ed Silverman, "The Number of Drug Shortages—and Patient Frustration—Keeps Growing," *Wall Street Journal*, June 1, 2015.

40 "Medicines Use and Spending Shifts: A Review of the Use of Medicines in the U.S. in 2014," *IMS Health*, 2015.

41 "Trends in Retail Prices of Generic Prescription Drugs Widely Used by Older Americans, 2006 to 2013," AARP Public Policy Institute, May 2015.

42 Robert Pear, "Obama Proposes That Medicare Be Given the Right to Negotiate the Cost of Drugs," *New York Times*, April 27, 2015.

6. Fuel Follies

1 *New York Times,* September 20, 2011.

2 Daniel LeDuc, "Business Leaders Call for National Energy Policy," Pew Charitable Trusts, Clean Energy Initiative, October 5, 2012.

3 Ibid.

4 D. C. Rice, R. Schoney, and K. Mahaffey, "Methods and rationale for derivation of a reference dose for methylmercury by the US EPA," *Risk Analysis: An Official Publication of the Society for Risk Analysis,* 2003, www.ncbi.nlm.nih.gov/pubmed/11181111.

5 U.S. Environmental Protection Agency, "Mercury Study Report to Congress: An inventory of anthropogenic mercury emissions in the United States," 1997.

6 *American Lawyer,* August 1, 2005. Referenced at Institute for Agriculture and Trade Policy, http://www.iatp.org.

7 Ibid.

8 "Fact Sheet: EPA's Clean Air Mercury Rule," March 15, 2005. For more information, see www.epa.gov/air/mercuryrule/factsheetfin.html.

9 Connor Gibson, "Jeffrey Holmstead: The Coal Industry's Mercury Lobbyist," Polluterwatch Blog, December 21, 2011 (updated November 2012).

10 *New York Times,* October 11, 2011.

11 http://fusion.net/story/142473/the-american-coal-industry-is-collapsing/.

12 "Marcellus Shale: New Research Surprises Geologists," Geology.com. http://frack.mixplex.com/content/marcellus-shale-gas-new-research-results-surprise-geologists.

13 R. W. Hoise, "New Thinking Needed: Pa. Must Back Natural Gas Tax That Helps Local Governments," TheDailyReview.com, August 29, 2010.

14 Kevin McNellis, "Names in the News: Pennsylvania's Marcellus Shale Advisory Commission," National Institute on Money in State Politics, July 28, 2012, http://classic.followthemoney.org/press/PrintReportView.phmtl?r=455.

15 Pennsylvania Land Trust Association, "Marcellus Shale Drillers in Pennsylvania Amass 1614 Violations Since 2008," October 1, 2010, http://conserveland.org/?s=marcellus.

16 Don Hopey, "Pennsylvania Environmental Secretary Mike Krancer to Step Down," *Pittsburgh Post-Gazette*, March 23, 2013, http://www.post-gazette.com/news/state/2013/03/23/Pennsylvania-environmental-secretary-Mike-Krancer-to-step-down/stories/201303230164.

17 Kristen Allen, *The Big Fracking Deal: Marcellus Shale—Pennsylvania's Untapped Resource,* 23 Villanova Envrionmental Law Journal 51 (2012).

18 McNellis, "Names in the News."

19 T. McDonnell, "Smelling a Leak: Is the natural gas industry buying academics?" *Grist,* July 30, 2012.

20 J. Efstathiou, "Penn State Faculty Snub of Fracking Study Ends Research," *Bloomberg,* October 3, 2012.

21 http://www.nytimes.com/2012/11/03us/pennsylvania-mitted-poison-data-in-water-report.html/.

22 http://stateimpact.npr.org/pennsylvania/2014/10/29/energy=companies-donate-more-than1-million-to-corbetts-campaign-coffers/.

23 http://www.marcellus-shale.us/political-contributions-htm/.

24 Ibid.

25 J. Elliott, "Another Layer to Rendell's Fracking Connections," *Pro Publica,* April 8, 2013.

26 http://www.elementpartners.com/team-edrendell.html.

27 http://www.Stateimpact.npr.org/pennsylvania/former-dep-chief-michael-krancer.

28 http://public-accountability.org/2013/02/fracking-and-the-revolving-door-in-pennsylvania/.

29 Personal interview with solar pioneer Neville Williams, July 14, 2015.

30 *International Business Times,* April 6, 2015.

31 Ibid.

32 See www.flsolarchoice.org.

33 *Wall Street Journal,* February 20, 2015.

34 www.heartland.org/newspaper-article/2015/03/02/solar-power-lobbyists-seek-subvert-florida-tea-party.

7. Fat Wallets, Expanding Waistlines

1 Cynthia Ogden, PhD, Margaret D. Carroll, MSPH, Brian K. Kit, MD, MPH, and Katherine M. Flegal, PhD, "Prevalence of Childhood and Adult Obesity in the United States, 2011–2012," *Journal of the American Medical Association,* February 26, 2014, http://jama.jamanetwork.com/article.aspx?articleid=1832542.

2 Ibid.

3 "Childhood Obesity in the United States: Facts and Figures," Institute of Medicine of the National Academies, September 2004, http://www.iom.edu

/~/media/Files/Reportpercent20Files/2004/Preventing-Childhood-Obesity-Health-in-the-Balance/FINALfactsandfigures2.pdf.

4 Arthur H. Rubenstein, "Obesity: A Modern Epidemic," *Transactions of the American Clinical and Climatological Association*, 2005, http://www.ncbi.nlm.nih.gov/pmc/articles/PMC1473136/?report=classic.

5 "Obesity Threatens to Cut U.S. Life Expectancy, New Analysis Suggests," National Institutes of Health, March 16, 2005, http://www.nih.gov/news/pr/mar2005/nia-16.htm.

6 Eliana Dockterman, "Study: Obesity May Shorten Life Expectancy by Up to 8 Years," *Time*, December 4, 2014, http://time.com/3619251/obesity-life-expectancy/.

7 "Early Childhood Obesity Prevention Policies: Goals, Recommendations, and Potential Actions," Institute of Medicine of the National Academies, June 23, 2011, http://www.iom.edu/Reports/2011/Early-Childhood-Obesity-Prevention-Policies/Recommendations.aspx.

8 "Vital signs: obesity among low-income, preschool-aged children—United States, 2008–2011," Centers for Disease Control and Prevention, August 9, 2013, http://www.ncbi.nlm.nih.gov/pubmed/23925173.

9 "Evaluating Obesity Prevention Efforts: A Plan for Measuring Progress," Institute of Medicine of the National Academies, August 2013, http://www.iom.edu/~/media/Files/Reportpercent20Files/2013/Evaluating-Obesity-Prevention-Efforts/EPOP_rb.pdf.

10 Elizabeth Mendes, "Americans' Concerns About Obesity Soar, Surpass Smoking," *Gallup*, July 18, 2012, http://www.gallup.com/poll/155762/americans-concerns-obesity-soar-surpass-smoking.aspx.

11 "Scientific Report of the 2015 Dietary Guidelines Advisory Committee: Advisory Report to the Secretary of Health and Human Services and the Secretary of Agriculture," Dietary Guidelines Advisory Committee, February 2015, http://www.health.gov/dietaryguidelines/2015-scientific-report/PDFs/Scientific-Report-of-the-2015-Dietary-Guidelines-Advisory-Committee.pdf.

12 Anahad O'Connor, "Nutrition Panel Calls for Less Sugar and Eases Cholesterol and Fat Restrictions," *New York Times*, February 19, 2015, http://well.blogs.nytimes.com/2015/02/19/nutrition-panel-calls-for-less-sugar-and-eases-cholesterol-and-fat-restrictions/.

13 Authors' analysis of Center for Responsive Politics records.

14 "Who needs lobbyists? See what big business spends to win American minds," Center for Public Integrity, January 15, 2015, http://www.publicintegrity.org/2015/01/15/16596/who-needs-lobbyists-see-what-big-business-spends-win-american-minds#!6.

15 Robert Pear, "Congress Approves Child Nutrition Bill," *New York Times*, December 2, 2010, http://www.nytimes.com/2010/12/03/us/politics/03child. html.

16 Authors' analysis of Center for Responsive Politics data.

17 Authors' analysis of Center for Responsive Politics data.

18 Nick Confessore, "How School Lunch Became the Latest Political Battleground," *New York Times*, October 7, 2014, http://www.nytimes. com/2014/10/12/magazine/how-school-lunch-became-the-latest-political-battleground.html.

19 Ibid.

20 Jim Spencer and Mike Hughlett, "Pizza still counts as a veggie in schools," *Minneapolis Star Tribune*, November 21, 2011, http://www.startribune.com/ lifestyle/health/134208058.html.

21 Brett Neely, "Washington pizza sauce fight has deep Minnesota ties," Minnesota Public Radio, November 18, 2011, http://www.mprnews.org/ story/2011/11/18/schwan-foods-pizza-as-vegetable-minnesota-delegation.

22 Duff Wilson and Janet Roberts, "Special Report: How Washington went soft on childhood obesity," Reuters, April 27, 2012, http://www.reuters.com/ article/2012/04/27/us-usa-foodlobby-idUSBRE83Q0ED20120427.

23 "School Meal Program Regulations," National Potato Council, http:// nationalpotatocouncil.org/issues/health-and-nutrition/.

24 Sam Rosen-Amy, "Congress Passes Year's First Spending Bill With Plenty of Riders, Declares Pizza a Vegetable," Center for Effective Government, November 21, 2011, http://www.foreffectivegov.org/node/11915.

25 Confessore, "How School Lunch Became the Latest Political Battleground."

26 Ron Nixon, "Nutrition Group Lobbies Against Healthier School Meals It Sought, Citing Cost," *New York Times*, July 1, 2014, http://www.nytimes .com/2014/07/02/us/nutrition-group-lobbies-against-healthier-school-meals-it-sought-citing-cost.html.

27 Authors' interview with spokesperson for the School Nutrition Association.

28 www.stateofobesity.org/states/al/.

29 www.americashealthrankings.org/AL/.

30 Peter Overby, "Lobbyists Loom Behind the Scenes of School Nutrition Fight," NPR, June 11, 2014, http://www.npr.org/blogs/thesalt/2014/06/11 /320753007/behind-the-scenes-of-school-nutrition-fight-big-food-money-flows.

31 Jay Sjerven, "Congress eases whole grain and sodium requirements in school meals," *Food Business News*, December 16, 2014, http://www

.foodbusinessnews.net/articles/news_home/Regulatory_News/2014/12/Congress_eases_whole_grain_and.aspx?ID=percent7B29827895-2A79-4F20-9ED5-CFD960523BE7 percent7D.

32 Letter to the Senate and House Members of Committees on Agriculture Appropriations, School Nutrition Association Past Presidents Initiative, May 27, 2014, http://www.democraticleader.gov/sites/democraticleader.house.gov/files/SNA percent20Past percent20Presidents.pdf.

33 "SNA President Testifies on School Meal Successes and Challenges," School Nutrition Association, April 15, 2015, https://schoolnutrition.org/PressReleases/SNAPresidentTestifiesonSchoolMealSuccessesandChallenges/.

34 http://www.fns.U.S.D.A.gov/pressrelease/2014/009814.

35 D. Ludwig, K. Peyterson, and S. Gortmaker, "Relation between consumption of sugar-sweetened drinks and childhood obesity: A perspective, observational analysis," *The Lancet,* 2001.

36 K. Brownell and K. Warner, "The Perils of Ignoring History: Big Tobacco Played Dirty and Millions Died. How Similar Is Big Food?" *Milbank Quarterly* 87(1): 259–94.

37 Kelly D. Brownell, PhD, and Thomas R. Frieden, MD, MPH, "Ounces of Prevention—The Public Policy Case for Taxes on Sugared Beverages," *New England Journal of Medicine,* April 30, 2009, http://www.nejm.org/doi/full/10.1056/NEJMp0902392.

38 Roberta R. Friedman, ScM and Kelly D. Brownell, PhD, "Sugar-Sweetened Beverage Taxes: An Updated Policy Brief," Yale Rudd Center for Food Policy and Obesity, October 2012, http://www.yaleruddcenter.org/resources/upload/docs/what/reports/Rudd_Policy_Brief_Sugar_Sweetened_Beverage_Taxes.pdf.

39 Erin Quinn, "Who needs lobbyists? See what big business spends to win American minds," Center for Public Integrity, January 15, 2015, http://www.publicintegrity.org/2015/01/15/16596/who-needs-lobbyists-see-what-big-business-spends-win-american-minds#!1.

40 *Washington Post,* June 25, 2014.

41 Americans Against Food Taxes Form 990s, https://www.citizenaudit.org/270514291/.

42 "Pennies," Americans Against Food Taxes TV ad, September 11, 2009, https://www.youtube.com/watch?v=sxIwwrO2JYg.

43 Christine Spolar and Joe Eaton, "The food lobby's war on a soda tax," Center for Public Integrity, November 4, 2009, http://www.publicintegrity.org/2009/11/04/2758/food-lobbys-war-soda-tax.

44 Swati Yanamadala et al., "Food industry front groups and conflicts of interests: The case of Americans Against Food Taxes," *Public Health Nutrition* 15, no. 8, 2012, http://journals.cambridge.org/download.php?file=percent2FPHN percent2FPHN15_08 percent2FS1368980012003187a.pdf&code=ebb31e0749a886 bc3a840b894cced959.

45 "The Masterminds Behind the Phony Anti-Soda Tax Coalitions," Nancy Huehnergarth, *Huffington Post*, September 2, 2012, http://www.huffington post.com/nancy-huehnergarth/soda-ban-new-york_b_1644883.html.

46 New York State lobbying records.

47 "2010 A $weet year for Albany lobbyists," NYPIRG, March 4, 2010, http:// www.nypirg.org/media/releases/goodgov/NYPIRG-percent202010percent20 Lobbying.pdf.

48 Duff Wilson and Janet Roberts, "Special Report: How Washington went soft on childhood obesity," Reuters, April 27, 2012, http://www.reuters.com/ article/2012/04/27/us-usa-foodlobby-idUSBRE83Q0ED20120427.

49 Anemona Hartocollis, "Failure of State Soda Tax Plan Reflects Power of an Antitax Message," *New York Times*, July 2, 2010, http://www.nytimes .com/2010/07/03/nyregion/03sodatax.html.

50 William Harless, "Beverage lobbyist funds 'community' campaign against soda tax," *California Watch*, June 13, 2012, http://californiawatch.org/dailyreport /beverage-lobbyist-funds-community-campaign-against-soda-tax-16585.

51 "Group Fighting Proposed Richmond Soda Tax Files Lawsuit," CBS San Francisco, September 5, 2012, http://sanfrancisco.cbslocal.com/2012/09/05 /group-fighting-proposed-richmond-soda-tax-files-lawsuit/.

52 Fernando Quintero, "Advocates bulking up for the next battle with Big Soda," Berkeley Media Studies Group, January 8, 2013, http://www.bmsg.org /blog/advocates-bulking-up-for-the-next-battle-with-big-soda.

53 http://articles.latimes.com/2012/dec/09/opinion/la-oe-zingale-soda-tax-campaign-funding-20121209.

54 Representative Marvin Jones of Texas, one of the sponsors of the bill, was later recognized with the industry's Dyer Memorial Award as "Sugar Man of the Year."

55 Alexandra Wexler, "Bulk of U.S. Sugar Loans Went to Three Companies," *Wall Street Journal*, June 26, 2013.

56 Brian Riley, "U.S. Trade Policy Gouges American Sugar Consumers," Heritage Foundation, June 5, 2014.

57 www.aei.org/AmericanBoondoggle.

58 Ibid.

59 *Wall Street Journal*, October 13, 2013.

60 Fran Smith, "Sugar—Congress' Favorite Sweetener," Competitive Enterprise Institute, December 9, 2013.

61 Jennifer Comiteau, "When Does Brand Loyalty Start?" *Adweek*, March 24, 2003, http://www.adweek.com/news/advertising/when-does-brand-loyalty-start-62841.

62 Kristen Harrison, PhD, and Amy L. Marske, MA, "Nutritional Content of Foods Advertised During the Television Programs Children Watch Most," *American Journal of Public Health*, September 2005, http://www.ncbi.nlm.nih.gov/pmc/articles/PMC1449399/#r6.

63 Mark Bittman, "The Right to Sell Kids Junk," *New York Times*, March 27, 2012, opinionator.blogs.nytimes.com/2012/03/27/the-right-to-sell-kids-junk/.

64 "Preliminary Proposed Nutrition Principles to Guide Industry Self-Regulatory Efforts," Interagency Working Group on Food Marketed to Children, https://www.ftc.gov/sites/default/files/documents/public_events/food-marketed-children-forum-interagency-working-group-proposal/110428foodmarketproposedguide.pdf.

65 Lyndsey Layton and Dan Eggen, "Industries lobby against voluntary nutrition guidelines for food marketed to kids," *Washington Post*, July 9, 2011, http://www.washingtonpost.com/politics/industries-lobby-against-voluntary-nutrition-guidelines-for-food-marketed-to-kids/2011/07/08/gIQAZSZu5H_story.html.

66 Katy Bachman, "Industry Group: Feds Would Muzzle Advertising of Popular Foods," *Adweek*, August 4, 2011, http://www.adweek.com/news/advertising-branding/industry-group-feds-would-muzzle-advertising-popular-foods-133878.

67 Kraft Foods lobbying report, http://soprweb.senate.gov/index.cfm?event=getFilingDetails&filingID=0697C58D-9493-4C44-AFFD-30384F45A76F&filingTypeID=69.

68 "Limiting Food Marketing to Children," Center for Science in the Public Interest, https://www.cspinet.org/new/pdf/limitingfood_marketing.pdf.

69 "Restore FTC Authority to Regulate Food and Beverage Marketing Aimed at Children," Partnership for Prevention, https://www.prevent.org/Prevention-Policy-Agenda-for-the-110th-Congress/Restore-FTC-Authority-to-Regulate-Food-and-Beverage-Marketing-Aimed-at-Children.aspx.

70 "Foods and Beverages That Meet the CFBAI Category-Specific Uniform Nutrition Criteria That May Be in Child-Directed Advertising," Better Business Bureau Children's Food and Beverage Advertising Initiative, http://www.bbb.org/globalassets/local-bbbs/council-113/media/cfbai/cfbai-product-list-january-2014.pdf.

71 http://www.fightchronicdisease.org/media-center/releases/new-data-shows-obesity-costs-will-grow-344-billion-2018.

72 "F as in Fat: How Obesity Threatens America's Future," Trust for America's Health, 2012, http://www.rwjf.org/content/dam/farm/reports/reports/2012/rwjf401318.

73 "The medical care costs of obesity: An instrumental variables approach," John Cawleya and Chad Meyerhoeferd, *Journal of Health Economics*, 2012.

74 "Economic Costs of Obesity," National League of Cities, http://www.healthycommunitieshealthyfuture.org/learn-the-facts/economic-costs-of-obesity/.

75 Eric Pianin and Brianna Ehley, "Budget Busting U.S. Obesity Costs Climb Past $300 Billion a Year," *Fiscal Times*, June 19, 2014, http://www.thefiscaltimes.com/Articles/2014/06/19/Budget-Busting-US-Obesity-Costs-Climb-Past-300-Billion-Year.

76 "10 Flabbergasting Costs of America's Obesity Epidemic," *PHIT America*, April 11, 2013, http://www.phitamerica.org/News_Archive/10_Flaggergasting_Costs.htm§hash.kHzrdOHp.dpuf.

77 "Adult Obesity Facts," Centers for Disease Control and Prevention, http://www.cdc.gov/obesity/data/adult.html.

78 Ross A. Hammond and Ruth Levine, "The economic impact of obesity in the United States," *Diabetes, Metabolic Syndrome and Obesity: Targets and Therapy*, August 17, 2010, http://www.brookings.edu/~/media/research/files/articles/2010/9/14 percent20obesity percent20cost percent20hammond percent20levine/0914_obesity_cost_hammond_levine.

79 Sharon Begley, "As America's waistline expands, costs soar," *Reuters*, April 30, 2012, http://www.reuters.com/article/2012/04/30/us-obesity-idUS-BRE83T0C820120430.

80 Ibid.

81 Whit Johnson, "Too fat to serve: Military wages war on obesity," *CBS News*, March 8, 2012, http://www.cbsnews.com/news/too-fat-to-serve-military-wages-war-on-obesity/.

82 Authors' analysis of comments submitted to Federal Trade Commission and lobbying records, https://www.ftc.gov/policy/public-comments/initiative-378.

83 "Accelerating Progress in Obesity Prevention: Solving the Weight of the Nation," Institute of Medicine, May 8, 2012, http://www.iom.edu/Reports/2012/Accelerating-Progress-in-Obesity-Prevention.aspx.

8. Enough to Make You Sick

1 "Lumber Liquidators Linked to Health and Safety Violations," *60 Minutes*, CBS News, March 1, 2015, http://www.cbsnews.com/news/lumber-liquidators-linked-to-health-and-safety-violations/.

2 *Lila Washington et al. v. Lumber Liquidators, Inc.* (N.D. Cali. 2015), http://www.hbsslaw.com/Templates/media/files/case_pdfs/Lumber_Liquidators/3_31_Filing.pdf.

3 David Heath, "How politics derailed EPA science on arsenic, endangering public health," Center for Public Integrity, June 28, 2014, http://www.publicintegrity.org/2014/06/28/15000/how-politics-derailed-epa-science-arsenic-endangering-public-health.

4 "Questions and Answers Regarding Laminate Flooring," United States Environmental Protection Agency, http://www2.epa.gov/formaldehyde/questions-and-answers-regarding-laminate-flooring-0.

5 "What Is Formaldehyde? Why Is Formaldehyde Chemistry So Special?" American Chemistry Council website.

6 "Answers to Frequently Asked Questions about the Health Effects of Formaldehyde," American Chemistry Council, April 6, 2011, http://www.americanchemistry.com/ProductsTechnology/Formaldehyde/Answers-to-FAQs-about-the-Health-Effects-of-Formaldehyde.PDF.

7 Liz Szabo, "Study links formaldehyde to more common cancers," *USA Today*, May 12, 2009, http://usatoday30.usatoday.com/news/health/2009-05-12-formaldehyde-cancer_N.htm; "Mortality From Lymphohematopoietic Malignancies and Brain Cancer Among Embalmers Exposed to Formaldehyde," Michael Hauptmann et al., *Journal of the National Cancer Institute*, November 20, 2009, http://jnci.oxfordjournals.org/content/101/24/1696.full#ref-1.

8 Authors' interview with Becky Gillette.

9 "Formaldehyde and Cancer Risk," National Cancer Institute, June 10, 2011, http://www.cancer.gov/about-cancer/causes-prevention/risk/substances/formaldehyde/formaldehyde-fact-sheet.

10 "Katrina, Rita victims get $42.6M in toxic FEMA trailer suit," Associated Press, *CBS News*, September 28, 2012, http://www.cbsnews.com/news/katrina-rita-victims-get-426m-in-toxic-fema-trailer-suit/.

11 "Prepared Testimony of Lindsay Huckabee: Government Reform and Oversight Committee, U.S. House of Representatives," NPR, July 19, 2007, http://www.npr.org/documents/2008/may/huckabeetestimony.pdf.

12 *Toxicological Profile for Formaldehyde*, Research Triangle Institute, Agency for Toxic Substances and Disease Registry of U.S. Department of Health and Human Services, July 1999.

13 Liz Szabo, "Study Links Formaldehyde to More Common Cancers," *USA Today*, May 12, 2009, http://usatoday30.usatoday.com/news/health/2009-05-12-formaldehyde-cancer_N.htm.

14 "Formaldehyde in Your Products," Occupational Health and Safety Administration, https://www.osha.gov/SLTC/hairsalons/formaldehyde_in_products.html.

15 "National Poll Shows Bipartisan Support for Stronger Protections from Toxic Chemicals," National Resources Defense Council, July 19, 2012, http://www.nrdc.org/media/2012/120719.asp.

16 "Poll of Small Business Owners on Toxic Chemicals," American Sustainable Business Council, September 2012, http://asbcouncil.org/toxic-chemicals-poll#.VUvGhNNVhBc.

17 "High-Risk Series: An Update," GAO-09-271, January 2009, Washington, DC: Government Accountability Office, http://www.gao.gov/new.items /d09271.pdf.

18 Daniel Stevens, "Chemical Industry Increases Contributions and Lobbying as Congress Takes Up Chemical Bill," MapLight, March 16, 2015, http://maplight.org/content/chemical-industry-increases-contributions-and-lobbying-as-congress-takes-up-chemical-bill.

19 Erin Quinn, "Who Needs Lobbyists? See what big business spends to win American minds," Center for Public Integrity, January 15, 2015, http://www .publicintegrity.org/2015/01/15/16596/who-needs-lobbyists-see-what-big-business-spends-win-american-minds.

20 Joaquin Sapien, "How Senator Vitter Battled the EPA Over Formaldehyde's Link to Cancer," *ProPublica*, April 15, 2010, http://www.propublica.org/article /how-senator-david-vitter-battled-formaldehyde-link-to-cancer.

21 Alex Knott, "Lobbyists bankrolling politics," Center for Public Integrity, May 6, 2004, http://www.publicintegrity.org/2004/05/06/7511/lobbyists-bankrolling-politics.

22 Sapien, "How Senator Vitter Battled the EPA."

23 Laura E. Beane Freeman et al., "Mortality from Lymphohematopoietic Malignancies Among Workers in Formaldehyde Industries: The National Cancer Institute Cohort," *Journal of the National Cancer Institute*, May 20, 2009, http://www.ncbi.nlm.nih.gov/pmc/articles/PMC2684555/.

24 "The Grizzle Company," The Grizzle Company, http://www.grizzleco.com/.

25 Jennifer Sass and Daniel Rosenberg, "The Delay Game: How the Chemical Industry Ducks Regulations of the Most Toxic Substances," Natural Resources Defense Council, October 2011, http://www.nrdc.org/health/files /irisdelayreport.pdf.

26 "EPA nomination held up amid debate over formaldehyde risks," Jonathan Tilive, *Times-Picayune*, September 24, 2009, http://www.nola.com/politics /index.ssf/2009/09/epa_nomination_held_up_amid_de.html.

27 "Fundraising Dinner for David Vitter," *Political Party Time*, March 24, 2010, http://politicalpartytime.org/party/19825/.

28 Richard Denison, PhD, "The chemical industry says formaldehyde and styrene don't cause cancer. Only one of 52 scientists agree," Environmental

Defense Fund, March 26, 2013, http://blogs.edf.org/health/2013/03/26/the-chemical-industry-says-formaldehyde-and-styrene-dont-cause-cancer-only-one-of-52-scientists-agree/.

29 David Heath, "Obama's EPA breaks pledge to divorce politics from science on toxic chemicals," Center for Public Integrity, January 23, 2015, http://www.publicintegrity.org/2015/01/23/16641/obamas-epa-breaks-pledge-divorce-politics-science-toxic-chemicals.

30 "Department of the Interior, Environment, and Related Agencies Appropriation Bill, 2012: Report, together with Dissenting Views," U.S. House of Representatives, July 19, 2011, http://www.gpo.gov/fdsys/pkg/CRPT-112hrpt151/pdf/CRPT-112hrpt151.pdf.

31 David Heath, "How politics derailed EPA science on arsenic, endangering public health," Center for Public Integrity, June 28, 2014, http://www.publicintegrity.org/2014/06/28/15000/how-politics-derailed-epa-science-arsenic-endangering-public-health.

32 Heath, "Obama's EPA breaks pledge."

33 Bruce Alpert, "American Chemistry Council 1st $100,000+ donor to David Vitter Super PAC," *Times-Picayune*, July 16, 2014, http://www.nola.com/politics/index.ssf/2014/07/american_chemistry_council_1st.html.

34 Eric Lipton and Rachel Abrams, "The Uphill Battle to Better Regulate Formaldehyde," *New York Times*, May 3, 2015, http://www.nytimes.com/2015/05/04/business/energy-environment/the-uphill-battle-to-better-regulate-formaldehyde.html.

35 Wendell Potter, *Deadly Spin: An Insurance Insider Speaks Out on How Corporate PR Is Killing Health Care and Deceiving Americans* (New York: Bloomsbury, 2010).

36 Bill Perdue, "Formaldehyde Emissions Standards for Composite Wood Products: Comments of the American Home Furnishings Alliance," American Home Furnishings Alliance, http://www.compositepanel.org/userfiles/filemanager/5266ea97165ad/.

37 Eric Lipton and Rachel Abrams, "The Uphill Battle to Better Regulate Formaldehyde," *New York Times*, May 3, 2015, http://www.nytimes.com/2015/05/04/business/energy-environment/the-uphill-battle-to-better-regulate-formaldehyde.html.

38 Richard Denison, "EDF comments at EPA's public stakeholder meeting on its IRIS program," Environmental Defense Fund, November 14, 2012, http://blogs.edf.org/health/2012/11/14/edf-comments-at-epas-public-stakeholder-meeting-on-its-iris-program/.

39 Lee Drutman, *The Business of America Is Lobbying: How Corporations Became Politicized and Politics Became More Corporate* (Oxford University Press, 2015), 45.

40 Ibid., 44–45.

41 Ibid.

42 Heath, "How politics derailed EPA science."

43 Ibid.

44 James Hamblin, "The Toxins That Threaten Our Brains," *Atlantic*, March 18, 2014, http://www.theatlantic.com/features/archive/2014/03/the-toxins-that-threaten-our-brains/284466/.

45 "Chemical Regulation: Observations on the Toxic Substances Control Act and EPA Implementation," U.S. Government Accountability Office, June 13, 2013, http://www.gao.gov/products/GAO-13-696T.

46 Kate Sheppard, "Senators Introduce Bill to Overhaul U.S. Chemical Regulations," *Huffington Post*, March 10, 2015, http://www.huffingtonpost.com/2015/03/10/toxic-chemicals-senate-bill_n_6842524.html.

47 Timothy Cama, "Chemical safety bill picks up support in Senate," *The Hill*, May 7, 2015, http://thehill.com/policy/energy-environment/241339-chemical-safety-bill-picks-up-support-in-senate.

48 David McCumber, "Questions raised on authorship of chemicals bill," *San Francisco Chronicle*, March 16, 2015, http://www.sfgate.com/nation/article/Questions-raised-on-authorship-of-chemicals-bill-6137823.php.

49 Return of Organization Exempt from Income Tax: American Chemistry Council, Internal Revenue Service, 2013, https://s3.amazonaws.com/s3.documentcloud.org/documents/1371629/american-chemistry-council-2013.pdf.

50 Eric Lipton, "Tom Udall's Unlikely Alliance with the Chemical Industry," *New York Times*, http://www.nytimes.com/2015/03/07/us/tom-udalls-unlikely-alliance-with-the-chemical-industry.html.

51 "Written Commentary of Lindsay Huckabee: Prepared for the Committee on Science and Technology," NPR, April 1, 2008, http://www.npr.org/documents/2008/may/huckabeetestimony08.pdf.

52 "Prepared Testimony of Lindsay Huckabee: Government Reform and Oversight Committee, U.S. House of Representatives," *NPR*, July 19, 2007, http://www.npr.org/documents/2008/may/huckabeetestimony.pdf.

53 Sarah Maslin Nir, "Perfect Nails, Poisoned Workers," *New York Times*, May 11, 2015, http://www.nytimes.com/2015/05/11/nyregion/nail-salon-workers-in-nyc-face-hazardous-chemicals.html.

54 "FDA Authority over Cosmetics," U.S. Food and Drug Administration, August 3, 2013, http://www.fda.gov/Cosmetics/GuidanceRegulation/LawsRegulations/ucm074162.htm.

55 "Personal Care Products Council: Report Images," OpenSecrets.com, 2015, http://www.opensecrets.org/lobby/client_reports.php?id=D000028328&year=2015.

56 Hamblin, "The Toxins That Threaten Our Brains."

57 Stefanie Knoll, "Harmful chemicals and neurotoxins: Slightly eroding intelligence, damaging societies," *Journalist's Resource*, March 21, 2015, http://journalistsresource.org/studies/environment/pollution-environment /neurobehavioral-effects-developmental-toxicity#.

Philippe Grandjean, MD, and Philip J. Landrigan, MD, "Neurobehavioral effects of developmental toxicity," *The Lancet*, February 14, 2014, http://www.thelancet. com/journals/laneur/article/PIIS1474-4422percent2813percent2970278-3 /abstract.

58 Leonardo Trasande, "Further Limiting Bisphenol A in Food Uses Could Provide Health and Economic Benefits," *Health Affairs*, January 2014, http:// content.healthaffairs.org/content/early/2014/01/16/hlthaff.2013.0686.

59 Lynne Peeples, "BPA Among Toxic Chemicals Driving Up Health Care Costs, Experts Say," *Huffington Post*, January 24, 2014, http://www.huffington-post.com/2014/01/22/bpa-health-care-costs_n_4644372.html.

60 Knoll, "Harmful chemicals and neurotoxins."

9. It's Fixable

1 http://reason.com/poll/2014/04/03/americans-say-75-percent-of-politicians.

2 http://www.demos.org/sites/default/files/publications/FreshStart_ PublicFinancingCT_0.pdf.

3 http://apr.sagepub.com/content/31/5/520.full.pdf.

4 Ibid.

5 http://www.demos.org/sites/default/files/publications/FreshStart_ PublicFinancingCT_0.pdf.

6 Ibid.

7 Ibid.

8 Ibid.

9 http://www.brennancenter.org/publication/donor-diversity-through-public-matching-funds.

10 http://www.brennancenter.org/press-release/study-public-financing-contributes-greater-diversity-participation-nyc-elections.

11 http://www.nydailynews.com/opinion/mouth-money-article-1.2011596.

12 http://missoulian.com/news/state-and-regional/montana-house-backs-bill-to-require-dark-money-groups-disclose/article_72bd75d5-6371-5b6b-b1d7-026d09be7d9f.html.

13 "Political Contribution Disclosure Survey Results," CFA Institute, August 2014, http://cfainstitute.org/Survey/political_contribution_survey_final.pdf.

14 http://www.usnews.com/opinion/articles/2015/04/23/obama-should-sign-order-to-force-contractors-to-disclose-political-spending.

15 http://www.washingtonpost.com/blogs/monkey-cage/wp/2015/04/16/what-we-get-wrong-about-lobbying-and-corruption/.

16 http://billmoyers.com/2015/04/07/living-high-life-congress/.

17 http://www.reddit.com/r/IAmA/comments/1qk2aa/we_are_dc_super_lobbyists_jack_quinn_and_john/cddkjnt.

18 Jack Abramoff, *Capitol Punishment: The Hard Truth About Washington Corruption From America's Most Notorious Lobbyist* (Washington, D.C., WND Books, 2011) 273.

19 http://www.politico.com/news/stories/0710/40207.html.

20 http://thehill.com/blogs/floor-action/house/238743-gop-lawmaker-proposes-permanent-lobbying-ban.

21 http://www.nytimes.com/2015/05/03/us/politics/fec-cant-curb-2016-election-abuse-commission-chief-says.html.

22 http://www.publicintegrity.org/2013/12/17/13996/how-washington-starves-its-election-watchdog.

23 Ibid.

24 Larry Noble, personal communication, May 28, 2015.

25 http://www.publicintegrity.org/2013/12/17/13996/how-washington-starves-its-election-watchdog.

26 Larry Noble, personal communication, May 28, 2015.

27 http://www.nytimes.com/2015/05/03/us/politics/fec-cant-curb-2016-election-abuse-commission-chief-says.html.

28 http://abcnews.go.com/Politics/jeb-bush-presidential-candidate-seconds-today/story?id=31027090.

29 Larry Noble, personal communication, May 28, 2015.

30 Kathay Feng, personal communication, May 28, 2015.

31 http://www.campaignlegalcenter.org/news/publications-speeches/californias-fppc-provides-example-dysfunctional-federal-agencies-follow.

32 Larry Noble, personal communication, May 28, 2015.

10. The Makings of an All-American Movement

1 Nick Kristof, "Polluted Political Games," *New York Times*, May 28, 2015, http://www.nytimes.com/2015/05/28/opinion/nicholas-kristof-polluted-political-games.html.

Index

Note: page numbers followed by *f* refer to figures.

A Note on the Authors

Wendell Potter is an author and journalist whose work has appeared in *Newsweek*, the *Guardian*, the *Nation*, the Center for Public Integrity, and at WendellPotter.com.

Nick Penniman is executive director of the organization Issue One. He was previously publisher of the *Washington Monthly* and director of the Huffington Post Investigative Fund.

Nick lives in D.C., a few miles from the U.S. Capitol Building; Wendell lives in Philadelphia, a few miles from Independence Hall.